T0198174

FUNDAMENTALS OF
PEDIATRIC IMAGING

FUNDAMENTALS OF
PEDIATRIC IMAGING

THIRD EDITION

EDITED BY
Lane F. Donnelly MD

Professor Radiology & Pediatrics
Associate Dean
Co-Executive Director, Stanford Medicine Center for Improvement
    Stanford University School of Medicine
Chief Quality Officer
Christopher G. Dawes Endowed Director of Quality
Pediatric Radiologist
    Stanford Children's Health
Palo Alto, CA, USA

CONTRIBUTORS
Monica Epelman

Robert J. Fleck Jr.

Carolina V. Guimaraes

Michael P. Nasser

Oscar M. Navarro

Alexander J. Towbin

Evan J. Zucker

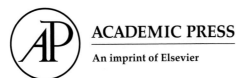

ACADEMIC PRESS

An imprint of Elsevier

ELSEVIER

Notices

Knowledge and best practice in this field are constantly changing. As new research and experience
broaden our understanding, changes in research methods, professional practices, or medical treatment
may become necessary.

Practitioners and researchers must always rely on their own experience and knowledge in evaluating
and using any information, methods, compounds, or experiments described herein. In using such
information or methods they should be mindful of their own safety and the safety of others, including
parties for whom they have a professional responsibility.

To the fullest extent of the law, neither the Publisher nor the authors, contributors, or editors,
assume any liability for any injury and/or damage to persons or property as a matter of products
liability, negligence or otherwise, or from any use or operation of any methods, products, instructions,
or ideas contained in the material herein.

Library of Congress Cataloging-in-Publication Data
A catalog record for this book is available from the Library of Congress

British Library Cataloguing-in-Publication Data
A catalogue record for this book is available from the British Library

ISBN: 978-0-12-822255-3

For information on all Academic Press publications visit our website at https://www.elsevier.com/
books-and-journals

Publisher: Nikki Levy
Acquisitions Editor: Joslyn Chaiprasert-Paguio
Editorial Project Manager: Tracy I. Tufaga
Production Project Manager: Selvaraj Raviraj
Cover Designer: Miles Hitchen

Typeset by TNQ Technologies

Printed in India

Last digit is the print number: 9 8 7 6 5 4 3

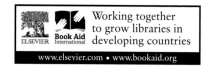

CONTRIBUTORS

Lane F. Donnelly MD
Professor Radiology & Pediatrics
Associate Dean
Co-Executive Director, Stanford Medicine
Center for Improvement
    Stanford University School of Medicine
Chief Quality Officer
Christopher G. Dawes Endowed Director of
Quality
Pediatric Radiologist
    Stanford Children's Health
Palo Alto, CA, USA

Monica Epelman
Professor of Radiology,
    University of Central Florida
Pediatric Radiologist
Vice-Chair, Department of Medical Imaging /
Radiology
    Nemours Children's Hospital
Orlando, FL, USA

Robert J. Fleck
Associate Professor of Radiology
    University of Cincinnati, College of
    Medicine
Pediatric Radiologist
    Cincinnati Children's Hospital
Cincinnati, OH, USA

Carolina V. Guimaraes
Clinical Associate Professor of Radiology
    Stanford University School of Medicine
Pediatric Neuroradiology
    Stanford Children's Health
Palo Alto, CA, USA

Michael P. Nasser
Assistant Professor of Clinical — Affiliate
    Department of Radiology, University of
    Cincinnati, College of Medicine
Pediatric Radiologist
Medical Director of Radiology, Liberty Campus
    Cincinnati Children's Hospital
Cincinnati, OH, USA

Oscar M. Navarro
Professor
    Department of Medical Imaging,
    University of Toronto
Pediatric Radiologist
Fellowship Program Director
Department of Diagnostic Imaging
    The Hospital for Sick Children Toronto,
Ontario, CA

Alexander J. Towbin
Professor of Radiology and Pediatrics University
    of Cincinnati, College of Medicine
Associate Chief, Department of Radiology
Neil. D. Johnson Chair of Radiology Informatics
Pediatric Radiologist
    Cincinnati Children's Hospital
Cincinnati, OH, USA

Evan J. Zucker
Clinical Associate Professor of Radiology
    Stanford University School of Medicine
Pediatric Radiologist
Medical Director, Pediatric Radiology
Operations
    Stanford Children's Health
Palo Alto, CA, USA

It is hard to believe that it has been 20 years since the first version of this book, *Fundamentals of Pediatric Radiology*, was published in 2001. It seems like forever ago. The next version of the book was *Pediatric Imaging: Fundamentals first Edition* in 2009 followed by *Fundamentals of Pediatric Imaging, second Edition* in 2016. We are now pleased to present *The Fundamentals of Pediatric Imaging, third Edition*—the fourth version of this book. I feel very fortunate to have been associated with this textbook throughout the years. By medical textbook standards, the book has been very successful—with over 25,000 copies sold. It has been particularly popular among radiology residents and fellows. Although I am very proud of many initiatives that I have been involved with both in pediatric radiology and in quality, safety, and service, often my name is most closely associated with this little book.

How this book came to be is a long story. When I was a radiology resident at the University of Cincinnati, there was a senior musculoskeletal imaging faculty member named Dr. Aaron Weinstein.

Every Thursday morning at 7a.m., he ran "Bone Conference." The format was the following: residents brought cases, often from the teaching files, and presented them as unknowns, which other residents had to "take." Dr. Weinstein would comment upon and critique the job done by the resident taking the unknown case (and often the resident who picked the case) as well as offer pearls of wisdom. Not only was Dr. Weinstein an expert in musculoskeletal imaging but he had also been at the University of Cincinnati for so long that he has already seen every interesting musculoskeletal case in the teaching files, usually multiple times, so he was nearly impossible to stump. He was also a cantankerous old man (much of it was a show) and he smoked constantly, even during conference, which gave the whole thing an added cinematic flare. We were all very fond of Dr. Weinstein, but the guy was intimidating. The entire process was terrifying to me as a young resident. I was continuously concerned about being humiliated at this conference in front of my peers and superiors. So, every single Wednesday evening of my residency I read the short *Fundamentals of Musculoskeletal Radiology* textbook by Clyde Helms—cover to cover. I figured if I had a very good grasp over the basics of musculoskeletal imaging, it would minimize the chance of me

looking like an idiot. I loved that book and I often wondered why well-written, short, practical books about the other radiology subspecialties did not really exist. I know that I retained more useful information when I read short and basic books over and over than when I read longer, more detailed texts once.

In the late 1990s, I was on faculty in the Department of Radiology at Duke University and had the opportunity to work with and learn from Clyde Helms. I shared with him my love for his book, the story of how I read this book every Wednesday evening when I was in residency, and my disappointment that there were no other high-quality fundamental books in the other subspecialties. He encouraged me to write such a book on pediatric radiology and put me in contact with the folks at what was then WB Sanders (now part of Elsevier). I was in my early 30s and just a couple of years out of training at the time and probably had no business writing a textbook about anything, but I proceeded and *Fundamentals of Pediatric Radiology* resulted. The intention of the book is to serve as a basic introductory text on pediatric imaging. The book is written in prose, rather than as an outline, and is intended to be readable. The emphasis is on commonly encountered imaging scenarios and pediatric diseases. The topics included reflect questions commonly asked by residents on the pediatric radiology service, important issues that the rotating residents often seem not to know, and commonly made mistakes. The book is intended to serve as an introduction or review for residents or medical students who are about to begin a rotation in pediatric radiology, a resource to general or pediatric radiologists who wish to brush up on pediatric radiology, or a guide for pediatric residents or pediatricians who want to learn more about pediatric radiology.

Although I authored the first two versions of this book, given the growing scope and complexity of pediatric imaging, authors with subspecialty expertise now write each of the chapters. In this edition, those contributing authors include Drs. Monica Epelman (Chest), Carolina Guimaraes (Neuro), Evan Zucker (Cardiac), Oscar Navarro (Genitourinary), Robert Fleck (Airway), and Alex Towbin (Musculoskeletal). I am deeply indebted to these authors for their expertise, contributions, and help. Dated portions of the text have been updated, figures replaced with more modern imaging, and new areas covered. I think you will find the same practicality and easy-to-read prose as in previous additions.

Finally, I would like to acknowledge that much of what appears in this book is the summation of what numerous radiologists have taught us, and I would like to thank them for their time and efforts. I have had the honor and privilege to work mostly at great organizations and with great leaders and mentors. The case material in this book is the result of the hard work of the faculty, technologists, and trainees in those departments and the referring physicians who care for these patients. I would like to acknowledge their efforts, without which this book would not be possible.

Best of luck with pediatric imaging.

Lane F. Donnelly, MD

CONTENTS

CHAPTER 1

SPECIAL CONSIDERATIONS IN PEDIATRIC IMAGING

Lane F. Donnelly

■ PEDIATRIC RADIOLOGY AS A POTENTIAL CAREER

A powerful and fulfilling aspect of becoming a pediatric healthcare provider is the satisfaction that comes from working with and for children. Few activities are more rewarding than helping children and their families. The sense of mission when working in a children's hospital is palpable and very different than what is often experienced in adult healthcare systems. In addition, there are many other attractive aspects of pediatric care. First, most kids recover from their illnesses, as compared with elderly adults. Most pediatric illnesses are not self-induced. Pediatric diseases are highly varied and interesting. In addition, pediatric conditions are being increasingly recognized as important precursors to adult illnesses that cause significant morbidity and mortality—for example obesity, osteoporosis, and glucose intolerance. Finally, children and their families are highly appreciative of pediatricians' help.

My impression has always been that most pediatric radiologists seem very happy with both their jobs and career choice. There are a number of attractive aspects about pediatric radiology. First, one of the most important elements of job satisfaction is the quality of the interactions with coworkers. In general, the physicians who choose to go into pediatric subspecialties, as well as other healthcare workers who choose to work at pediatric institutions, tend to be nice people. Aggressive, power-hungry people tend not to want to work with children. This makes a huge difference in the quality of daily work life. In addition, pediatric subspecialists seem to rely on the opinions of pediatric radiologists more than many of their adult subspecialist counterparts. Similarly, pediatric radiology does not seem to have the same number of turf battles that many adult-oriented departments have.

Another unique feature of pediatric radiology is that one gets to be a "general specialist." Pediatric radiology is a small part of medical imaging overall, and in this sense, the pediatric radiologist is very much a subspecialist. Compared with general radiologists who must have a working knowledge of a daunting amount of information, most pediatric radiologists feel comfortable that they have an adequate command of the knowledge they need to provide outstanding care. That being said, I am continuously surprised of how often my colleagues and I encounter cases that are unlike any we have previously experienced. Things certainly never get boring. At the same time, pediatric radiologists are generalists in the sense that many pediatric radiologists deal with most modalities and organ systems. We get the best of both worlds. It is also possible in pediatric radiology to become a subsubspecialist, such as a pediatric neuroradiologist, pediatric interventional radiologist, pediatric cardiac imager, or pediatric fetal imager.

■ INTRODUCTION: SPECIAL CONSIDERATIONS IN PEDIATRIC IMAGING

Many issues are unique to the imaging of children as compared with that of adults. Imaging examinations that are easily carried out in adults require special adjustments to be successfully achieved in children. The rotating resident on a pediatric imaging rotation and the general radiologist who occasionally images children must be prepared to deal with these issues and to adjust imaging techniques to safely and successfully obtain imaging examinations. In this introductory chapter, several of the general issues that can arise when imaging children are briefly addressed.

Relationship Between Imager and Parents

In both pediatric and adult patient care situations, there are often family members with whom the imager must interact. However, in the pediatric setting, there are several unique features in the relationship among imager, patient, and family. When caring for children, communication more often takes place between the radiologist and parent than between the radiologist and patient. Obviously, age-appropriate communication directly with the child is also paramount to success. In addition, the degree of interaction between the imager and the child–parent unit may be greater in the pediatric setting than in the adult setting because of associated issues, such as the potential need for sedation, the need for consent from the parent rather than the child (if the child is a minor), and the need for intense explanation of the procedure on the levels of both the child and the parent. Most people are also much more inquisitive and protective concerning occurrences when their children are involved. Because of these reasons, descriptions of what to expect during the visit to the imaging area may have to be more detailed and nuanced when dealing with pediatric patients and their parents.

The stress level of parents when their child is or may be ill is immense, and such stress often brings out both the best and worst in people. Because of the intense bonds between most parents and their children, the relationship between imager and parents is most successful when the radiologist exercises marked empathy, patience, professionalism, and effective communication.

Professionalism and Effective Communication

It is interesting to note that in pediatric health care most of the complaints by parents and families are not related to technical errors; they are more commonly related to issues of professionalism and communication. Of reported parent complaints, 30% are related to poor communication and unprofessional behavior. In addition, practicing effective communication has been shown to have multiple positive effects, including better patient outcome, decreased cost, increased patient and family satisfaction, and decreased chance of litigation in the presence of adverse events.

Although physicians are referred to as healthcare professionals, historically they have not received formal training in professionalism and communication, have had poor role models, and have been seen as individual practitioners rather than as members of healthcare teams. Radiology departments and individual radiologists must be proactive in making improvements

in this area. Having a program to improve and standardize interactions with families can be helpful. Scripting expected interactions can help improve patient and family interactions, such as defining how physicians introduce themselves to patients and families (including stating position and role in the upcoming procedure), as well as behaviors to avoid (for example, stating that the patient's ordering physician does not know how to order or that one does not have time to talk to a referring physician because one is too busy). A commonly used approach to interaction with patients is AIDET, described on the Studer Group website. A = acknowledge, I = Introduce, D = Duration, E = Explanation, and T = Thank you. Use of such an approach has been shown to improve the patient and family's impression of the quality of care rendered. Scripting both the type of conversation and process in general is also very helpful for the delivery of difficult news, such as defining the process for communicating with the family when a child is diagnosed with a new tumor, for example.

Inability to Cooperate

Infants and young children are commonly unable to cooperate with requirements for imaging commonly met by adults. For example, they may be unable to keep still, remain in a certain position, concentrate for more than a brief moment, or breath hold. Children of various ages have unique limitations. Infants and toddlers may be unable to stay still, whereas 3-year-olds are more apt to refuse to cooperate. These limitations affect almost all pediatric imaging examinations: radiography, fluoroscopy, ultrasound, computed tomography (CT), magnetic resonance imaging (MRI), nuclear imaging, and interventional radiology. There are a number of potential solutions that can be helpful in these situations. Commonly employed techniques include distracting the child, providing child-friendly surroundings (Figs. 1-1 through 1-6), immobilization, and sedation.

Distracting the child with something other than the procedure is often a simple and easy tactic to use. Talking to older children about school and other activities can be helpful. Certified child life specialists are very successful in helping to coach and distract children so that they can complete imaging exams without sedation. They often use rattles and noise-making toys with very young children. Video players are a very useful distraction technique for ultrasound, fluoroscopy, and CT. Video goggles (Fig. 1-7) have been very successful in decreasing sedation for MRI. Children are often able to

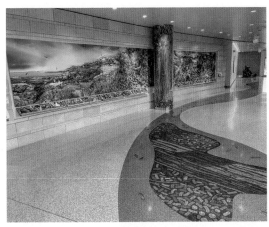

■ FIGURE 1-1 Colorful, child-friendly décor in pediatric hospital hallway. Note educational mural about coastal nature on wall, colorful tiles on floor, and bear with cub statue down hall. Many children's hospitals are now being decorated with modern, brightly colored, open areas without "cartoonish"themes.

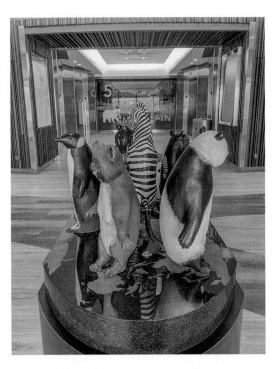

■ FIGURE 1-3 Elevator lobby with child-friendly animal stature and mountain themed redwood decorations.

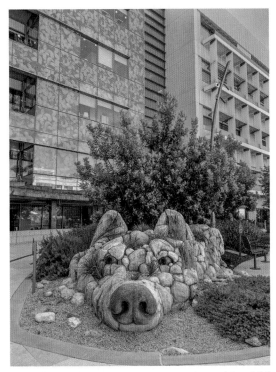

■ FIGURE 1-2 Intrahospital garden area with child-friendly coyote head formed out of rocks. Many hospitals are using gardens and other natural settings to help in healing process.

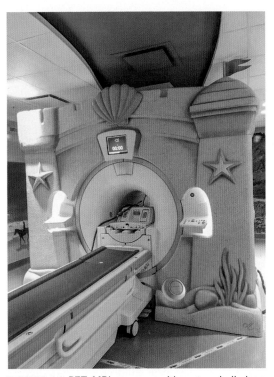

■ FIGURE 1-4 PET MRI scanner with outer shell decorated as a sand castle.

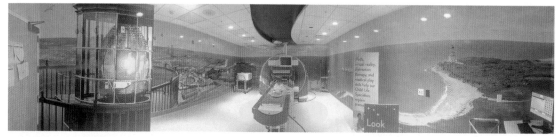

■ FIGURE 1-5 Nuclear medicine room decorated with décor indicative of the Northern California coast and Bay Area landmarks.

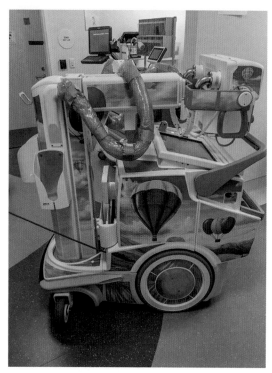

■ FIGURE 1-6 Portable radiograph unit decorated with child-friendly decals.

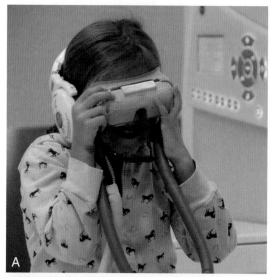

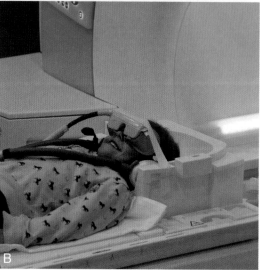

■ FIGURE 1-7 Video goggles can help young children to cooperate for MR examination, thus avoiding sedation. **A,** Video goggles on a child preparing for an MR examination. **B,** Video goggles with audio headphones in place as child is slid into scanner. Note happy demeanor.

cooperate with undergoing an MRI when watching a movie or cartoon on the video goggles. It is amazing how cooperative many children will be when they are able to watch television. Using a combined program that includes the introduction of a child life specialist, a combination of the tactics discussed earlier to calm infants and young children, and the promotion of a culture that avoids sedation whenever possible was shown to reduce the frequency of need for sedation in children less than 7 years of age by 34.6% for MRI and 44.9% for CT.

Providing child-friendly surroundings may help to ease a young child's anxiety and increase cooperation. Paintings on the walls and equipment and cartoonish figures in the examination rooms can be helpful. Eliminating or minimizing painful portions of the examination can also be very helpful in keeping a young child cooperative. The placement of an intravenous line often causes a great deal of patient anxiety and renders the child uncooperative for a subsequent imaging study, such as a CT scan. Using topical analgesia to decrease the pain of the intravenous line placement commonly makes this portion of the examination less traumatic. In addition, it is helpful to schedule appropriate sequencing of imaging examinations so that the most difficult exam is performed last. For example, it can be much easier to perform a renal ultrasound before rather than after the child has experienced a voiding cystourethrogram.

Immobilization is also a helpful technique. Infants who are bundled or "papoosed" in a blanket are more apt to stay still than infants who are not. This may make the difference between needing or not needing sedation to obtain an examination. There are also a number of commercially available immobilization devices that are helpful when performing certain examinations. Imaging departments that image children should consider making such equipment available.

In certain situations, distraction and immobilization may not be successful, and sedation or general anesthesia may be necessary to obtain imaging studies. Because of the prolonged nature of the examination and the need for the patient to be completely still, many children younger than 6 years of age require sedation or anesthesia for MRI studies. Because of the increased speed of acquisition by the newer CT scanners and the previously mentioned sedation reduction programs, sedation is needed much less often now than in the past for children undergoing CT examination. Other procedures that might require sedation include some nuclear medicine studies and most interventional procedures.

Standards of care for sedation and anesthesia are required by the Center for Medicare and Medicaid Services and The Joint Commission. Any imaging department planning to sedate children must have a defined sedation program that is in concordance with these guidelines. The sedation program must have protocols for pre-sedation preparation, sedative agents used, monitoring during sedation and during post-sedation recovery, and discharge criteria. At most children's hospitals, sedation and anesthesia programs are run by nonradiologists, typically anesthesiologists, emergency physicians, or intensive care physicians. At many institutions, such physicians have access to sedatives that are better for imaging sedation, such as propofol or dexmedetomidine.

Variable Size and Physiology

Because of the size variability from infant to adult-sized children, many adaptations must be considered for pediatric imaging studies in relation to size. The doses of contrast and drugs used in imaging examinations need to be adjusted according to a child's size, often on a per weight (mg/kg) basis. Oral contrast dosing is also based on patient weight or age. Using CT as an illustrative example, other variables may also be affected by patient size. In small children, the largest possible intravenous line may be very small, often 22 gauge or 24 gauge. The intravenous line may be placed in the foot or hand. The length of the region of interest to be imaged is variable, and the lengths of the patient's veins are variable. Physiologic parameters, such as the patient's cardiac output, are also more variable in children than in adults. These factors affect parameters such as the time between contrast injection and onset of scanning, as well as choices in contrast administration technique (hand bolus vs. power injector). Slice thickness should be smaller in younger children because of the smaller anatomic parts. Similar adjustments must be considered in all other imaging modalities when applied to children. Radiation dose reduction is discussed in Patient Safety.

Age-Related Changes in Imaging Appearance

Another factor that makes imaging in children different from that in adults is the continuous changes in the normal imaging appearance of multiple organ systems during normal childhood development. The normal imaging appearance of certain aspects of organ systems can be different both at varying ages during childhood and between children and adults. For example, the kidneys look different on ultrasound in neonates from the way they look in a 1-year-old child. The developing brain demonstrates differences in signal at varying ages on MRI, which is related to changes in myelination. A large mediastinal shadow related to the thymus may be normal or severely abnormal depending upon the child's age. The skeleton demonstrates marked changes at all ages of childhood; this is related to the maturation of apophyses and epiphyses and the progressive ossification of structures. Knowledge of the normal age-related appearances of these organ systems is vital to appropriate interpretation of imaging studies. Lack of this knowledge is one of the most common causes of errors made in the interpretation of pediatric imaging studies.

Age-Related Differential Diagnoses

The types of diseases that affect children are vastly different from those that commonly affect adults. Therefore, the differential diagnosis and significance of a particular imaging finding in a child are dramatically different from those determined by the identical imaging finding in an adult. In addition, the diseases that affect specific age groups within the childhood years are different. Therefore, the differential diagnosis and significance of a particular imaging finding in a 2-month-old infant may differ dramatically from those determined by the identical imaging finding in a 10-year-old child.

Quality, Safety, Service, and Improvement

There has been incredible progress over the past 20 years in the attention to improvement in the areas of quality, safety, and service both in medicine in general as well as in the specific area of pediatric radiology. There is still much work to do. A full review of improvement science or high reliability is beyond the scope of this book, but we will review some of the highlights.

Data suggest that quality improvement is difficult but very rewarding work. Approximately 70% of initiatives to launch organizational change are not sustained. One study showed that even as short as 1 year post implementation that a third of improvement initiatives are not successfully sustained. This is potentially not surprising. Health care has been described as one of the most complicated sociotechnical systems. In order to be successful in introducing improvement change in health care, one needs to create a culture conducive of accelerating improvement. I think that most people understand and believe that culture is important in implementing change. The challenge is often where to get started to change that culture? It can seem like an amorphous target. We would advocate that in order to create such a culture, you must focus both on the social domain, or way that people interact, as well as the technical domain or how the processes to achieve the work are designed. Focus on either

the technical or social domains alone typically is unsuccessful. One way to change the social domain is to take it into consideration when designing your technical domain or processes. Focusing on the processes can help create the social culture to enhance improvement. You can build your cultural expectations for your leaders and team members into your process such a well-designed system for daily management, problem solving accountability, goal setting and deployment, and staff and physician recognition.

Let us take one of those processes as an example—Daily Management Systems. Daily management systems are designed to quickly identify issues, empower front-line areas to solve those issues, and, when the front line cannot resolve them, escalate the issues to those who can help. Increasingly, in medicine, as well as other fields, tiered huddle systems are used to create daily readiness. Radiologists, technologists, and managers come together in a brief huddle each morning in front of a visual board to make sure that they are ready to care for the patients scheduled for that day (Fig. 1-8). Such processes often have three parts: daily readiness, problem accountability, and metrics evaluation. One approach to daily readiness is evaluating the volume scheduled for that day and organizing the approach to concerns around safety and the acronym MESA (Methods, Equipment, Supplies, Associates). Does anyone have any safety concerns? Do we have the right *M*ethods to take care of the patients today (does anyone have questions around protocols or atypical patients?)? Do we have the right *E*quipment to take care of the patients today (is there any planned downtime, broken equipment, or information technology issues?)? Do we have the *S*upplies we need to take care of the patients today? Do we have the right *A*ssociates to take care of the patients today (did anybody call in sick, do we have the right people with the right expertise?)? Going through a set of such questions leads to a list of issues. Having a defined problem accountability process that assigns each issue a single owner and defines the immediate countermeasure and the date at which the owner will come back to report an update at the huddle is important so that issues do not go unresolved or only partially remedied. Such daily management systems emphasize many of the aspects needed to create a high reliability system: safety is everyone's responsibility, people should speak up in the face of uncertainty, and processes should be standardized. Ideally, the only variation in a healthcare system should be that related to the condition of the patient. There should not be variability related to technologists, protocols, care sites, or physicians. Radiologists need to work

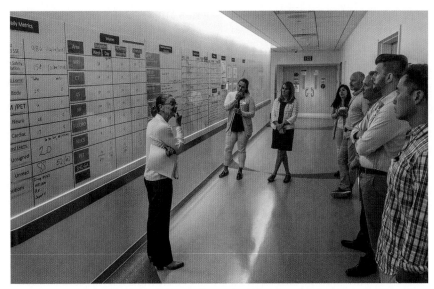

■ **FIGURE 1-8** Image of radiology daily readiness huddle occurring in front of a visual board.

together to create evidence-based standardized imaging protocols and procedures, as well as reports, and continuously strive to improve them. In order to foster improvement, we want to create a culture where healthcare providers see two aspects to their clinical work: 1. To work within the created system of providing care and 2. To constantly improve that system of care.

When setting up an improvement initiative for success, dedicating effort to create a "SMART" goal is foundational. SMART is a mnemonic to help create goals to position a project for success. S = specific, M = measurable, A = attainable, R = relevant, and T = timely. In my experience, the letter that often gets left off is the "T" for timely. In order to set the appropriate pace and to drive accountability, it is incredibly important to focus on the timelines for the key drivers for the initiative. In our experience, the key drivers for many improvement initiatives fall into one of four categories: standardization, data transparency, accountability, and coordination. We have found that reviewing these four areas when crafting key drivers has served us well in accurately planning our action plans.

RADIATION SAFETY

Safety issues specific to radiology include, among others, radiation safety, MRI safety, and correct effective communication of the information in and interpretation of imaging examinations. Radiation safety will be partially covered here because it is germane to pediatric radiology. Children are much more sensitive to the potential harmful effects of radiation than are adults, and children also have a longer expected life span during which to develop potential complications of radiation, such as cancer. Therefore, attention to radiation safety in all areas of pediatric radiology is paramount. CT delivers higher doses of radiation than do other diagnostic imaging modalities, except Positron Emission Tomography. Given the small but real risk associated with the radiation dose from a CT in a child, it is essential for all radiologists to practice dose reduction techniques in pediatric CT. Such tactics include avoiding CT when unnecessary; using alternative diagnostic methods that do not use radiation, such as ultrasound, when possible; and adjusting CT parameters to minimize dose when CT is performed. Because children are smaller than adults and need less radiation to create the same signal-to-noise ratios, the tube current (mA), as well as kilovolts and other factors, can be greatly reduced when imaging a small child. Many other factors can be adjusted to reduce dose as well.

It is also very important not to overreact to this potentially small risk related to radiation dose for CT. For any truly clinically indicated examination, the risk of not doing the CT and not having that information is often magnitudes greater than that related to radiation risk.

SUGGESTED READING

Bomher ST, Munguia JM, Albert MS, Nelson KW, Barmann-Losche J, Paltchek TS, Donnelly LF: The approach to improving patient experience at children's hospitals: a primer for pediatric radiologists, *Pediatr Radiol* 50:1482–1491, 2020.

Donnelly LF, Lee GM, Sharek PJ: Costs of quality and safety in radiology, *Radiographics* 38:1682−1687, 2018.

Donnelly LF: Avoiding failure: tools to successful sustainable quality improvement projects, *Pediatr Radiol* 47:793−797, 2017a.

Donnelly LF, Cherian SS, Chua KB, Thankachan S, Millecker LA, Koroll AG, Bisset III GS: The daily readiness huddle − a process to rapidly identify issues and foster improvement through problem solving accountability, *Pediatr Radiol* 47:22−30, 2017.

Donnelly LF: Aspirational characteristics for effective leadership of improvement teams, *Pediatr Radiol* 47:17−21, 2017b.

Donnelly LF, Dickerson JM, Goodfriend MA, Muething SE: Improving patient safety: effects of a safety program on performance and culture in a department of radiology, *Am Journal Rev* 193:165−171, 2009.

Donnelly LF, Strife JL: How I do it: establishing a program to promote professionalism and effective communication in radiology, *Radiology* 283:773−779, 2006.

Frush DP: Overview of CT technologist for children, *Pediatr Radiol* 44:422−426, 2014.

Frush DP, Bisset GS: Pediatric sedation in radiology: the practice of safe sleep, *Am Journal Rev* 167:1381−1387, 1996.

Frush DP, Goske MJ: Image gently: toward optimizing the practice of pediatric CT through resources and dialogue, *Pediatr Radiol* 45:471−475, 2015.

Greer MC, Vasanawala SS: Invited commentary: reducing sedation and anesthesia in pediatric patients at MRI, *Radiographics* 40:503−504, 2020.

Larson DB, Kruskal JB, Kreche KN, Donnelly LF: Key concepts of patient safety in radiology, *Radiographics* 35:1677−1693, 2015.

Pichert JW, Miller CS, Hollo AH, et al.: What health professionals can do to identify and resolve patient dissatisfaction, *Jt Comm J Qual Improv* 124:303−312, 1998.

Snyder EJ, Zhang W, Jasmin KC, Thankachan S, Donnelly LF: Gauging potential risk for patients in pediatric radiology by review of over 2,000 incident reports, *Pediatr Radiol* 48:1867−1874, 2018.

Thrall JH: Quality and safety revolution in health care, *Radiology* 233:3637−3640, 2004.

CHAPTER 2

AIRWAY

Robert J. Fleck

Signs and symptoms referable to the airway are much more common in children than in adults. For practical purposes, abnormalities of the airway can be divided into acute upper airway obstruction, lower airway obstruction (extrinsic compression, intrinsic obstruction), obstructive sleep apnea (OSA), and congenital high airway obstruction syndrome (CHAOS).

Clinically, children with acute upper airway obstruction (above the thoracic inlet) tend to present with inspiratory stridor, whereas children with lower airway obstruction (below the thoracic inlet) are more likely to present with expiratory wheezing. However, the categorization of a child with noisy breathing into one of these two groups can be very difficult. The primary imaging evaluation of the pediatric airway for acute conditions should include frontal and lateral high-kilovolt radiography of the airway and frontal and lateral views of the chest.

■ ACUTE UPPER AIRWAY OBSTRUCTION

Acute stridor in a young child is the most common indication for imaging the pediatric airway. The most common causes of acute upper airway obstruction in children include laryngomalacia, inflammatory disorders, and foreign bodies. Laryngomalacia accounts for 60% of the cases of stridor in pediatric patients and is characterized by positional inspiratory stridor, which often disappears with crying. Although radiographs are often obtained, laryngomalacia is not a diagnosis that can be made on radiographs. Direct visualization with a nasopharyngoscope provides a definitive diagnosis. The most common inflammatory disorders causing stridor include croup, epiglottitis, exudative tracheitis, and retropharyngeal cellulitis and abscess. Anatomic structures that are especially important to evaluate on radiographs of children with acute upper airway obstruction include the epiglottis, aryepiglottic folds, subglottic trachea, and retropharyngeal soft tissues.

Croup

Croup (acute laryngotracheobronchitis) is the most common cause of acute upper airway obstruction in young children. The peak incidence occurs between 6 months and 3 years of age. The mean age at presentation of croup is 1 year of age. In children older than 3 years, other causes of airway obstruction should be suspected. Croup is viral and is usually a benign, self-limited disease. In children with croup, redundant, loosely attached mucosa in the subglottic region becomes inflamed, swells, and encroaches upon the airway. The children present with a barky cough and intermittent inspiratory stridor. Croup usually occurs following or during other symptoms of lower respiratory tract infection. Most affected children are diagnosed clinically in the physician's office and never receive imaging. Children with croup are managed supportively as outpatients, and the parents are managed by reassurance. Inhaled corticosteroids are becoming a popular therapy in children with croup. They have been shown to reduce the length and severity of illness.

The purpose of obtaining radiographs in a patient with suspected croup is not so much to confirm the diagnosis but rather to exclude other, more serious causes of upper airway obstruction that require intervention.

The normal configuration of the subglottic airway has been likened to a Port wine bottle, with the subglottic airway appearing rounded, with "shoulders" that are convex outward (Fig. 2-1 and 2-2). In croup, the immediate subglottic airway becomes narrowed and thin due to edema in the mucosal tissue between the vocal folds and the cricoid cartilage. This swelling obscures the normal shoulders of the subglottic airway and creates a smooth funnel-shaped subglottic airway which blends with the slight outward angel of the pediatric cricoid cartilage and projects like the neck of a Riesling wine bottle (Fig. 2-1) on X-ray (Fig. 2-3). Lateral radiographs may demonstrate a narrowing or loss of definition of the lumen of the subglottic trachea (see Fig. 2-3) and often hypopharyngeal overdistention. With croup, the epiglottis and aryepiglottic folds appear normal.

Epiglottitis

In contrast to croup, epiglottitis is a life-threatening disease that can potentially require

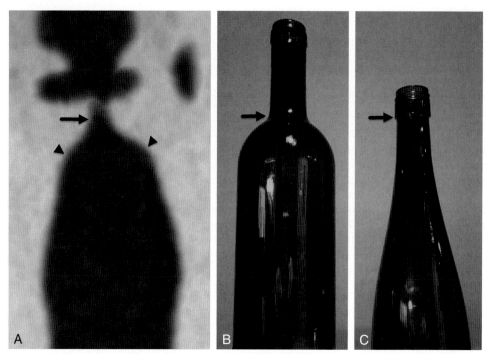

■ FIGURE 2-1 Subglottic configuration: normal and croup. **A,** Coronal computed tomography (CT) reformat through a normal pediatric airway demonstrates the shoulders (*arrowheads*) immediately below the glottis (*arrows* mark the glottis). **B,** The shoulders of the normal glottis have an appearance similar to a Port wine bottle. **C,** With croup, subglottic edema obscures the normal shoulder, and on frontal projection, the subglottic airway assumes a funnel-shaped, narrowed airway, resembling the appearance of a Riesling bottle.

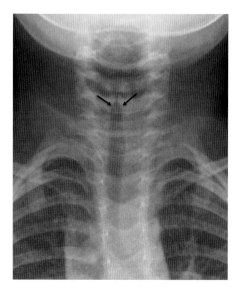

■ FIGURE 2-2 Normal frontal radiograph of the airway. The subglottic airway demonstrates rounded shoulders (*arrows*) that are convex outward.

emergent intubation. The possibility that a child with epiglottitis might arrive in a deserted radiology department was historically a constant source of anxiety for on-call radiology residents. However, most cases of epiglottitis were historically caused by *Haemophilus influenzae* and are now preventable by immunization (HiB vaccine or combination vaccine), so the incidence of epiglottitis has dramatically decreased. The causes of epiglottitis are now also more diverse. Related to this, care of children with epiglottitis is now more of a challenge because healthcare workers are less attuned to recognize and treat patients with this disorder. Children with epiglottitis are usually toxic appearing and present with an abrupt onset of stridor, dysphagia, fever, restlessness, and an increase in respiratory distress when recumbent. In the pre-HiB vaccine era, the classically described peak age of incidence was 3.5 years. However, since the introduction of the HiB vaccine, there has been a marked increase in the mean age of presentation to 14.6 years. Because of the risk for complete airway obstruction and respiratory failure, no maneuvers should be performed that make the patient uncomfortable. If the diagnosis is not made on physical examination, a single lateral radiograph of the neck should be obtained, usually with the patient erect or in whatever position that allows the patient to breathe comfortably. Children with epiglottitis should never be made to lie supine against their will to obtain a radiograph because it can result in acute airway obstruction and potentially, death.

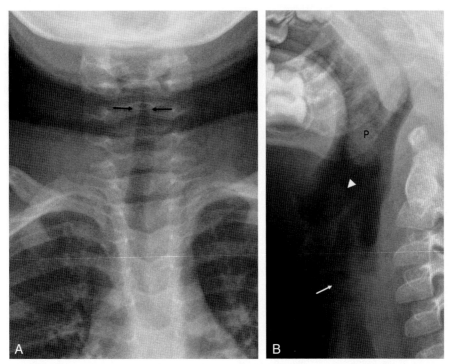

■ **FIGURE 2-3** Croup. **A,** Frontal radiograph showing symmetric subglottic narrowing (*arrows*) with loss of normal shouldering. The narrowing extends more inferiorly than the piriform sinuses. **B,** Lateral radiograph showing poorly marginated inferior border of the laryngeal ventricle (*arrow*). Note furled epiglottis (*arrowhead*), which is normal, and thin aryepiglottic folds. Also note mildly enlarged palatine (P) tonsils.

With epiglottitis, on the lateral radiograph, there is marked enlargement of the epiglottis. A normal epiglottis typically has a thin appearance with the superior aspect being sharply pointed. The swollen epiglottis has been likened to the appearance of a thumb. With epiglottitis, there is also thickening of the aryepiglottic folds (Figs. 2-4 and 2-5). The aryepiglottic folds are the soft tissues that extend from the epiglottis posterior-inferiorly to the arytenoid cartilage and normally are convex downward. When the aryepiglottic folds become abnormally thickened, they appear convex superiorly. Symmetric sub-glottic narrowing, similar to croup, may be seen on frontal radiography (if obtained).

An obliquely imaged, or omega-shaped, epiglottis may artifactually appear wide because both the left and right sides of the epiglottis are being imaged adjacent to each other. This should not be confused with a truly enlarged epiglottis. The absence of thickening of the aryepiglottic folds can be helpful in making this differentiation. With an omega-shaped epiglottis (normal variant), often both the left and right walls of the epiglottis are visible.

In current times, related to both the uncommon occurrence of epiglottitis and the frequent reliance on computed tomography (CT) to evaluate more common inflammatory neck conditions (such as retropharyngeal abscess), it is increasingly more common to see and diagnose epiglottitis on CT rather than on radiography. Although not classically advocated as a diagnostic tool for epiglottitis (given the risks of laying such patients supine and giving them intravenous [IV] contrast), the findings of epiglottitis are easily identified on CT (Fig. 2-5). Findings include swelling and low-attenuation edema of the epiglottis and aryepiglottic folds associated with inflammatory stranding in adjacent fat.

Exudative Tracheitis

Exudative tracheitis (also known as bacterial tracheitis, membranous croup, or membranous laryngotracheobronchitis) is another uncommon but potentially life-threatening cause of acute upper airway obstruction. The disorder is characterized by a purulent infection of the trachea in which exudative plaques form along the tracheal walls (much like those seen in diphtheria). Affected children are usually older and more ill than those with standard croup; typically, their ages range from 6 to 10 years. Although initial reports described most cases to be secondary to infection by *Staphylococcus aureus*, other reports

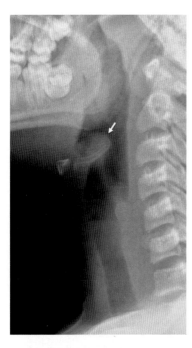

■ **FIGURE 2-4** Epiglottitis. Lateral radiograph showing marked thickening of the epiglottis (*arrow*). The aryepiglottic folds are only mildly thickened in this case.

finding. A plaque-like irregularity of the tracheal wall is also highly suspicious (Fig. 2-6). Nonadherent mucus may mimic a membrane radiographically. In cooperative patients, having them cough and then repeating the film may help to differentiate mucus from a membrane. Other findings include symmetric or asymmetric subglottic narrowing or irregularity or loss of definition of the tracheal wall in a child with a high fever and age older than that typical of croup. Membranes and tracheal wall irregularities may be seen on frontal or lateral radiographs only; therefore, it is important to get both views. Treatment includes IV antibiotics, possible stripping of exudative membranes, and endotracheal intubation.

A number of controversies regarding exudative tracheitis exist. First, it is seen with great frequency at some institutions and not at all at others. Second, although it is considered a life-threatening condition, to my knowledge, no patient has ever died at home of this disease—which seems odd. In our opinion, there are definitive cases of this disease, but it is likely overdiagnosed and overtreated in some organizations.

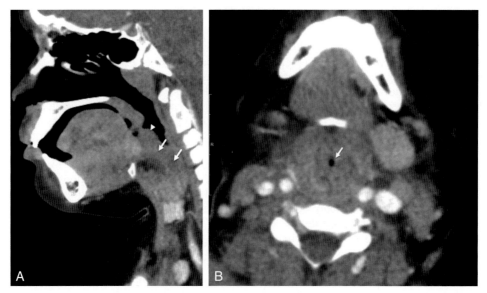

■ **FIGURE 2-5** Epiglottitis. **A,** Sagittal CT image showing low-attenuation swelling of the epiglottis (*arrowhead*). Also note marked thickening and low-attenuation edema of the aryepiglottic folds (*arrows*). **B,** Axial CT image shows the marked narrowing of the subglottic airway (*arrow*).

have noted multimicrobial infections. It is unclear whether the disease is a primary bacterial infection or a secondary bacterial infection that occurs following damage to the respiratory mucosa by a viral infection. A linear soft tissue filling defect (a membrane) seen within the airway on radiography is the most characteristic

Retropharyngeal Cellulitis and Abscess

Retropharyngeal cellulitis is a pyogenic infection of the retropharyngeal space that usually follows a recent pharyngitis or upper respiratory tract infection. Children present with sudden onset of fever, stiff neck, dysphagia, and occasionally

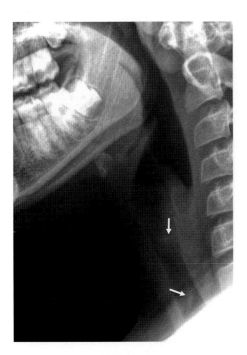

■ FIGURE 2-6 Exudative tracheitis. Lateral radiograph showing irregular plaque-like filling defects (*arrows*) and airway wall irregularities within trachea. Again, note the normal appearance of the nonthickened epiglottis in this patient.

stridor. Most affected children are young, with more than half of the cases occurring between 6 and 12 months of age. On lateral radiography, there is thickening of the retropharyngeal soft tissues (Fig. 2-7). In a normal infant or young child, the soft tissues between the posterior aspect of the aerated pharynx and anterior aspect of the vertebral column should not exceed the anterior-to-posterior diameter of the cervical vertebral bodies. If these soft tissues are thicker, an abnormality should be suspected. Apex anterior convexity of the retropharyngeal soft tissues provides supportive evidence that there is true widening of the retropharyngeal soft tissues (Fig. 2-7).

However, in infants, who have short necks, it is common to see pseudothickening of the retropharyngeal soft tissues when the lateral radiograph is obtained without the neck being well extended (Fig. 2-8). If it is unclear on the initial lateral radiograph whether the soft tissues are truly rather than artifactually widened, it is best to repeat the lateral radiograph with the neck placed in full extension (Fig. 2-8). Fluoroscopy can also be used to evaluate whether the pseudothickening is persistent. The only radiographic feature that can differentiate abscess from cellulitis is the identification of gas within the retropharyngeal soft tissues.

CT is commonly performed to define the extent of disease and to help to predict cases in which a drainable fluid collection is present (Fig. 2-7). On CT, a low-attenuation, well-defined area with an enhancing rim is suggestive for a drainable fluid collection (Fig. 2-7). Cellulitis without abscess is actually more common than the presence of a drainable abscess on early CT. Therefore, it is recommended that use of CT imaging in the early presentation be reserved for toxic appearing patients, suspicion for extension, or when IV antibiotics do not seem to be effective. The advantage of this approach is that when the CT is performed the cellulitis may have become more organized to become a drainable collection.

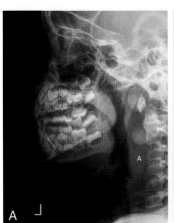
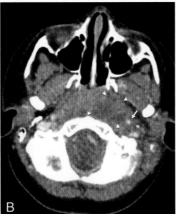
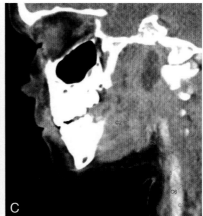

■ FIGURE 2-7 Retropharyngeal abscess. **A,** Lateral radiograph showing thickening of the retropharyngeal soft tissues (A), which are wider than the adjacent vertebral bodies. **B,** Contrast-enhanced CT in axial plane shows ill-defined low-attenuation thickening of the retropharyngeal soft tissues (*arrowheads*) compatible with inflammation and associated narrowing of the left carotid artery (*arrow*). **C,** Contrast-enhanced CT in the sagittal plane off midline shows a well-defined low-attenuation collection after 3 days of antibiotics.

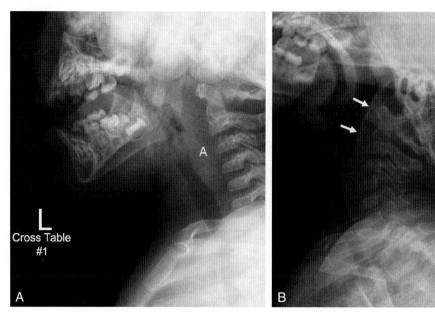

■ **FIGURE 2-8** Pseudoretropharyngeal soft tissue thickening secondary to lack of extended neck positioning. **A,** Initial lateral radiograph, obtained in a supine position, showing apparent thickening of retropharyngeal soft tissues mimicking potential retropharyngeal abscess (A). **B,** Repeat lateral radiograph, while sitting-up with neck extended, shows normal thickness of retropharyngeal soft tissues (*arrows*), much narrower in thickness than adjacent vertebral bodies.

■ LOWER AIRWAY OBSTRUCTION

The most common cause of wheezing in children is small airway inflammation, such as is caused by asthma and viral illness (bronchiolitis). When the wheezing persists, presents at an atypical age for asthma, or is refractory to treatment, other reasons for lower airway obstruction are entertained. Other causes of lower airway obstruction can be divided into those that are intrinsic to the airway (such as bronchial foreign body, tracheomalacia, or intrinsic masses) and those that cause extrinsic compression of the trachea (such as vascular rings). The initial radiologic screening procedure for wheezing is frontal and lateral radiography of the airway and chest. Radiographs are used to exclude acute causes of upper airway obstruction, evaluate for other processes that can cause wheezing (such as cardiac disease), and help to categorize the abnormality as being more likely to be an intrinsic or an extrinsic airway process. Important findings to look for on the radiographs include evidence of tracheal narrowing, position of the aortic arch, asymmetric lung aeration, radiopaque foreign body, and lung consolidation. When tracheal compression is present on radiography, it is important to note both the superior to inferior level of the compression and whether the compression comes from the anterior or posterior aspect of the trachea because various

vascular rings present with different patterns of tracheal compression (Fig. 2-9).

If the radiographs suggest an intrinsic abnormality, bronchoscopy is the next procedure of choice. If the radiographs suggest an extrinsic compression, cross-sectional imaging is performed. CT and magnetic resonance imaging (MRI) can be used to evaluate the airway. The advantages of CT over MRI are that most infants can be scanned without sedation on CT (which is a significant factor in an infant with airway difficulties) and that better evaluation of the lungs is possible. The disadvantages of CT are the radiation exposure and dependence upon IV contrast. With modern technology, both CT and MRI can be used to create dynamic cine images to depict abnormal airway motion (malacia).

Extrinsic Lower Airway Compression

Almost any process that causes either a space-occupying mass within the mediastinum or the enlargement or malposition of a vascular structure can lead to compression of the airway. The classically described vascular causes of lower airway compression include double aortic arch, anomalous left pulmonary artery, and innominate artery compression syndrome. However, other causes of airway compression include middle mediastinal masses, such as a bronchogenic cyst (Fig. 2-10) or large anterior

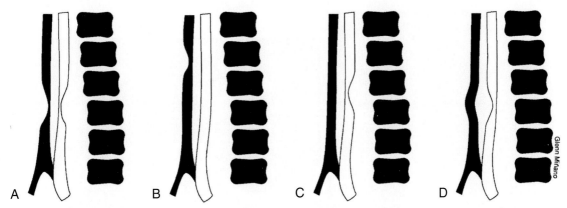

FIGURE 2-9 Patterns of compression of the trachea and esophagus in common vascular rings. The diagrams are comparable to a lateral radiograph of the chest. The trachea is black; the esophagus is white. **A,** Double aortic arch. The trachea is compressed on its anterior aspect, and the esophagus is compressed on its posterior aspect. **B,** Innominate artery compression. The trachea is compressed on its anterior aspect. The level of compression is just below the thoracic inlet, higher than other vascular causes of compression. **C,** Left arch with aberrant right subclavian artery or right arch with aberrant left subclavian artery. There is compression of the posterior aspect of the esophagus. The trachea is not compressed. **D,** Aberrant left pulmonary artery (pulmonary sling). The trachea is compressed on its posterior aspect and the esophagus is compressed on its anterior aspect.

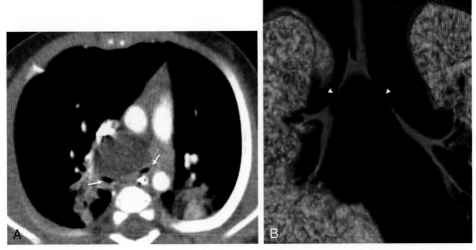

FIGURE 2-10 Bronchogenic cyst causing compression of the trachea and bronchi. **A,** Axial contrast-enhanced CT shows mass anterior to the airway at the level of the carina compressing and narrowing the main bronchi (*arrows*). **B,** 3D surface—rendered image of the airways emphasizes the severe narrowing of the bilateral main bronchi (*arrowheads*).

mediastinal masses (Fig. 2-11); enlargement of the ascending aorta, such as is seen in Marfan syndrome; enlargement of the pulmonary arteries, as in congenital absence of the pulmonary valve; malposition of the descending aorta, as in midline descending aorta-carina-compression syndrome; enlargement of the left atrium; or abnormal chest wall configuration, such as a narrow thoracic inlet. With the congenital vascular causes of airway compression, in addition to the obvious anatomic extrinsic compression, there is also often a component of intrinsic malacia related to the long-term nature of the airway being compressed. This can cause persistent symptoms even after the extrinsic compression has surgically been remedied.

On axial imaging, the trachea is normally rounded in configuration (Fig. 2-12), sometimes with a flattened posterior wall related to the noncartilaginous portion. A normal trachea cross-section is never oval or oblong, with a greater left-to-right than anterior-to-posterior diameter (never "pancake shaped"). When the airway appears pancake shaped, it is abnormal. An oval-shaped appearance of the trachea on CT or MRI is a much more sensitive finding for tracheomalacia than attempting to identify a 50% change in cross-sectional area.

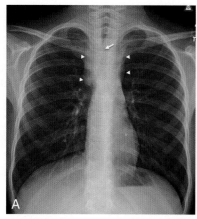
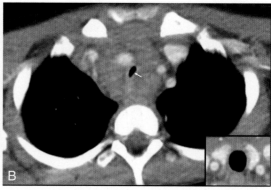

■ **FIGURE 2-11** Lymphoma causing compression of the trachea. **A,** Chest X-ray shows a modest anterior mediastinal mass (*arrowheads*) with severe narrowing of the trachea (*arrow*). **B,** Axial CT of the chest shows the severe narrowing (*arrow*) is caused by a mass of lymph nodes surrounding the trachea. The inset in the right lower corner shows the normal caliber of this patient's trachea more superiorly at the level of the thyroid gland.

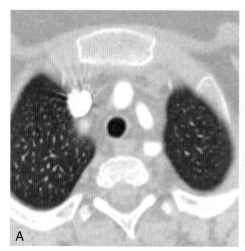
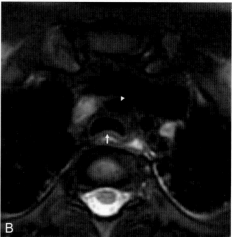

■ **FIGURE 2-12** Normal and Abnormal trachea on CT and MRI. **A,** Normal: Axial CT showing the normal configuration of trachea is round. **B,** Abnormal: An oval or pancake-shaped intrathoracic trachea is not normal. Flattening of the trachea by the right brachiocephalic artery (*arrowhead*) and invagination of the posterior membrane (*arrow*) on this T2 magnetic resonance imaging (MRI) indicates tracheomalacia.

DOUBLE AORTIC ARCH

Double aortic arch is a congenital anomaly related to the persistence of both the left and right fourth aortic arches. It is the most common symptomatic vascular ring. Usually an isolated lesion, it typically presents with symptoms early in life (soon after birth). Anatomically, the two arches surround and compress the trachea anteriorly and esophagus posteriorly. Typically, the right arch is dominant, both larger and positioned more superiorly (Fig. 2-13). In such cases, the left arch is ligated by performing a left thoracotomy. When the left arch is dominant, a right thoracotomy is performed, and the right arch is ligated. Related to surgical planning, determining the dominant arch is one of the

goals of cross-sectional imaging. With double aortic arch, the level of compression is the mid-to-lower intrathoracic trachea. In addition, there is symmetric takeoff of four great arteries from the superior aspect of the arches.

ANOMALOUS ORIGIN OF THE LEFT PULMONARY ARTERY (PULMONARY SLING)

In cases of anomalous origin of the left pulmonary artery (pulmonary sling), the left pulmonary artery arises from the right pulmonary artery rather than from the main pulmonary artery and passes between the trachea and esophagus as it courses toward the left lung. The resultant sling

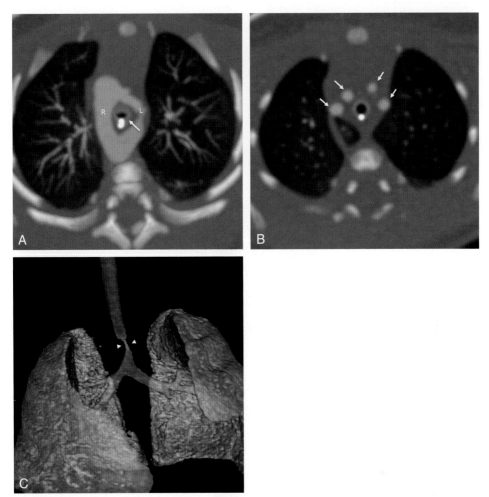

■ **FIGURE 2-13** Double aortic arch. **A,** CT image shows right and left arches (R, L) surrounding endotracheal tube (*arrow*). The left arch is nearly atretic but rejoins to form the descending aorta posteriorly. The right arch is larger than the left. **B,** Symmetry of the aortic branches (*arrows*) is associated with the double aortic arch. **C,** Follow-up dynamic CT performed for persistent symptoms shows severe tracheal collapse (*arrowheads*) during tidal breathing expiration compatible with tracheomalacia.

compresses the trachea. Pulmonary sling is the only vascular anomaly to course between the trachea and esophagus (Fig. 2-14). Therefore, compression of the posterior aspect of the trachea and the anterior aspect of the esophagus on lateral imaging is characteristic. It is the only vascular cause of airway compression that is associated with asymmetric lung inflation on chest imaging (see Fig. 2-14). Pulmonary sling can be associated with congenital heart disease, complete tracheal rings (an additional cause of airway problems), and anomalous origin of the right bronchus (see Fig. 2-14). On CT, the trachea is compressed at the level of the sling and appears flattened in the anterior-to-posterior direction—like a pancake. If complete tracheal rings are present, the rings are typically superior to the pulmonary sling, and the trachea appears very small in caliber and very round at the level of the rings (see Fig. 2-14).

RIGHT AORTIC ARCH WITH ABERRANT LEFT SUBCLAVIAN ARTERY

Right aortic arch with an aberrant left subclavian artery (RAA-ALSCA) is another arch anomaly that can be associated with airway compression (Fig. 2-15). Airway compression typically occurs when there is a persistent ductus ligament completing the ring. However, identifying a persistent ductus ligament is not possible by direct findings on imaging. There are several mechanisms by which RAA-ALSCA contributes to airway compression in addition to compression by the completed ring. Often there is dilatation of the subclavian artery at the origin from the right aorta (called a Kommerell diverticulum), which can contribute to airway compression. In addition, the descending aorta may lie in the midline, immediately anterior to the vertebral bodies, as the descending aorta passes

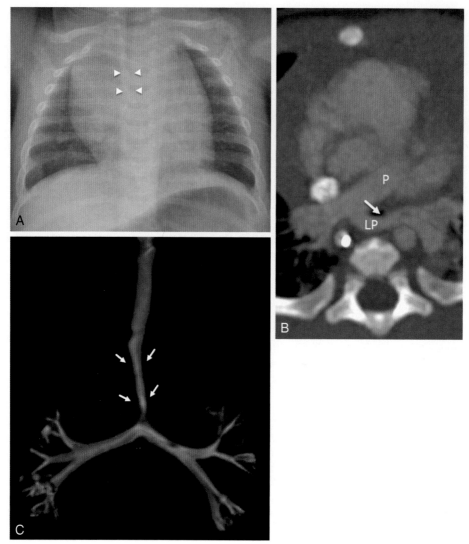

■ **FIGURE 2-14** Pulmonary sling. **A,** Chest X-ray shows the loss of the distal tracheal lumen (*arrowheads*). **B,** CT in axial plane shows anomalous origin of left pulmonary artery (LP) from the right pulmonary artery, rather than from the main pulmonary artery (P). The pulmonary sling wraps around and compresses the trachea (*arrow*) as it passes into the left hemithorax. Note the enteric tube in the esophagus (dense round structure), posterior to the sling. **C,** 3D surface–rendering CT image shows airway narrowing. The distal trachea is very small and round in caliber (*arrows*), consistent with complete tracheal rings.

from right to left as it descends (see Fig. 2-15). This midline descending aorta can contribute to airway compression as the result of the abnormal stacking of anatomic structures in the limited space between the sternum and vertebral bodies and typically causes that compression at the level of the distal tracheal carina. There is often a component of dynamic airway collapse (malacia) associated.

INNOMINATE ARTERY COMPRESSION SYNDROME

The innominate artery passes immediately anterior to the trachea just inferior to the level of

the thoracic inlet. In infants, in whom the innominate artery arises more to the left than in adults and in whom the mediastinum is crowded by the relatively large thymus, there can be narrowing of the trachea at this level. There is a spectrum from normal to severe narrowing; the term *syndrome* is reserved for cases that are symptomatic. The compression and resultant symptoms decrease with time as the child grows, and surgical therapy is reserved for cases in which symptoms are severe or the associated tracheomalacia, persistent. On lateral radiography, there is indentation of the anterior aspect of the trachea at or just below the thoracic inlet. CT demonstrates the abnormality as anterior compression of

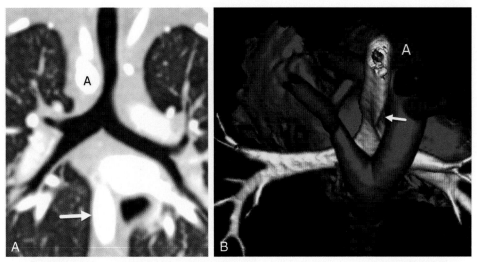

■ **FIGURE 2-15** Double aortic arch with dominant right arch and associated airway narrowing. **A,** Coronal reformatted CT shows dominant right aortic arch (A) and a small left aortic arch with moderate narrowing of the trachea. A midline descending aorta is visualized (*arrow*). **B,** 3D surface–rendered CT from posterior superior view shows the complete ring and the dominant right arch (A) that is indenting and narrowing the trachea (*arrow*).

the trachea at the level of the crossing of the innominate artery and excludes other causes of the airway compression (Fig. 2-16).

Intrinsic Lower Airway Obstruction

Intrinsic abnormalities of the lower airway include dynamic processes, such as tracheomalacia, tracheal stenosis, foreign bodies, and focal masses. Tracheomalacia is tracheal wall softening related to abnormality of the cartilaginous rings of the trachea. It can be a primary or secondary condition and results in intermittent collapse of the trachea. The diagnosis cannot be

made on a single static radiograph. However, lateral fluoroscopy or endoscopy can demonstrate dynamic changes in the caliber of the trachea, and they are diagnostic. Cine imaging with MRI or CT may also be helpful.

The most common soft tissue masses in the trachea are hemangiomas, which most commonly occur in the subglottic region, are often associated with facial hemangiomas in a beard distribution, and appear on frontal radiographs with asymmetric subglottic narrowing. Other tracheal masses include tracheal papilloma and tracheal granuloma (Fig. 2-17).

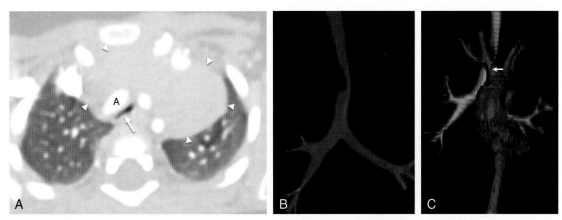

■ **FIGURE 2-16** Innominate artery compression syndrome. **A,** CT in axial plane shows innominate artery (A) compressing the trachea (*arrow*). The trachea is oblong and nearly completely compressed along the right side. Note the large thymus (*arrowheads*). **B,** 3D reconstructed CT of the trachea shows narrowing of the trachea. **C,** 3D reformatted CT shows the aorta and trachea. The innominate artery (*arrow*) compresses the trachea.

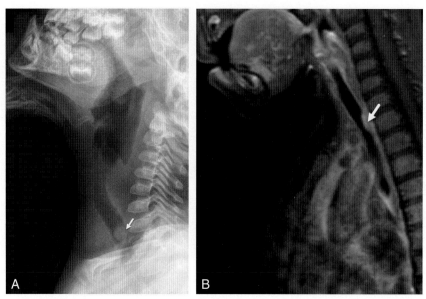

■ **FIGURE 2-17** Intrinsic mass in airway. **A,** Lateral radiograph shows a mass (*arrow*) along the posterior trachea. **B,** Sagittal T1-weighted, postcontrast MRI shows enhancement of the mass (*arrow*) which was Ewing sarcoma, an extremely unusual cause of intrinsic airway obstruction.

AIRWAY FOREIGN BODY

Infants and toddlers explore their environments with their mouths and will put almost anything into them. When such foreign bodies are aspirated, the bronchus is the most common site of lodgment. The aspiration commonly is not witnessed, and symptoms may be indolent, leading to an occult presentation. Radiographic findings of bronchial foreign bodies include asymmetric lung aeration, hyperinflation, oligemia, atelectasis, lung consolidation, pneumothorax, and pneumomediastinum. Most bronchial foreign bodies (as much as 97%) are nonradiopaque. Inspiratory films alone can be normal in as much as one third of patients in whom bronchial foreign bodies are present. Because the volume of the affected lung segments can be normal, increased, or decreased, the key radiographic feature is the lack of change in lung volume demonstrated at different phases of the respiratory cycle. Evaluation at varying phases of the respiratory cycle is easily accomplished in cooperative children by taking expiratory and inspiratory films. In infants and uncooperative children, the population most at risk for foreign body aspiration, air trapping can be detected in bilateral decubitus views of the chest or by fluoroscopy. Some articles propose noncontrast-enhanced CT for the diagnosis of bronchial foreign bodies, but it is not a widespread practice currently. The differential diagnoses for an asymmetric lucent lung include bronchial foreign body, Swyer–James syndrome, and pulmonary hypoplasia.

Laryngeal or tracheal foreign bodies are far less common than bronchial foreign bodies and usually present with abrupt stridor or respiratory distress. Radiographic findings include a radiopaque foreign body, soft tissue density within the airway, and loss of visualization (silhouetting) of the airway wall contours. Foreign bodies lodged within the proximal esophagus, most commonly coins, may also present with airway compression. This is especially true when the foreign body is not expected and been present for some time.

Obstructive Sleep Apnea

One of the most common clinical problems involving the pediatric airway is the presence of OSA. This disorder affects 3% of children (millions in the United States alone) and is increasingly being associated with significant morbidities, such as poor performance in school, attention deficit disorder, excessive daytime sleepiness, and failure to thrive. Most children with OSA are otherwise healthy children in whom there is enlargement of the adenoid and palatine tonsils, causing OSA. When the adenoid and palatine tonsils are removed, the OSA-related symptoms typically resolve.

The palatine tonsils can be evaluated on physical examination. In these children, imaging is limited to a lateral radiograph of the airway, obtained to evaluate the adenoid tonsils. On radiography, adenoids appear as a soft tissue mass in the posterior nasopharynx. Criteria for enlargement include diameter greater than

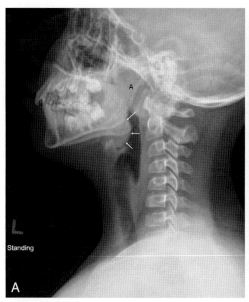
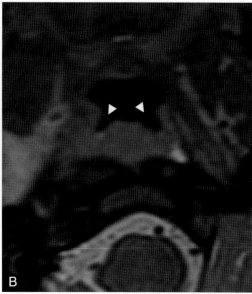

■ **FIGURE 2-18** Enlargement of the adenoid and palatine tonsils. **A,** Lateral radiograph showing enlarged, recurrent adenoid (A) tonsils causing obstruction of the nasopharynx. Posterior bulging at the level of the posterior tongue, nearly filling the vallecular, suggests enlarged lingual tonsils (*arrows*). Note normal epiglottis and aryepiglottic folds. **B,** Axial T2-weighted MRI show the torus tubarius and location of Eustachian tubes (*arrowheads*) in a patient with regrowth of the adenoids. Effort to not damage the Eustachian tubes is why the adenoid tonsil tissue cannot be completely removed and often regrow.

12 mm and a convex outward anterior boarder (Fig. 2-18). Markedly enlarged adenoid tissues may completely obstruct the posterior nasopharynx. Enlarged palatine tonsils can also be seen radiographically, appearing as a large soft tissue mass projecting over the posterior aspect of the soft palate on lateral radiography. Palatine tonsils are generally removed in their entirety. Adenoids cannot be entirely removed because of the adjacent torus tubarius which is the opening of the Eustachian tube. Removing adenoidal tissue too far laterally could cause damage to the cartilage of the Eustachian tube. Recurrent adenoids are a consequence of this tonsillar tissue regrowing (Fig. 2-18).

Certain children with OSA have more complicated airway issues. In these children, a magnetic resonance (MR) sleep study may be helpful for future planning. Such studies have been shown to influence management decisions and help to plan surgical interventions in most cases. Sequences performed include T1-weighted (for anatomy) images, T2-weighted images with fat saturation (depicts tonsillar tissue as bright on a dark background), and fast gradient echo images that can be displayed in a cine, or movie, fashion to depict patterns of airway motion and collapse. Indications for MR sleep studies include persistent OSA despite previous airway surgery (most commonly tonsillectomy and adenoidectomy); predisposition to

multilevel obstruction, such as in Down and other syndromes; OSA and severe obesity; and preoperative evaluation before complex airway surgery. Commonly encountered diagnoses include recurrent enlarged adenoid tonsils, enlarged palatine tonsils, enlarged lingual tonsils, glossoptosis, hypopharyngeal collapse, and abnormal soft palate. Cine CT has also been advocated as a way to evaluate these patients but does not provide as much soft tissue detail, especially about lingual tonsil thickness, and allows evaluation of only one respiratory cycle.

Recurrent and Enlarged Adenoid Tonsils

The adenoid tonsils are absent at birth, rapidly proliferate during infancy, and reach their maximal size when children are between 2 and 10 years of age. During the second decade of life, they begin to decrease in size. It is surprising how commonly the adenoids grow back. This is due to avoidance of damage to the adjacent eustachian tube and not being able to completely remove the adenoid tissue and tonsils related to the eustachian tubes. It is one of the most common causes of recurrent OSA after tonsillectomy and adenoidectomy. Adenoid tonsils are recurrent and enlarged (Fig. 2-19) if they are greater than 12 mm in anterior-to-posterior diameter and are associated with intermittent collapse of the posterior nasopharynx on cine images. There

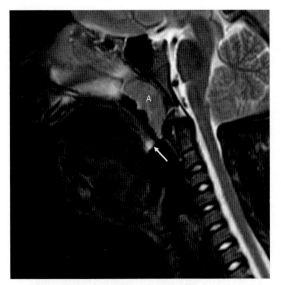

■ FIGURE 2-19 Recurrent and enlarged adenoid tonsils. Sagittal fast spin-echo inversion recovery (FSEIR) image showing enlarged, recurrent adenoid tonsils (A) causing severe obstructive sleep apnea despite prior tonsillectomy and adenoidectomy. Edematous uvula (*arrow*) and distal soft palate from chronic trauma related to snoring.

may also be associated collapse of the hypopharynx because the relatively superior obstruction generates negative pressure in the hypopharynx during inspiration. On axial images, the postsurgical appearance of a V-shaped defect in the midportion of the adenoid tonsil is typically seen (Fig. 2-20).

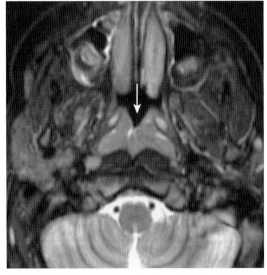

■ FIGURE 2-20 Recurrent and enlarged adenoid tonsils shown on axial FSEIR MR image. Note wedge-shaped central defect (*arrow*) in adenoid tonsil, typical of postoperative appearance.

Enlarged Palatine Tonsils

Unlike the adenoid tonsils, which commonly grow back after surgical removal, the palatine tonsils do not. Therefore, because most MR sleep studies are performed after tonsillectomy, absence of the palatine tonsils is depicted in most cases. When present and enlarged (Fig. 2-21), the palatine tonsils appear as round, high T2 signal structures in the palatine fossa, and they bob inferiorly and centrally, intermittently obstructing the airway. There is no published range of normal size for palatine tonsils on imaging.

Enlarged Lingual Tonsils

Enlargement of the lingual tonsils is being recognized as a common cause of persistent OSA following previous tonsillectomy and adenoidectomy. Lingual tonsils are enlarged if they are greater than 5 mm thick. In such patients, the lingual tonsils can become quite large and obstruct the retroglossal airway. Enlarged lingual tonsils appear as high-signal masses (Fig. 2-22) that are round or that have grown together and appear as a single dumbbell-shaped mass immediately posterior to the tongue. It is an important diagnosis to make on imaging because it is not readily seen on physical examination and is one of the most easily surgically curable causes of persistent OSA. Additionally, MRI clearly shows the thickness of the lingual tonsils and size and shape of the tongue. Endoscopy only shows the surface and the lingual tonsils and they may appear to be enlarged when the underlying tongue is actually what is enlarged. Enlargement of the lingual tonsils appears to be particularly common after tonsillectomy and adenoidectomy in obese children and in children with Down syndrome. On radiography, enlarged lingual tonsils can appear as a soft tissue mass continuous with the posterior aspect of the tongue and filling the vallecula.

Glossoptosis

Glossoptosis is defined as posterior motion of the tongue during sleep. The posterior aspect of the tongue intermittently falls posteriorly and abuts the posterior pharyngeal wall, obstructing the retroglossal airway (Fig. 2-23). It is associated with large tongues (macroglossia), small jaws (micrognathia), and decreased muscular tone. It is commonly seen in children with Down syndrome, Pierre Robin sequence, and neuromuscular disorders, such as cerebral palsy. On axial imaging, intermittent posterior motion of the tongue in the anterior-to-posterior direction is depicted on cine images.

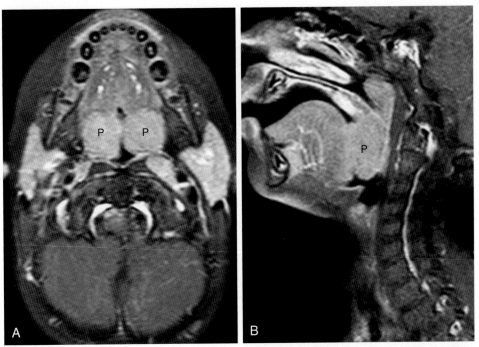

■ **FIGURE 2-21** Enlarged "kissing" bilateral palatine tonsils. **A,** Axial T2-weighted image shows bilateral markedly enlarged palatine tonsils (P) touching in the midline and obstructing airway. **B,** Sagittal T2-weighted image shows enlarged palatine tonsil (P).

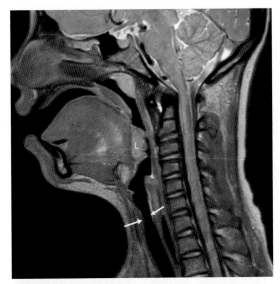

■ **FIGURE 2-22** Enlarged lingual tonsils. Sagittal proton density image showing enlarged lingual tonsils (L) obstructing the retroglossal pharynx. Subglottic stenosis (*arrows*) from prolonged intubation as a premature infant is also present.

Hypopharyngeal (Retroglossal) Collapse

Hypopharyngeal collapse can be a primary phenomenon caused by decreased muscle tone, or it may occur secondary to negative pressure generated by a more superior obstruction (typically enlarged adenoid tonsils). With hypopharyngeal collapse, there is cylindrical collapse of the retroglossal airway, with the anterior, posterior, left, and right walls of the airway all collapsing centrally (Fig. 2-24). In contrast, with glossoptosis, the tongue moves anteriorly and posteriorly, and the lateral diameter of the airway remains unchanged. This differentiation is easiest to observe on axial cine images at the level of the midportion of the tongue, from superior to inferior. It is important to characterize the pattern of collapse of the retroglossal airway as hypopharyngeal collapse or glossoptosis because the surgical options for the two groups of patients are quite different. Additionally, glossoptosis diagnosed by endoscopy is the current indication for implantation of a hypoglossal nerve stimulator (HGNS). The HGNS is not as efficacious in treating hypopharyngeal collapse.

Abnormal Soft Palate

A prominent soft palate is one of the contributing factors in some cases of OSA, and there are surgical procedures that decrease the size of the soft palate. As you can imagine, there are no published criteria for abnormal soft palate enlargement. If the soft palate is prominent in size, is draped over the tongue and hangs more inferiorly than the midportion of the tongue, and

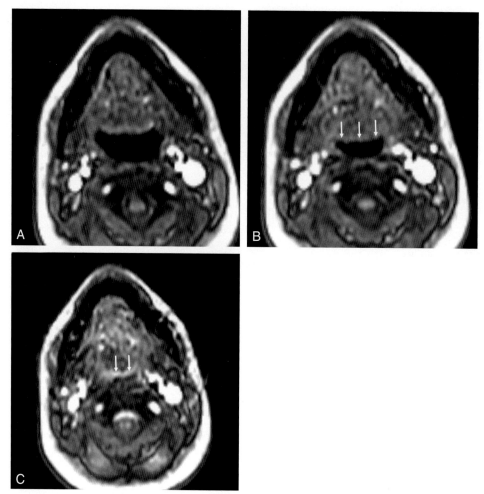

■ **FIGURE** 2-23 Glossoptosis. **A,** Axial cine MR image of the retroglossal airway during expiration showing airway ballooning open. **B,** Axial Cine MR image obtained at a time of transition from expiration to inspiration just before complete collapse. Arrows indicated the primary direction of motion. **C,** Complete collapse of the retroglossal airway due to anterior posterior motion of the tongue. Arrows indicate location of collapsed airway.

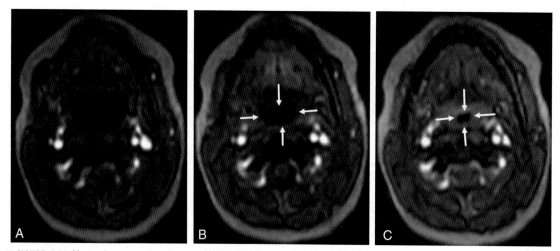

■ **FIGURE** 2-24 Hypopharyngeal collapse. **A,** Axial cine image during expiration showing open, ballooning retroglossal airway. **B,** Axial cine image during inspiration showing partial collapse of the retroglossal airway (*arrows*).**C,** Axial cine image showing complete collapse (*arrows*). Note that lateral left and right, anterior, and posterior walls all collapse cylindrically to the center of airway, in contrast to tongue moving posteriorly, as seen in glossoptosis.

is associated with intermittent collapse of the posterior nasopharynx or retroglossal airway, we consider it enlarged.

The soft palate can be edematous, as seen on physical examination in patients with significant OSA. This is thought to be related to the repeated trauma of snoring. On T2-weighted MR sequences, the edema is depicted as an increased signal throughout the soft palate; in patients without OSA, the soft palate is similar in signal to that of the musculature of the tongue.

■ CONGENITAL AIRWAY OBSTRUCTION

With the increase in fetal surgery centers and associated increased use of fetal ultrasound and MRI, pediatric radiologists are beginning to see an increasing number of cases of CHAOS, although it remains a rare entity. CHAOS is the term given to a constellation of findings resulting from this form of airway obstruction. Causes of this airway obstruction include in utero laryngeal atresia, subglottic stenosis, and head and neck masses obstructing the upper airway, most commonly lymphatic malformations or teratomas. Fetal imaging findings in CHAOS (Fig. 2-25) include massive increases in lung volumes, flattened or everted hemidiaphragms,

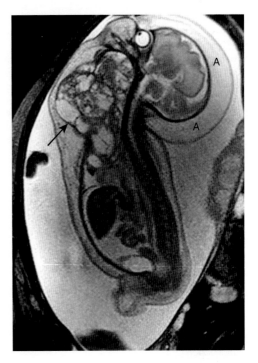

■ **FIGURE 2-26** Teratoma of the neck. Fetal MRI sagittal to fetal head and neck showing large complex cystic mass (*arrow*) in the region of the neck. Mass is obstructing the airway.

hydrops, and polyhydramnios. Infants with airway obstruction secondary to masses (Fig. 2-26) or other causes, with or without associated CHAOS findings, may be delivered via ex utero intrapartum treatment (EXIT). In EXIT, the head of the infant is delivered via a cesarean section, and the airway is established by tracheotomy or intubation before the child is being taken off placental circulation. Once the airway has been established, the child can be completely delivered.

SUGGESTED READING

Berdon WE, Baker DH: Vascular anomalies and the infant lung: rings, slings, and other things, *Semin Roentgenol* 7:39–63, 1972.

Capitanio MA, Kirkpatrick JA: Obstruction of the upper airway in infants and children, *Radiol Clin* 6:265–277, 1968.

Donnelly LF, Frush DP, Bisset GS: The multiple presentations of foreign bodies in children, *Am Journal Rev* 170:471–477, 1998.

Donnelly LF, Strife JL, Bisset GS: The spectrum of extrinsic lower airway compression in children: MR imaging, *Am Journal Rev* 168:59–62, 1997.

Fleck RJ, Shott SR, Mahmoud M, Ishman SL, Amin RS, Donnelly LF: Magnetic resonance imaging of obstructive sleep apnea in children, *Pediatr Radiol* 48:1223–1233, 2018.

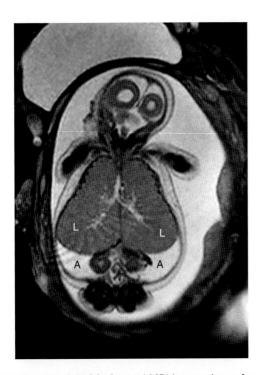

■ **FIGURE 2-25** CHAOS. Coronal MRI image shows fetus with markedly enlarged lung volumes (L) with inverted diaphragms, ascites (A), and polyhydramnios. There is also anasarca.

Dunbar JS: Upper respiratory tract obstruction in infants and children, *Am Journal Rev* 109:227–246, 1970.

Guimaraes CV, Linam LE, Kline-Fath BM, et al.: Prenatal MRI findings of fetuses with congenital high airway obstruction sequence, *Korean J Radiol* 10:129–134, 2009.

Heyer CM, Nuesslein TY, Jung D, et al.: Tracheobronchial anomalies and stenoses: detection with low-dose multidetector CT with virtual tracheobronchoscopy: comparison with flexible tracheobronchoscopy, *Radiology* 242:542–549, 2007.

John SD, Swischuk KE: Stridor and upper airway obstruction in infants and children, *Radiographics* 12:625–643, 1992.

Pacharn P, Poe SA, Donnelly LF: Low-tube-current CT for children with suspected extrinsic airway compression, *Am Journal Rev* 179:1523–1527, 2002.

Yedururi S, Guillerman RP, Chung T, et al.: Multimodality imaging of tracheobronchial disorders in children, *Radiographics* 28:e29, 2008.

CHAPTER 3

CHEST

Monica Epelman

The chest radiograph is one of the most commonly obtained examinations in pediatric imaging. It is also the examination most likely to be encountered by radiology residents, pediatric residents, general radiologists, and pediatricians. In this chapter, topics such as chest imaging in neonates and the evaluation of suspected pneumonia are discussed in detail.

■ NEONATAL CHEST

Causes of respiratory distress in newborn infants can be divided into those that are secondary to diffuse pulmonary disease (medical causes) and those that are secondary to a space-occupying mass compressing the pulmonary parenchyma (surgical causes).

Diffuse Pulmonary Disease in the Newborn

Diffuse pulmonary disease causes respiratory distress much more commonly than surgical diseases, particularly in premature infants, who make up the majority of cases of respiratory distress in the newborn. A simple way to evaluate these patients and try to offer a limited differential diagnosis is to evaluate the lung volumes and to characterize the pulmonary opacities.

Lung volumes can be categorized as high, normal, or low. Normally, the apex of the dome of the diaphragm is expected to be at the level of approximately the 10th posterior rib. If present, lung opacity can be characterized as either streaky, perihilar (central) densities that have a linear quality or as diffuse, granular opacities that have an almost sand-like character. Classically, cases fall into one of the following two categories: (1) cases with high lung volumes and streaky perihilar densities and (2) cases with low lung volumes and granular opacities (Table 3-1). This is more of a guideline rather than a rule because many neonates with diffuse pulmonary disease have normal lung volumes. The differential diagnosis for cases with high lung volumes and streaky perihilar densities includes meconium aspiration, transient tachypnea of the newborn (TTN), and neonatal pneumonia.

Most of the neonates in this group are term. The differential for cases with low lung volumes and granular opacities includes surfactant deficiency and one specific type of infection—group B streptococcal (GBS) pneumonia. Most of these neonates are premature.

Meconium Aspiration Syndrome

Meconium aspiration syndrome results from intrapartum or intrauterine aspiration of meconium. It usually occurs secondary to stress, such as hypoxia, and more often occurs in term or postmature neonates. The aspirated meconium causes both obstruction of small airways secondary to its tenacious nature as well as chemical pneumonitis. The degree of respiratory failure can be severe and may also lead to pulmonary air leaks and persistent pulmonary hypertension. Radiographic findings include hyperinflation (high lung volumes), which may be asymmetric and patchy, and asymmetric lung densities that tend to have a ropy appearance and a perihilar distribution (Fig. 3-1). Commonly, there are areas of hyperinflation alternating with areas of atelectasis. Pleural effusions can be present. Because of the small airway obstruction by the meconium, air-block complications are common, with pneumothorax occurring in 20%–40% of cases. Meconium aspiration syndrome is relatively common; it occurs in approximately 2%–10% of infants whose birth is associated with meconium-stained amniotic fluid. In the United States, a retrospective multicenter study reported that approximately 2% of infants had an admission diagnosis of meconium aspiration syndrome annually. Although meconium-stained amniotic fluid occurs in approximately 10%–15% of deliveries, meconium aspiration syndrome develops in less than 5% of them.

Transient Tachypnea of the Newborn

TTN is also referred to by a variety of other names, including wet lung disease and transient respiratory distress. It occurs secondary to delayed clearance of fetal lung fluid. Physiologically, the clearing of fetal lung fluid is facilitated by the "thoracic squeeze" during vaginal

✴ **TABLE 3-1** Differential Diagnosis of Diffuse Pulmonary Disease in the Newborn	
High Lung Volumes, Streaky Perihilar Densities	**Low Lung Volumes, Granular Opacities**
Meconium aspiration syndrome	Surfactant deficiency
Transient tachypnea of the newborn	Group B streptococcal pneumonia
Neonatal pneumonia	

deliveries; therefore, most cases of TTN are related to cesarean section, in which the thoracic squeeze is bypassed. Other causes include maternal diabetes and use of maternal anesthesia or analgesia during delivery. The hallmark of TTN is a benign course. Respiratory distress develops by 6 h of age, peaks at 1 day of age, and is resolved by 2–3 days. There is a spectrum of radiographic findings similar to those seen with mild-to-severe pulmonary edema. There is a combination of airspace opacification, interstitial edema, prominent and indistinct pulmonary vasculature, fluid in the fissures, pleural effusion, and cardiomegaly (Fig. 3-2). Lung volumes are normal to increased.

Neonatal Pneumonia

Neonatal pneumonia can be caused by a large number of infectious agents that can be acquired intrauterine, during birth, or soon after birth. With the exception of GBS pneumonia, which will be discussed separately, the radiographic

appearance of neonatal pneumonia is that of patchy, asymmetric perihilar densities and hyperinflation (Fig. 3-3). Pleural effusions may be present (Fig. 3-4). Such cases of neonatal pneumonia may have a similar radiographic appearance to and be indistinguishable from meconium aspiration syndrome or TTN on imaging alone.

Surfactant-Deficient Disease

Surfactant-deficient disease (SDD), also known as *respiratory distress syndrome* (RDS) or *hyaline membrane disease*, is a common disorder, with approximately 24,000 new cases annually in the United States. The incidence of RDS increases with decreasing gestational age at birth. The risk of SDD increases with decreasing gestational age. In a study from the Child Health and Human Development (NICHD) Neonatal Research Network centers, approximately 98% of the neonates born at 24 weeks had RDS, while the incidence was 5% in those born at 34 weeks. SDD is also the most common cause of death in live newborns. SDD is related to the inability of premature type II pneumocytes to produce surfactant. Normally, surfactant coats the alveolar surfaces and decreases surface tension, which allows the alveoli to remain open. As a result of the lack of surfactant, there is alveolar collapse. The radiographic findings reflect these pathologic changes (Fig. 3-5). Lung volumes are low. There are bilateral granular opacities that represent collapsed alveoli interspersed with open alveoli. Because the larger bronchi do not collapse, there are prominent air bronchograms. When the process is severe enough and the majority of alveoli are collapsed, there may be

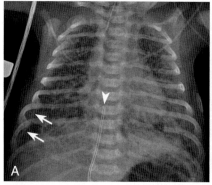 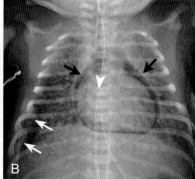 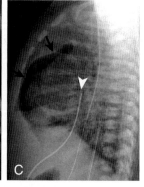

■ **FIGURE 3-1 Meconium aspiration syndrome. A,** Newborn chest radiograph shows normal-to-large lung volumes and bilateral, coarse, ropy markings. Note right pleural effusion (*white arrow*). Also note umbilical venous catheter with tip (*arrowhead*) into right atrium. Tip should be at the junction of the right atrium and inferior vena cava. **B,** Frontal and **C,** Lateral views of the chest obtained a few days later due to clinical deterioration show interval development of pneumopericardium (*black arrows*). Note that the umbilical venous catheter tip terminates deep in the right atrium (*arrowhead*). Tip should be at the inferior cavoatrial junction. Right pleural effusion persists (*white arrows*).

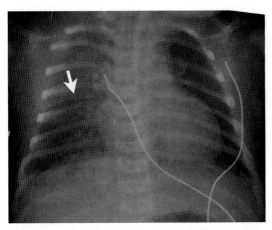

■ FIGURE 3-2 **Transient tachypnea of the newborn.** Newborn chest radiograph shows normal lung volumes, mild cardiomegaly, indistinct pulmonary vascularity, mild diffuse haziness, although more pronounced in the right upper lung field, and fluid in the minor fissure (*arrow*). Within 24 h the patient was asymptomatic.

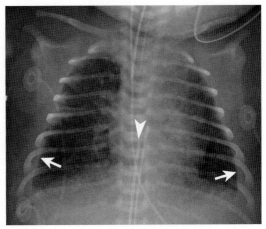

■ FIGURE 3-4 **Neonatal pneumonia.** Newborn chest radiograph shows normal-to-large lung volumes and coarse, perihilar markings. The remainder of the lungs shows diffuse ground-glass granularity with more confluent retrocardiac opacities with some air bronchograms. Note bilateral small pleural effusions (*arrows*). The granularity associated with this case raises a differential diagnosis of surfactant deficiency disease. However, the bilateral pleural effusions favor infection because pleural effusions are quite uncommon with surfactant deficiency disease. Also note umbilical venous catheter with tip in the right atrium (*arrowhead*). Tip should be at the junction of the right atrium and inferior vena cava.

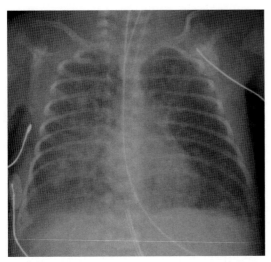

■ FIGURE 3-3 **Neonatal pneumonia.** Newborn chest radiograph shows large lung volumes and coarse, bilateral perihilar markings and patchy areas of opacity.

coalescence of the granular opacities, resulting in diffuse lung opacity. Imaging findings may not be prominent at birth, but a normal film at 6 h of age excludes the presence of SDD.

Surfactant Replacement Therapy

One of the therapies for SDD is surfactant administration. Surfactant can be administered via nebulized or aerosol forms. It is administered into the trachea via a catheter or an adapted endotracheal tube. The administration of surfactant in neonates with SDD is associated with decreased oxygen and ventilator setting requirements, decreased air-block complications, decreased incidence of intracranial hemorrhage and bronchopulmonary dysplasia (BPD), also known as chronic lung disease of prematurity, and decreased death rate. However, there is an associated increased risk for development of patent ductus arteriosus, pulmonary hemorrhage, as well as an acute desaturation episode in response to surfactant administration. Surfactant administration can be given on a rescue basis when premature neonates develop respiratory distress or can be given prophylactically in premature infants who are at risk. Prophylactic administration is commonly given immediately after birth and has become common practice. In response to surfactant administration, radiography may demonstrate complete, central, or asymmetric clearing of the findings of SDD (Fig. 3-5). There is usually an increase in lung volumes. Neonates without radiographic findings of a response to surfactant have poorer prognoses than those who have radiographic evidence of a response. A pattern of alternating distended and collapsed acini may create a radiographic pattern of bubble-like lucencies that can mimic pulmonary interstitial emphysema (PIE). Knowledge of the timing of surfactant delivery is helpful to render accurate interpretation of chest radiographs taken in the neonatal intensive care unit (NICU).

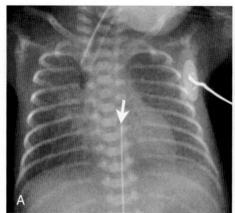
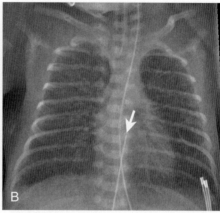

■ **FIGURE 3-5** **SDD responding to surfactant therapy. A,** Radiograph shortly after birth shows low-normal lung volumes, confluent densities, and air bronchograms. There is an umbilical arterial catheter with its tip (*arrow*) at the level of T6–7. **B,** Radiograph obtained immediately following surfactant administration shows increased lung volumes and decreased lung opacities. An enteric tube has been inserted in the interim.

Group B Streptococcal Pneumonia

GBS pneumonia is the most common type of pneumonia in neonates. The infection is acquired during birth, and approximately 10% −30% of women in labor are colonized by the organism. Premature infants are more commonly infected than are term infants. In contrast to the other types of neonatal pneumonia, the radiographic findings include bilateral granular opacities and low lung volumes (Fig. 3-6), the identical findings in SDD. The presence of pleural fluid is a helpful differentiating factor because it is very uncommon in surfactant deficiency but has been reported in between 25% and 67% of cases of GBS pneumonia.

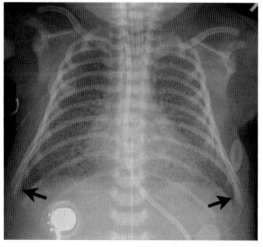

■ **FIGURE 3-6** **Group B streptococcal pneumonia.** Radiograph shows low-normal lung volumes and diffuse granular opacities, similar in appearance to cases of surfactant deficiency. However, the small bilateral pleural effusions (*arrows*) favor infection.

Persistent Pulmonary Hypertension of the Newborn

Persistent pulmonary hypertension of the newborn (PPHN), also known as *persistent fetal circulation*, is a term often used in the NICU and is addressed here because it can be a source of confusion. The high pulmonary vascular resistance that is normally present in the fetus typically decreases during the newborn period. In normal conditions, after clamping the cord and with the first breaths, there is a drastic drop in pulmonary vascular resistance permitting the circulation that in utero bypasses the lungs, to perfuse the lungs. If this drastic decrease in pulmonary vascular resistance does not take place, blood would continue to bypass the lungs and pulmonary pressures would remain abnormally high; the condition is termed *persistent pulmonary hypertension*. It is a physiologic finding rather than a specific disease. It can be a primary phenomenon or it can occur secondary to causes of hypoxia, such as meconium aspiration syndrome, neonatal pneumonia, or pulmonary hypoplasia associated with congenital diaphragmatic hernia (CDH). These patients are quite ill. The radiographic patterns are variable and are more often reflective of the underlying cause of hypoxia than the presence of persistent pulmonary hypertension. Occasionally, it may be seen in neonates with clear chest radiographs, and in these cases, it is referred as primary PPHN.

Neonatal Intensive Care Unit Support Apparatus

One of the primary roles of chest radiography in the NICU is to monitor support apparatus, including endotracheal tubes, enteric tubes, central venous lines, umbilical arterial and venous catheters, and extracorporeal membrane oxygenation (ECMO) catheters. The radiographic evaluation of many of these tubes is the same as that seen in adults and is not discussed here. When evaluating the positions of endotracheal tubes in premature neonates, it is important to consider that the length of the entire trachea may be only approximately 1 cm. Keeping the endotracheal tube in the exact center of such a small trachea is an impossible task for caregivers, and phone calls and reports suggesting that the tube needs to be moved 2 mm proximally may be more annoying than helpful. Direct phone communication may be more appropriately reserved for times when the tube is in a main bronchus or above the thoracic inlet. There is an increased propensity for inadvertent esophageal intubation to occur in neonates as compared with in adults. Although it would seem that esophageal intubation would be incredibly obvious clinically, this is not always the case. The authors have experienced cases in which a child has in retrospect been discovered to have been esophageally intubated for more than 24 h. Therefore, the radiologist may be the first to recognize esophageal intubation. Obviously, when the course of the endotracheal tube does not overlie the path of the trachea, the use of esophageal intubation is fairly obvious. Other findings of esophageal intubation include a combination of low lung volumes, gas within the esophagus, and gaseous distention of the bowel (Fig. 3-7).

Umbilical Arterial and Venous Catheters

Umbilical lines are commonly used in the NICU. The pathway of the umbilical venous catheter is umbilical vein to left portal vein to ductus venosus, the most superior portion of the ductus venosus joins, or becomes part of, one of the hepatic veins as they enter the inferior vena cava (Fig. 3-8). In contrast to umbilical arterial catheters, the course is in the superior direction from the level of the umbilicus. The ideal position of an umbilical venous catheter is with its tip at the junction of the right atrium and the inferior vena cava at the level of the hemidiaphragm. The umbilical venous catheter may occasionally deflect into the portal venous system rather than passing into the ductus venosus. Complications of such positioning can include hepatic hematoma or abscess.

Umbilical arterial catheters pass from the umbilicus inferiorly into the pelvis via the umbilical artery to the iliac artery. The catheters then turn cephalad within the aorta (Fig. 3-9). These catheters can be associated with thrombosis of the aorta and its branches. Therefore, it is important to avoid positioning the catheter with the tip at the level of the branches of the aorta (celiac, superior mesenteric, and renal arteries) or at the origin of the great arteries (arch). There are two acceptable umbilical arterial catheter positions: *high lines* have their tips at the level of the descending thoracic aorta (T8–T10) and *low lines* have their tips below the level of L3. The catheter tip should not be positioned between T10 and L3 because of the risk for major arterial thrombosis.

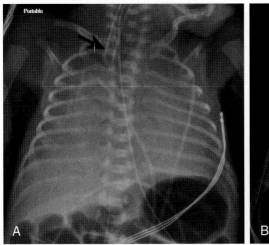
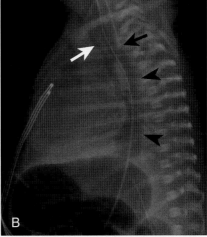

■ FIGURE 3-7 **Esophageal intubation in a 7-day-old. A,** Frontal chest radiograph after reintubation shows the endotracheal tube tip (*black arrow*) lateral to the expected location of the mid trachea. There are low lung volumes. There is gaseous distention of the stomach and bowel. **B,** Lateral view of the chest shows the endotracheal tube (*black arrow*) posterior to the enteric tube. The airway is displaced anteriorly and is decreased in caliber (*white arrow*). The esophagus (*arrowheads*) is quite air distended. The visualized bowel loops are also moderately air distended.

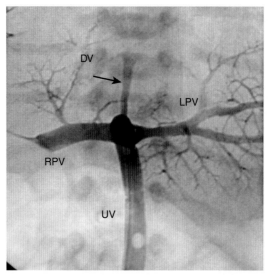

■ **FIGURE 3-8 Anatomy of the course of the umbilical vein (*UV*) catheter as demonstrated by contrast injection of umbilical catheter performed because of inability to advance UV catheter.** Note course of UV to portal vein to ductus venosus (*DV; arrow*). *LPV*, Left portal vein; *RPV*, right portal vein.

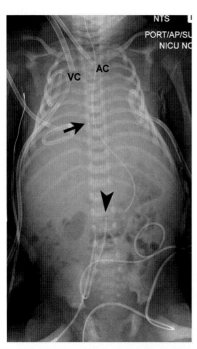

■ **FIGURE 3-9 Extracorporeal membrane oxygenation (ECMO) catheter placement for meconium aspiration syndrome and persistent air leak.** Note venous ECMO cannula (*VC*) has a radiopaque proximal portion and a lucent distal portion. The tip of the venous catheter is marked by a small radiopaque metallic marker (*arrow*) and is actually in the right atrium. Note the arterial ECMO cannula (*AC*) with tip in region of aortic arch. In addition, note "low"-type umbilical arterial catheter with tip overlying the abdominal aorta at the level of the lower endplate of L 2/3 (*arrowhead*). It should be repositioned. Enteric tube terminates in the stomach, and bilateral pleural pigtail catheters are seen overlying both hemithoraces. The lungs are completely opacified, not unexpected in an infant on ECMO.

There is no clear consensus as to whether a high or low umbilical artery catheter line is better, and both positions are still currently used, although some authors advocate that the high position has fewer complications.

Peripherally Inserted Central Catheters in Children

One of the more common lines now seen in children, as in adults, is peripherally inserted central catheters (PICCs). In contrast to adults, in whom some of the PICCs can be as large as 6F, the PICC lines used in children, particularly infants, are often small in caliber (2F or 3F) so that they can be placed into their very small peripheral veins. These small-caliber PICCs can be very difficult to see on chest radiography, so some of them must be filled with contrast to be accurately visualized. The tip of the PICC line that enters the child from the upper extremity should be positioned with the tip in the midlevel of the superior vena cava or superior cavoatrial junction. It is essential that PICC lines not be left in place with the tip well into the right atrium. Particularly, with the small-caliber lines, the atrium can be lacerated, leading to pericardial tamponade, free hemorrhage, or death. Many such cases have been reported nationally. In addition, the PICC should not be too proximal in the superior vena cava because the distal portion of the line can flip from the superior vena cava into the contralateral brachiocephalic or jugular vein. At many children's hospitals, the PICC lines are inserted in a dedicated suite by a team of nurses, with supervision by pediatric interventional radiologists or other physicians. Ultrasound (US) is often used to guide vein cannulation, and certified child life specialists may coach many kids through the procedure without sedation. Fluoroscopy is used at the end of the procedure to adjust and document tip position in the cavoatrial junction.

Extracorporeal Membrane Oxygenation

ECMO is a last resort therapy usually reserved for respiratory failure that has not responded to other treatments. ECMO is essentially a prolonged form of circulatory bypass of the lungs and is used only in patients who have reversible disease and a chance for survival. The majority of neonates who are treated with ECMO have respiratory failure as a result of meconium aspiration, persistent pulmonary hypertension (resulting from a variety of causes), severe congenital heart disease, or CDH. ECMO seems to be used less commonly now for diffuse pulmonary disease than it was in the 1990s.

There are two types of ECMO: arteriovenous and venovenous. In arteriovenous ECMO, the right common carotid artery and internal jugular veins are sacrificed. The arterial catheter is placed via the carotid and positioned with its tip overlying the aortic arch. The venous catheter is positioned with its tip over the right atrium (Fig. 3-9). One of the main roles of a chest radiograph of children on ECMO is to detect any potential migration of the catheters. Careful comparison with previous studies to make sure that the catheters have not moved proximally or distally is critical. These patients have many bandages and other items covering the external portions of the catheters, so migration may be hard to detect on physical examination. In addition, anasarca is invariable during ECMO because the increasing soft tissue edema may result in accidental dislodgment and subsequent accidental decannulation. Note that there are various radiographic appearances of the ECMO catheters. Some catheters end where the radiopaque portion of the tube ends, and others have a radiolucent portion with a small metallic marker at the tip (Fig. 3-9). It is common to see white-out of the lungs soon after a patient is placed on ECMO as a result of sudden decrease in airway pressure, decreased ventilator settings, and third-space shifting of fluid (Fig. 3-9). Patients on ECMO are anticoagulated and are therefore at risk for hemorrhage. They are often monitored by head US to exclude development of intracranial hemorrhage.

Types of Ventilation: High-Frequency Oscillator versus Conventional Ventilation

High-frequency oscillators are commonly used to treat neonates in the NICU. In contrast to conventional ventilation, high-frequency oscillators use supraphysiologic rates of ventilation with very low tidal volumes. Conventional ventilation has been likened to delivering a cupful of air approximately 20 times a minute. In contrast, high-frequency oscillation is like delivering a thimbleful of air approximately 1000 times per minute. The air is vibrated in and out of the lung, and appropriate gas exchange occurs at significantly lower peak inspiratory pressures than those required with conventional ventilation. The mechanism of how oscillators work is poorly understood. In conventional ventilation, the diaphragm moves up and down, whereas during high-frequency ventilation the diaphragm stays "parked" at a certain anatomic level. This level can be adjusted by changing the mean airway pressure of the oscillator. Caregivers usually like to maintain the diaphragm at approximately the level of the 10th posterior ribs. In general, the radiographic appearance of neonatal pulmonary diseases is not affected by whether the patient is being ventilated by conventional or high-frequency ventilation.

Complications in the Neonatal Intensive Care Unit

As in adult intensive care units, major complications detected by chest radiographs include those related to air leak complications, lobar collapse, or acute diffuse pulmonary consolidation. Another type of complication seen in neonates is the development of chronic lung disease of prematurity. Imaging findings of lobar collapse and air-block complications, such as pneumothorax, pneumomediastinum, and pneumopericardium, are similar in neonates and adults and will not be discussed here. One type of air-block complication that is unique to neonates is pulmonary interstitial emphysema (PIE).

Pulmonary Interstitial Emphysema

In patients with severe surfactant deficiency, ventilatory support can result in marked increases in alveolar pressure, leading to perforation of alveoli. The air that escapes into the adjacent interstitium and lymphatics is referred to as PIE. PIE appears on radiographs as bubble like or linear, nonbranching lucencies, and can be focal or diffuse (Fig. 3-10). The involved lung

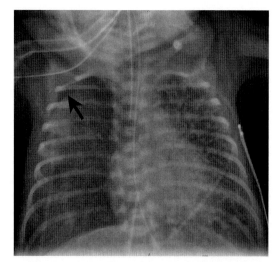

■ FIGURE 3-10 **Pulmonary interstitial emphysema in a premature infant with surfactant deficiency disease.** Chest radiograph shows asymmetric bubble like, non-branching lucencies within the left lung consistent with PIE. A small apical pneumothorax is seen on the right lung (*arrow*), which shows diffuse ground-glass opacification.

is usually noncompliant and seen to have a static volume on multiple consecutive chest radiographs. The finding is typically transient. The importance of detecting PIE is that it serves as a warning sign for other impending air-block complications, such as pneumothorax, and its presence can influence caregivers in decisions, such as switching from conventional to high-frequency ventilation.

It can be difficult to differentiate diffuse PIE from the bubble-like lucencies that are associated with developing BPD. When encountering this scenario, the patient's age can help to determine which is more likely. Most cases of PIE occur in the first week of life, prior to when most cases of

BPD develop. In patients older than 4 weeks, BPD is more likely. In addition, in patients who have undergone a series of daily films, PIE may be noted to occur abruptly, whereas BPD tends to occur gradually. As previously mentioned, SDD partially treated by surfactant replacement can cause a pattern of lucencies that may mimic PIE as well.

Rarely, PIE can persist and develop into an expansive, multicystic mass. The air cysts can become large enough to cause mediastinal shift and compromise pulmonary function. Often the diagnosis is indicated by sequential radiography showing evolution of the cystic mass from original findings typical of PIE. In unclear cases, computed tomography (CT) demonstrates that the air cysts are in the interstitial space by showing the broncho-vascular bundles positioned within the center of the air cysts. The broncho-vascular bundles appear as linear or nodular densities in the center of the lucent cysts.

Causes of Acute Diffuse Pulmonary Consolidation

Acute diffuse pulmonary consolidation is nonspecific in neonates, as it is in adults, and can represent blood, pus, or water. In the neonate, the specific considerations include edema, which may be secondary to the development of patent ductus arteriosus (Fig. 3-11); pulmonary hemorrhage, to which surfactant therapy predisposes; worsening surfactant deficiency (during the first several days of life but not later); or developing neonatal pneumonia (Table 3-2). Diffuse microatelectasis is another possibility because neonates have the propensity to artifactually demonstrate diffuse lung opacity on low lung volume radiographs obtained with expiratory

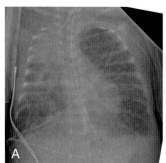
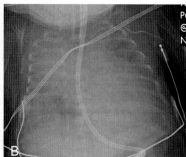
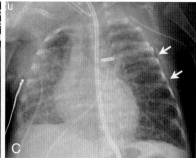

■ FIGURE 3-11 **Patent ductus arteriosus (PDA) leading to congestive heart failure in a 1-month-old premature. A,** Before development of PDA, radiograph shows normal-sized heart and right upper lobe atelectasis over a background of chronic lung disease. **B,** After development of PDA, radiograph shows cardiac enlargement and more extensive airspace opacification. **C,** Radiograph obtained immediately following ductus ligation shows decrease in heart size and improvement in lung aeration. Notice a very small amount of subcutaneous emphysema along the left lateral chest wall (*arrows*).

TABLE 3-2 Causes of Acute Diffuse Pulmonary Consolidation in Neonates

- Edema: patent ductus arteriosus
- Hemorrhage
- Diffuse microatelectasis: artifact
- Worsening surfactant deficiency (only during first days of life)
- Pneumonia

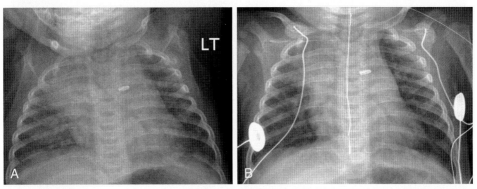

■ **FIGURE 3-12 Expiratory chest radiograph mimicking heart failure in infant. A,** Initial radiograph shows prominent size of cardiothymic silhouette, indistinctness and prominence of the central pulmonary vascularity, and low lung volumes. **B,** Repeat radiograph obtained immediately after **A** shows better expanded lungs and normal heart size.

technique (Fig. 3-12); this should not be mistaken for another cause of consolidation. Such radiographs showing low lung volumes offer little information concerning the pulmonary status of the patient and should be repeated when clinically indicated.

Bronchopulmonary Dysplasia

BPD, or *chronic lung disease of prematurity*, is a common complication, seen in premature infants and is associated with significant morbidity rates. BPD typically occurs in neonates treated with oxygen and positive pressure ventilation for respiratory failure, usually SDD. BPD is uncommon in children born at greater than 32 weeks of gestational age, but it occurs in more than 50% of premature infants born at less than 1000 g. BPD is the most common chronic lung disease of infancy.

The definition of BPD has evolved over time; currently, one of the most accepted definition is that of oxygen dependence for at least 28 days after birth, whereas the severity is graded in proportion to the respiratory support required at term. The most recent revision (2019), based on a prospective NICHD (National Institute of Child Health and Human Development) network study, again includes the presence of persistent parenchymal lung disease confirmed by radiography and the need of some form of respiratory support at 36 weeks of age.

BPD is related to injury to the lungs that is thought to result from some combination of mechanical ventilation and oxygen toxicity. Although four discrete and orderly stages of the development of BPD were originally described, they are not seen commonly and are probably not important to know. BPD typically occurs in a premature infant who requires prolonged ventilator support. At approximately the end of the second week of life, persistent hazy density appears throughout the lungs. Over the next weeks to months, a combination of coarse lung markings, bubble-like lucencies, and asymmetric aeration can develop (Fig. 3-13). Eventually, focal lucencies, coarse reticular densities, and band-like opacities develop. In childhood survivors of BPD, many of these radiographic findings decrease in prominence over the years and only hyperaeration may persist. The radiographic findings may completely resolve. Clinically, many children with severe BPD during infancy may eventually improve to normal pulmonary function or may only have minor persistent problems such as exercise intolerance, predisposition to infection, or asthma.

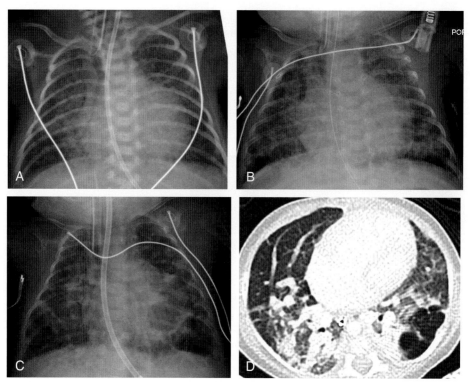

■ **FIGURE 3-13 Bronchopulmonary dysplasia in a premature girl. A,** Chest radiograph at 20 days of life shows persistent hazy bilateral lung opacities. **B,** Chest radiograph at 33 days of life shows coarsening of the lung markings. **C,** Chest radiograph and D, Chest CT at 70 days of life shows increased coarse lung markings and development of cystic lucencies at the left base. Notice the heterogenous lung aeration with focal areas of air trapping, architectural distortion, and subpleural parenchymal bands.

Focal Pulmonary Lesions in the Newborn

In contrast to diffuse pulmonary disease in newborns, focal masses can present with respiratory distress due to compression of otherwise normal lung. Most of these focal masses are related to congenital lung lesions. Congenital lung lesions may appear solid, as air-filled cysts, or as mixed cystic and solid. The differential for a focal lung lesion can be narrowed on the basis of whether the lesion is lucent or solid appearing on chest radiography (Table 3-3). The most likely considerations for a lucent chest lesion in a newborn are congenital lobar emphysema, congenital pulmonary airway malformation (CPAM), persistent PIE, and CDH. CT may be helpful in differentiating among these lesions by demonstrating whether the abnormal lucency is related to air in distended alveoli, in the interstitium, or in abnormal cystic structures. CPAM may appear solid or partially solid during the first days of life, as the cysts may be fluid filled. The fluid in these cystic components becomes replaced by air overtime. Lesions that typically appear solid during the neonatal period include

TABLE 3-3 Focal Lung Lesions in Neonates on Radiography	
Lucent Lesions	**Solid Lesions**
Congenital lobar overinflation	Sequestration
Congenital pulmonary airway malformation	Bronchogenic cyst
Pulmonary interstitial emphysema	Congenital pulmonary airway malformation (if imaged early in life, when cystic components are fluid filled)
Congenital diaphragmatic hernia	

sequestration and bronchogenic cyst. Many of these lesions can present in children beyond the neonatal period and have a different appearance (see below).

We think of and teach about specific congenital lung lesion entities. However, these lesions can be mixed or hybrid, in which characteristics of more than one type of lesion are present. The most common mixed lesions are those that show characteristics of both CPAM and sequestration. Congenital lung lesions are believed to be the result of fetal airway obstruction with varying degree of associated dysplastic changes. This explains the significant overlap of imaging findings of the various lesions. Bronchial atresia is commonly identified on resected specimens—found in nearly 70% of CPAM lesions and 100% of bronchopulmonary sequestrations.

Currently, these lesions now often present on prenatal US and magnetic resonance imaging (MRI) rather than when the infant became symptomatic. Historically, the most common clinical presentation in cases of bronchopulmonary sequestration was a young adult with recurrent pyogenic pneumonia of progressive severity. Currently, most of the congenital lung lesions we see are identified and followed through fetal life, with additional postnatal imaging obtained shortly after birth. A significant number of these children are asymptomatic. This has raised issues related to when and whether to perform surgical treatment in infants with asymptomatic lesions.

Congenital Lobar Overinflation

Also referred to as *congenital lobar emphysema* and *infantile lobar emphysema*, congenital lobar overinflation is related to overexpansion of alveoli. The etiology is debated. As the alveolar walls are maintained, there is not true emphysematous change. Some reports suggest a ball valve type of anomaly in the bronchus causing progressive air trapping. Most cases present with respiratory distress during the neonatal period; 50% within the first month and 75% within the first 6 months of life. In a minority of cases, there can be associated anomalies, usually cardiac. There is a lobar predilection; the most common site is the left upper lobe (43%), followed by the right middle lobe (35%) and right upper lobe (21%), with less than 1% in each of the other lobes. On chest radiography, a hyperlucent, hyperexpanded lobe is seen (Fig. 3-14). On initial radiographs, the lesion may appear to be a soft tissue density because of retained fetal lung fluid. This density resolves and is replaced by progressive hyperlucency. On CT, the air is in the alveoli, so the interstitial septa and broncho-vascular bundles are at the periphery (not the center) of the lucency (Fig. 3-14). The air spaces are larger than those in the adjacent normal lung, and the pulmonary vessels appear attenuated. The treatment is lobectomy.

Congenital Pulmonary Airway Malformation

CPAMs, also known as CCAM (congenital cystic adenomatoid malformation), are dysplastic lesions caused by overgrowth of mesenchymal elements and airway maldevelopment. It is a congenital adenomatoid proliferation that replaces normal alveoli. The majority are detected prenatally but can also present with respiratory distress at birth. Most involve only one lobe and, in contrast to congenital lobar emphysema, there is no lobar predilection. CPAMs were originally classified by Stocker into three types based on cyst size and microscopic similarities to presumed sites of origin of the malformation along the airway. Type 1 shows cysts greater than 2 cm; type 2 shows more uniform cysts measuring less than 2 cm; and type 3 appears solid or shows very small cysts (<0.2 cm). Subsequently, Langston developed a more comprehensive pathologic classification of all congenital lung malformations, which is the most accepted at present. In this classification, the type 1 CPAM is named large cyst type and the type 2 CPAM is named small cyst type based on similar cyst size and histologic criteria. In this classification, type 3 CPAM is excluded because it is considered to represent a form of pulmonary hyperplasia. Stocker later expanded his CPAM classification to include five types; however, the Langston classification is the most currently accepted because it correlates well with imaging findings. In fetal imaging, the classification of these anomalies is also mainly based on cyst size as microcysts (<5 mm) and macrocysts (>5 mm). Given the controversial and confusing terminology, it is best to thoroughly describe the imaging findings that characterize the malformation to guide management. It is best to describe: the gross number of cysts (e.g., single, several, or multiple), size of the largest cyst, lobe or lobes involved, degree of aeration of the CPAM, and presence or absence of an aberrant, systemic vessel. CPAMs communicate with the bronchial tree at birth and therefore fill with air within the first days of life. On radiography and CT, a completely cystic, mixed cystic and solid, or completely solid mass is seen. depending on the number and size of cysts and whether those cysts contain air or fluid (Figs. 3-15 and 3-16). The management of symptomatic CPAM is surgical resection. The management of asymptomatic CPAM is currently somewhat controversial. Many caregivers advocate elective resection because of the risk for infection and rarely malignancy.

A scenario encountered with increasing frequency is a prenatally diagnosed lung mass that

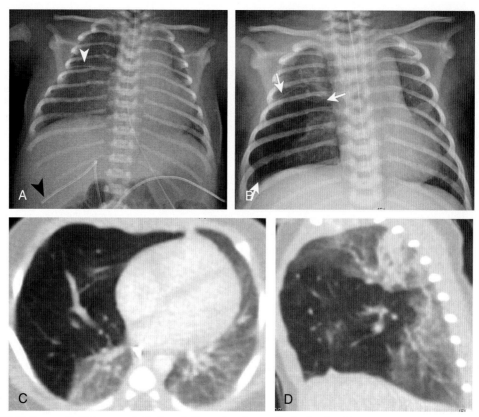

■ **FIGURE 3-14 Congenital lobar overinflation. A,** Frontal radiograph obtained at birth in a near term with respiratory distress shows findings initially attributed to transient tachypnea of the newborn, as there is a small amount of fluid in the minor fissure (*white arrowhead*). Notice the tip of the umbilical catheter in the right portal vein (*black arrowhead*) should be repositioned. **B,** Chest radiograph obtained a week later shows diffuse lucency in the right mid lung field (*arrows*). **C,** Axial and **D,** sagittal reformatted CT images obtained the following day show a hyperlucent and enlarged right middle lobe with asymmetric attenuation of vascular structures and increased space between the septa. Presumably, at initial radiograph obtained at birth, the right middle lobe was fluid filled and the overinflation occurred over time.

becomes less prominent on serial prenatal USs or magnetic resonance (MR) examinations and demonstrates only subtle findings or is not detected on a chest radiograph obtained soon after birth. In most of such cases, there are abnormalities on CT, even in light of a normal chest radiograph.

Many CPAMs identified prenatally are followed with fetal MRI (Fig. 3-15), and much has been learned about the nature of these lesions. CPAMs tend to increase in size until approximately 25 weeks of gestation. The mass of the CPAMs then tends to regress over time, sometimes dramatically. Compression of the contralateral lung by a large mass and development of fetal hydrops are associated with high mortality rates. Fetal intervention is typically reserved for cases with hydrops; management options include dominant cyst aspiration and fetal surgery with resection of the lesion. Trials using maternal steroids have shown promise in shrinking the

CPAM volumes and avoiding the need for other interventions.

Congenital Diaphragmatic Hernia

CDHs are usually secondary to posterior defects in the diaphragm (Bochdalek hernia) and are more common on the left side by a ratio of 5 to 1. CDH prevalence is estimated at approximately 1−4 cases per 10,000 live births. CDHs are isolated in 30%−70% of cases, but may occur as part of genetic syndrome or a complex nonsyndromic set of findings. Associated congenital heart disease can occur in as many as 50% of patients. Most infants with CDHs present at birth with severe respiratory distress. The hernia may contain stomach, small bowel, colon, or liver. The radiographic appearance depends on the hernia contents and on whether there is air within the herniated viscera. On initial radiographs, before the introduction of air into the

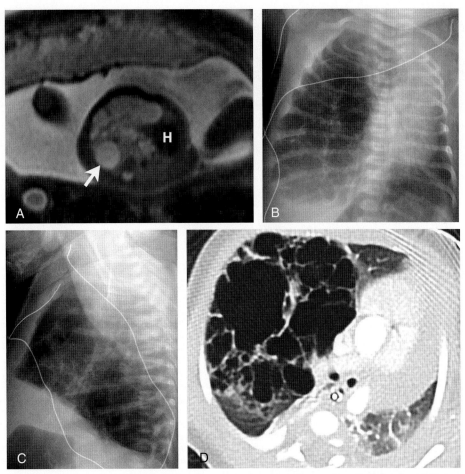

■ **FIGURE 3-15 Large cyst or type 1 congenital pulmonary airway malformation. A,** Axial fetal MR image shows hyperexpanded, high-signal, macrocystic lesion in the right lung. The *arrow* indicates a large cyst measuring more than 5 mm. There is associated mediastinal shift and the heart (*H*) is displaced to the left. **B,** Frontal and **C,** lateral postnatal chest radiographs, and **D,** axial CT image shows a large, lucent, multicystic lesion in the right lung. Notice the mass effect on the mediastinum and the flattening of the diaphragm.

viscera, the appearance may be radiopaque. Later, and more commonly, the herniated viscera contain air and the hernia appears as an air-containing cystic mass. Fewer air-filled viscera in the abdomen than expected and an abnormal position of support apparatus, such as a naso-gastric tube within a herniated stomach, are obvious clues that support the diagnosis (Fig. 3-17). Often a nasogastric tube becomes lodged at the esophagogastric junction because of the acute turn in the herniated stomach. This can be a supportive finding of the diagnosis.

The diagnosis of CDH is commonly made prenatally by US and further evaluated by fetal MRI (Fig. 3-18). The mortality rate for CDH is related to the degree of associated pulmonary hypoplasia. Systems of calculating lung volumes and predicting mortality have been devised for use with fetalUS, fetal MRI, and postnatal radi-ography. Radiographic predictors of poor prognoses include lack of aerated ipsilateral lung, low percentage of aerated contralateral lung, and severe mediastinal shift. Treatment includes support of respiratory failure, often by high-frequency ventilation or ECMO, and surgical repair. Multisystem morbidity is high among survivors, and almost all CDH patients have some degree of pulmonary hypoplasia and neu-rodevelopmental dysfunction. The main issues at birth are related to respiratory insufficiency and persistent pulmonary hypertension. Abnormal pulmonary vascular development and function can occur bilaterally, although these abnormal-ities are more commonly seen in the ipsilateral, hypoplastic lung. The reported mortality rates associated with CDH range from 20% to 60%. One factor contributing to mortality is the presence of associated abnormalities. By the na-ture of the herniated bowel into the chest, most patients with CDH have associated malrotation.

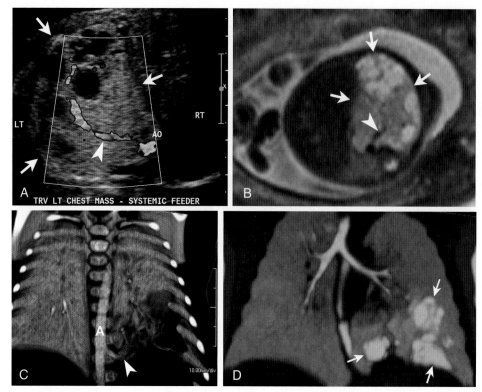

■ **FIGURE 3-16 Hybrid lesion with components of both CPAM and sequestration seen at pathology. A,** Prenatal US shows a large lesion (*arrows*) in left lower lobe with cystic components in the periphery and a feeding aortic vessel (*arrowhead*). **B,** Fetal MR image in axial plane shows a high-signal, multicystic lesion. **C,** Postnatal coronal 3D volume-rendered CT image shows a large systemic arterial feeder (*arrowhead*) arising from aorta (*A*) and extending into the lesion. Findings are characteristic of sequestration. **D,** Coronal minimum intensity projection CT image depicts the cystic components of the lesion to better advantage (*arrows*). Overall findings are consistent with a hybrid lesion with CPAM and sequestration components.

Sequestration

The term *pulmonary sequestration* refers to an area of congenital abnormal pulmonary tissue that does not have a normal connection to the bronchial tree. The characteristic imaging feature of sequestration is the demonstration of an anomalous arterial supply to the abnormal lung via a systemic artery arising from the aorta or its branches (Fig. 3-19). All modalities that can demonstrate this abnormal systemic arterial supply, including MRI, CT, US, and arteriography, have been advocated in making the diagnosis of sequestration. However, contrast-enhanced CT angiography is preferred because it both visualizes the systemic arterial supply when a sequestration is present (Fig. 3-16) and further characterizes the lung abnormality if a sequestration is not present.

Sequestration can present on prenatal imaging, with respiratory distress during the newborn period or with recurrent pneumonia in later childhood. Because sequestrations do not communicate with the bronchial tree unless they become infected, they usually appear as radiopaque masses during the neonatal period. After infection has occurred, air may be introduced and sequestration may appear as a multiloculated cystic mass. The most common location is within the left lower lobe.

There has been much discussion concerning differentiation between intralobar and extralobar sequestrations. Extralobar sequestrations have a separate pleural covering, whereas intralobar sequestrations, which are believed to be more common, do not; however, the presence or absence of pleural covering cannot be determined at imaging. Extralobar sequestrations are commonly associated with other abnormalities, whereas intralobar sequestrations are not. Differences in venous drainage patterns between intralobar and extralobar sequestrations have been emphasized as a differentiating factor but are actually variable with both types. Visualization of the supplying systemic artery is the characteristic finding and is what surgeons seek to document before surgically removing the lesion.

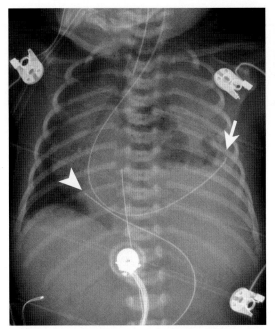

■ **FIGURE 3-17 Congenital diaphragmatic hernia.** Radiograph shows the tip of the nasogastric tube (*arrow*) in the left hemithorax indicating gastric herniation into the hernia sac. There is a generalized paucity of bowel gas in the visualized abdomen. There is mediastinal shift to the right. Contralateral right lung poorly aerated related to mediastinal shift to the right. Notice the tip of the umbilical venous line (*arrowhead*) is also seen above the diaphragm, presumably reflecting some left lobe liver herniation into the hernial sac.

Bronchogenic Cyst

Bronchogenic cysts occur secondary to abnormal budding of the tracheobronchial tree during development and occur in the lung parenchyma or the middle mediastinum (Fig. 3.20). Mediastinal lesions are reportedly more common, making up between 65% and 90% of cases and are most commonly subcarinal or paratracheal in location. Lung lesions are also most commonly central in location, often perihilar. Bronchogenic cysts are almost always solitary lesions; multiple bronchogenic cysts are very uncommon. Because of the propensity for middle mediastinal and perihilar locations, associated compression of the distal trachea or bronchi is not uncommon, resulting in air trapping in the lung distal to the lesion. Like sequestrations, they do not contain air until they become infected and appear as well-defined soft tissue attenuation or cystic air–fluid-containing masses. They can be quite large.

■ ROLES OF IMAGING IN PEDIATRIC PNEUMONIA

Respiratory tract infection is the most common cause of illness in children and continues to be a significant cause of morbidity and mortality. Worldwide respiratory infections are the most

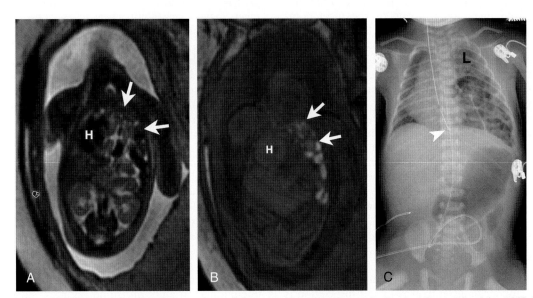

■ **FIGURE 3-18 Congenital diaphragmatic hernia. A,** Coronal T2-weighted and B, Coronal T1-weighted fetal MR images show multiple bowel loops (*arrows*) in left hemithorax. Notice the high T1 meconium on B. The heart (H) and mediastinum are shifted to the right. **B,** Chest radiograph after birth shows multiple bubble-like lucencies in left hemithorax consistent with herniated bowel loops. There is paucity of bowel gas in the abdomen. Note that in this case the stomach and nasogastric tube tip are not in the hernia. There is mediastinal shift to the right. **C,** The hypoplastic left lung (*L*) shows diffuse hazy opacification. Notice that the tip of the enteric tube terminates in the distal esophagus (*arrowhead*) and is not decompressing the stomach, which is markedly air distended.

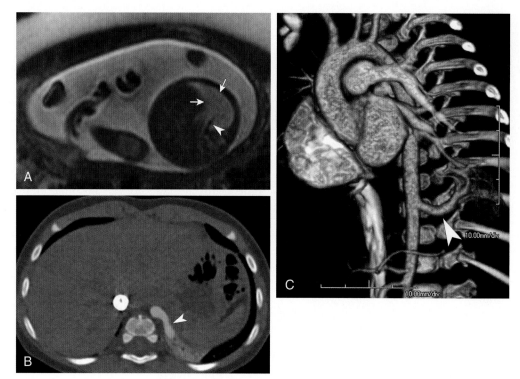

■ **FIGURE 3-19 Sequestration. A,** Fetal MR image shows a large, relatively homogeneous lung lesion (*arrows*) in the left lower lobe with discrete aortic feeder (*arrowheads*). Axial (**B**) and 3D volume-rendered and (**C**) Sagittal oblique CT images performed at 4 months of age show feeding systemic arterial supply (*arrowheads* in **B** and **C**) arising from the aorta and extending to the unaerated lesion in left lower lobe.

common cause of death in children under the age of 5 years. Evaluation of suspected community-acquired pneumonia is one of the most common indications for imaging in children, and it is one of the most common causes for hospitalization in children under the age of 18, second only to trauma. Because of the frequency with which this scenario arises, knowledge of the issues concerning the imaging of children with community-acquired pneumonia is important. The roles of imaging in these children are multiple: confirmation or exclusion of pneumonia, characterization and prediction of infectious agents, exclusion of other cause of symptoms, evaluation when there is failure to resolve, and evaluation of related complications.

Confirmation or Exclusion of Pneumonia

Making the diagnosis of pneumonia and consequently deciding on treatment and disposition is a common but complex and difficult issue. The symptoms and physical findings in children with pneumonia are sometimes nonspecific, especially in infants and young children. Many children present with nonrespiratory symptoms, such as fever, malaise, irritability, headaches, chest pain, abdominal pain, vomiting, or decreased appetite. Findings on physical examination are also less reliable in children than in adults because young children are less cooperative with exams and have smaller anatomy and smaller respiratory cycles. Because of the inaccuracy of physical examination, radiography is often requested to evaluate children with suspected pneumonia. Several studies have shown that in a large percentage of cases, findings on chest radiography change caregivers' diagnoses and treatment plans (antibiotics, bronchodilators, and patient disposition) for children being evaluated for potential pneumonia. At our institution, we obtain both a frontal and a lateral film in the evaluation of a child with suspected pneumonia. It has been shown that obtaining both views increases the negative predictive value of chest radiography for pneumonia. In addition, some findings, such as hyperinflation in an infant, are much more easily evaluated on the lateral than on the frontal views (Figs. 3-21 and 3.22).

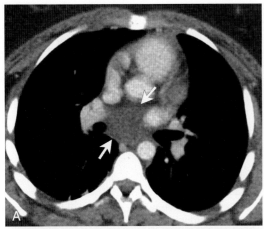

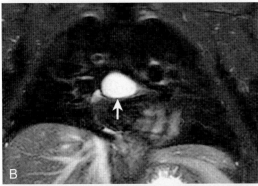

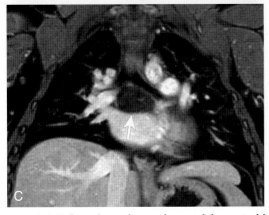

■ FIGURE 3-20 **Bronchogenic cyst in an adolescent girl.** **A,** CT obtained for initial metastatic work-up shows a fluid attenuation mass (*arrows*) in subcarinal location. **B,** Coronal T2-weighted fat-suppressed and (**B**), Coronal T1-weighted fat-suppressed postcontrast image confirm the cystic nature of the lesion (*arrows*) with minimal enhancement of the cyst wall.

Characterization and Prediction of Infectious Agent

The historic emphasis in textbooks and articles concerning pneumonia has been on radiographic patterns that suggest a specific infectious agent, such as staphylococcal or streptococcal

pneumonia. However, because of the limited ways in which the lung can respond to inflammation, findings suggestive of a specific diagnosis are usually not encountered on the radiograph of a child with suspected community-acquired pneumonia. The more general issue in the evaluation of suspected pneumonia is whether the infectious agent is likely to be bacteria or viral, which determines whether the patient should be placed on antibiotics. To answer this question, it is helpful to review the epidemiology of lower respiratory infections in children, the classic radiographic patterns of viral and bacterial pneumonia in children, and what is known about the accuracy of chest radiography in differentiating viral from bacterial infection.

The common causal agents of lower respiratory tract infections in children vary greatly with age. In all age groups, viral infections are much more common than bacterial infections. In infants and preschool-age children (4 months—5 years of age), viruses cause 95% of all lower respiratory tract infections. The epidemiology is much different in school-age children (6—16 years of age). In school-age children, although viral agents remain the most common cause of lower respiratory tract infections, the incidence of bacterial infection by *Streptococcus pneumoniae* increases. What is most striking is that *Mycoplasma pneumoniae*, which is an uncommon cause of pneumonia in preschool infants and children, is the cause of approximately 30% of lower respiratory tract infections in school-age children. Therefore, the odds that a child should be administered antibiotics for a respiratory tract infection are greatly influenced by the child's age. In addition, there has been a recent increase in the incidence of pneumonia secondary to multidrug-resistant *Staphylococcus aureus* infections. These can occur at any age.

Viral infections affect the airways, causing inflammation of the small airways and peribronchial edema. This peribronchial edema appears on radiography as increased peribronchial opacities—symmetric coarse markings that radiate from the hila into the lung (Fig. 3-21; Fig. 3-22). The central portions of the lungs appear to be "dirty" or "busy." It is one of the most subjective findings in radiology. In addition, the combination of the bronchial wall edema, narrowed airway lumen, and necrotic debris and mucus in the airway leads to small airway occlusion. This results in both hyperinflation and areas of subsegmental atelectasis. Hyperinflation is evident on chest radiographs in children in the presence of hyperlucency, the depression of the hemidiaphragm to more than 10 posterior ribs, and the increased anterior-to-posterior

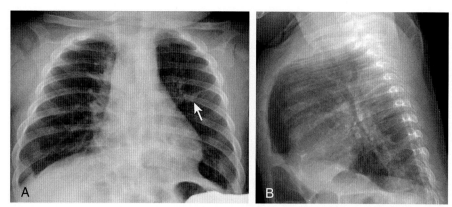

■ FIGURE 3-21 **Viral lower respiratory infection in a young child. A,** Frontal view shows increased perihilar markings and band-like density (*arrow*) in left mid lung field, representing subsegmental atelectasis. **B,** Lateral view better shows marked hyperinflation with flattened hemidiaphragms, increased anterior-to-posterior diameter of the chest, and barrel-shaped chest. Increased perihilar markings make hila appear prominent.

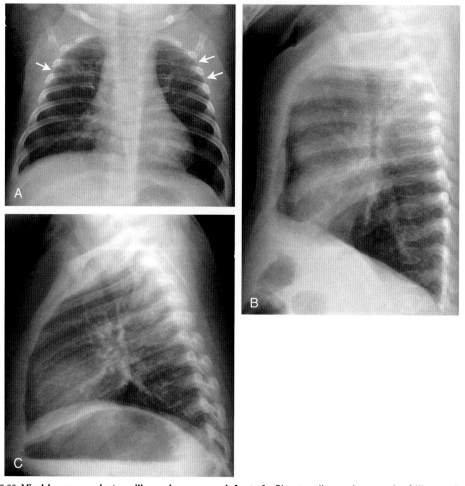

■ FIGURE 3-22 **Viral lower respiratory illness in a young infant. A,** Chest radiograph at peak of illness shows ropy increased perihilar markings and areas of subsegmental atelectasis. Hyperinflation can be hard to identify on the frontal view at this young age. One clue is the bulging of lung tissue between the ribs (*arrows*). **B,** Lateral radiograph shows marked hyperinflation. Note the flattening of the diaphragms. **C,** Radiograph obtained a week earlier in the same child shows a convex diaphragmatic contour, as expected. Note the smaller AP dimension of the upper thorax when compared to **B**.

chest diameter. Hyperinflation is often much better appreciated on lateral than on frontal radiographs in infants and small children (Fig. 3-22). Subsegmental atelectasis appears as wedge-shaped or linear areas of density, most commonly in the lower and mid lung fields (Fig. 3-21). There are several anatomic differences that render small children more predisposed to air trapping and collapse secondary to viral infection than adults: small airway luminal diameter, poorly developed collateral pathways of ventilation, and more abundant mucus production. The misinterpretation of areas of atelectasis as focal opacities suspicious for bacterial pneumonia is thought to be one of the more common misinterpretations in pediatric radiology.

In contrast to the airway involvement in viral pneumonia, bacterial pneumonia occurs secondary to inhalation of the infectious agent into the air spaces. There is a resultant progressive development of inflammatory exudate and edema within the acini, resulting in consolidation of the air spaces. On chest radiography, localized air space consolidation (Fig. 3-23) occurs with air bronchograms. The typical distribution is either lobar or segmental, depending on when in the course of development of the pneumonia the radiograph is obtained. Associated pleural effusions are not uncommon. In addition, there is a propensity for pneumonia to appear "round" in younger children (Fig. 3-24). Round pneumonia is more common in children younger than 8 years of age and is most often caused by *S. pneumoniae*. The occurrence of this pattern is thought to be related to poor development of pathways of collateral ventilation. Round pneumonia tends to be solitary and occurs more commonly posteriorly and in the lower lobes. When such a lung mass is seen in a child with cough and fever, round pneumonia should be suspected. The child should be treated with antibiotics, and the chest radiograph should be repeated. It is best to avoid unnecessary CT examination in this clinical scenario. When a round opacity is seen in a child older than 8 years of age, other pathology should be suspected.

Do these classic patterns of viral and bacterial infections accurately differentiate between children who have bacterial infection and need antibiotics and those who do not? Studies have shown that these radiographic patterns do have a high negative predictive value (92%) for excluding bacterial pneumonia. However, the positive predictive value is low (30%). In other words, 70% of children who have radiographic findings of bacterial infection actually have viral infection. In regard to decisions about administering antibiotics to children with suspected pneumonia, the goals are to treat all children who have bacterial pneumonia with antibiotics while minimizing the treatment of children with viral illnesses. Therefore, the high negative predictive value of chest radiography for bacterial pneumonia is useful in identifying those children who do not need antibiotics.

Exclusion of Other Pathologic Processes

Many of the presenting symptoms of pneumonia in children are nonspecific, and the spectrum of presentations overlaps with a number of other pathologic processes involving the chest or other

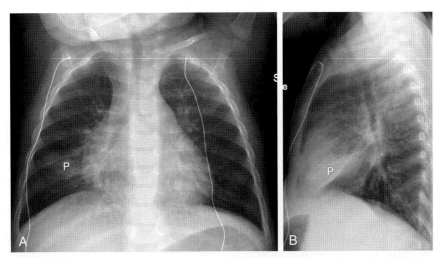

■ **FIGURE 3-23 Bacterial pneumonia.** Frontal (**A**) and Lateral (**B**) Chest radiographs show focal lung consolidation (*P*) with air bronchograms in the right middle lobe, consistent with early/developing bacterial pneumonia.

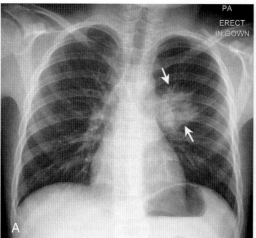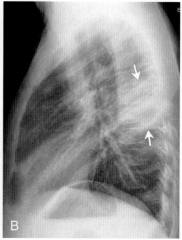

■ **FIGURE 3-24 Round pneumonia.** Frontal (**A**) and Lateral (**B**) Radiographs show rounded opacity overlying the left hilum consistent with round pneumonia (*arrows*). This is the location of the superior segment of the left lower lobe.

anatomic regions. Therefore, one of the other roles of chest radiography in the evaluation of a child who potentially has pneumonia is the exclusion of other processes. Two areas that are often blind spots for radiologists and may be involved by conditions that mimic pneumonia are the airway and chest wall. Processes that cause extrinsic compression of the trachea and bronchi can mimic pneumonia by causing noisy breathing, lobar collapse, and recurrent infection. Evaluation of the diameter of the airway should be stressed as a routine part of evaluating radiographs. Rib abnormalities may be evidence that a lung opacity seen on chest radiography does not represent pneumonia. The presence of rib erosion or asymmetric intercostal spaces helps to differentiate neuroblastoma from chest opacity secondary to pneumonia.

Failure to Resolve

Unlike in adults, in whom postobstructive pneumonia secondary to bronchogenic carcinoma is a concern, follow-up radiography to ensure resolution of radiographic findings is not routinely necessary in an otherwise healthy child. There is a tendency to obtain follow-up radiographs both too early and too often. Follow-up radiographs should be reserved for children who have persistent or recurrent symptoms and those who have an underlying condition, such as immunodeficiency. The radiographic findings of pneumonia can persist for 3–4 weeks, even when the patient is recovering appropriately clinically. When follow-up radiographs are indicated, it is ideal to avoid obtaining them until at least 2–3 weeks have passed, if clinical symptoms allow.

Causes of failure of suspected pneumonia to resolve include infected developmental lesions, bronchial obstruction, gastroesophageal reflux and aspiration, and underlying systemic disorders. The most common developmental lung masses that may become infected and present as recurrent or persistent pulmonary infection include sequestration and CPAM. These entities have been discussed previously.

Complications of Pneumonia

The evaluation of complications related to pneumonia can be divided into several clinical scenarios: primary evaluation of parapneumonic effusions, evaluation of a child who has persistent or progressive symptoms despite medical or surgical therapy, and the chronic sequelae of pneumonia.

PRIMARY EVALUATION OF PARAPNEUMONIC EFFUSIONS

Parapneumonic effusions occur commonly in patients who have bacterial pneumonia. Multiple therapeutic options are available in the management of parapneumonic effusions, including antibiotic therapy alone, repeated thoracentesis, chest tube placement, thrombolytic therapy, and thoracoscopy with surgical debridement. Great differences in opinion exist among caregivers regarding the timing and aggressiveness of management of parapneumonic effusions. Traditionally, the aggressiveness of therapy has been based on categorizing parapneumonic effusions as empyema or transudative effusion, as determined by needle aspiration and analysis of the pleural fluid.

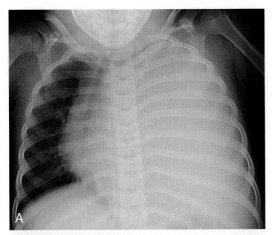

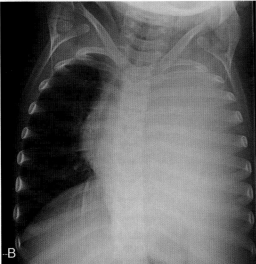

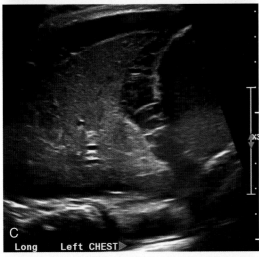

Several imaging modalities have been advocated to differentiate empyema from transudative effusion without the use of an invasive diagnostic thoracentesis, including decubitus radiographs, US, and CT. If there is a significant change in the position and appearance of the pleural fluid on the decubitus images as compared with the upright radiograph, the fluid is considered to be free flowing and nonloculated. If there is no change in position of the pleural fluid, the fluid is considered to be loculated However, decubitus views are not helpful in cases in which the entire hemithorax is opacified because the layering fluid cannot be adequately delineated without any adjacent air (Fig. 3.25). In the authors' experience, these decubitus radiographs have been more confusing than helpful, and we do not advocate the use of decubitus radiographs to evaluate pleural effusions. On CT, findings such as thickening or enhancement of the parietal pleura and thickening or increased attenuation of the extrapleural fat were previously thought to favor empyema (Fig. 3.26) over transudative effusion, but this has been shown to be inaccurate. The primary role of US in these instances is to identify, quantify, and characterize the effusion and empyema. US has also been advocated as an aid in making therapeutic decisions for parapneumonic effusions because it may provide image guidance for drainage or identify any residual collection. In one study, parapneumonic effusions were categorized as low grade (anechoic fluid without internal heterogeneous echogenic structures) or high grade (fibrinopurulent organization demonstrated by the presence of fronds, septations, or loculations) (Figs. 3-25 and 3-26). In children in whom effusions were high grade, hospital stay was reduced by nearly 50% when operative intervention was performed. The length of hospital stay in children with low-grade effusions was not affected by operative intervention. Therefore, US plays a more useful role than CT in the early evaluation of parapneumonic effusions. It is not uncommon for US to show multiple septations and in the same case to show no evidence of septations on CT (Fig. 3-26). US, rather than CT or decubitus radiographs, is the primary imaging modality to evaluate parapneumonic effusions.

■ **FIGURE 3-25 Parapneumonic effusion (empyema) evaluated by decubitus radiographs and ultrasound. A,** Radiograph shows a large left pleural effusion in child with pneumonia. **B,** Decubitus radiograph with left side down shows no change in pleural effusion. Lack of change is supposed to suggest loculation but is probably not that helpful to be a diagnostic tool, particularly in cases with complete or near complete opacification of a hemithorax with or without associated contralateral mediastinal shift. **C,** Sagittal ultrasound of left pleural fluid demonstrating innumerable septations and debris—a high-grade effusion, predictive of benefit from aggressive drainage. Ultrasound is extremely helpful in these cases because it can speedily differentiate a parapneumonic effusion from extensive consolidation or an underlying mass.

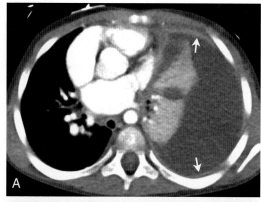

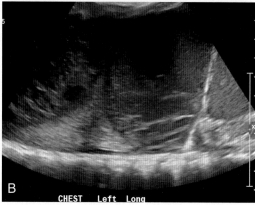

■ **FIGURE 3-26 Parapneumonic effusion (empyema) evaluated by CT and ultrasound. A,** CT shows left parapneumonic effusion. There are no septations seen by CT. There may be some peripheral enhancement, so-called pleural split sign (*arrows*), a finding suggestive of empyema. **B,** Sagittal ultrasound shows complex pleural fluid, with extensive debris and septations.

EVALUATION OF PERSISTENT OR PROGRESSIVE SYMPTOMS

When children exhibit persistent or progressive symptoms (fever, respiratory distress, sepsis) despite appropriate medical management of pneumonia, there is commonly an underlying suppurative complication. Potential suppurative complications include parapneumonic effusions (such as empyema), inadequately drained effusions, and persistent effusion due to malpositioned chest tube; parenchymal complications, such as cavitary necrosis or lung abscess; and purulent pericarditis. Although chest radiography is the primary imaging modality for detecting such complications, a significant percentage of such complications are not demonstrated by radiography. In a child who has had a noncontributory radiograph and who has not responded appropriately to therapy, contrast-enhanced CT has been shown to be useful in detecting clinically significant suppurative

complications. CT can help to differentiate whether there is a pleural or a parenchymal reason for persistent illness. Administration of intravenous contrast is vital to maximize the likelihood of detection and the characterization of both parenchymal and pleural complications.

LUNG PARENCHYMAL COMPLICATIONS

On contrast-enhanced CT, both non-compromised consolidated lung parenchyma and atelectasis enhance diffusely. Large areas of decreased or absent enhancement are indicative of underlying parenchymal ischemia or impending infarction. Suppurative lung parenchymal complications include a spectrum of abnormalities, such as cavitary necrosis, lung abscess, pneumatocele, bronchopleural fistula, and pulmonary gangrene. The name given to the suppurative process is determined by several factors, including the severity, distribution, condition of the adjacent lung parenchyma, and temporal relationship with disease resolution. Lung abscess represents a dominant focus of suppuration surrounded by a well-formed fibrous wall. Lung abscess is actually uncommon in otherwise healthy children and typically occurs in children who are immunocompromised. On contrast-enhanced CT, lung abscesses appear as fluid- or air-filled cavities with definable enhancing walls (Fig. 3-27). Typically, there is no evidence of necrosis in the surrounding lung. *Pneumatocele* is a term given to thin-walled cysts seen at imaging and may represent a later or less severe stage of resolving or healing necrosis (Fig. 3-28).

Cavitary necrosis is the most commonly encountered suppurative complication. It is characterized by a dominant area of necrosis of a consolidated lobe that is associated with a variable number of thin-walled cysts (Fig. 3-29). CT findings of cavitary necrosis include loss of normal lung architecture, decreased parenchymal enhancement, loss of the lung–pleural margin, and multiple thin-walled cavities containing air or fluid and lacking an enhancing border (Fig. 3-30). Although historically described as a complication of staphylococcal pneumonia, cavitary necrosis was much more commonly seen as a complication of streptococcal pneumonia during the 1990s. Cavitary necrosis in association with multidrug-resistant *S. aureus* infection has been occurring with increased frequency. The presence of cavitary necrosis is indicative of an intense and prolonged illness. However, unlike in adults in whom the mortality rate in cavitary necrosis is high and early surgical removal of the affected lung has been advocated, the long-term

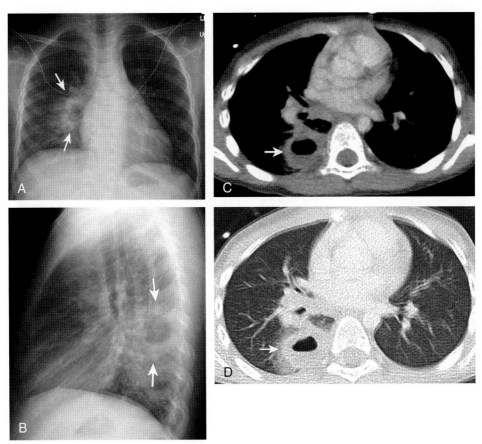

■ **FIGURE 3-27 Lung abscess.** Frontal (**A**) and Lateral (**B**) Chest radiographs in a 7-year-old show airspace consolidation in the superior segment of the right lower lobe with a large internal cavity (*arrows*) with an air–fluid level best seen on the lateral projection. Axial contrast-enhanced CT images in soft tissue (**C**) and Lung windows (**D**) Show a well-defined cavity (*arrows*) with thickened, irregular walls, containing an air–fluid level. *Streptococcus intermedius* grew in cultures.

outcome for children with cavitary necrosis is favorable in most cases with medical management alone. It is amazing that in children with cavitary necrosis, follow-up radiographs obtained more than 40 days after the acute illness are most often normal or show only minimal scarring.

It may sometimes be difficult on a single imaging study to differentiate a suppurative lung parenchymal complication of pneumonia from an underlying cystic congenital lung lesion that has become secondarily infected. Infected CPAMs may appear very similar to cavitary necrosis. Obviously, historical imaging studies showing a lack of a cystic lesion exclude underlying CPAM, but such historical examinations often do not exist or are not available. Observable resolution of the cystic lesion on follow-up studies ensures that the lesion is no longer clinically relevant and makes cavitary necrosis much more likely. However, some CPAMs have been reported to scar down and resolve after becoming infected.

CHRONIC LUNG COMPLICATIONS OF PNEUMONIA

Acute pneumonia can lead to parenchymal damage and long-term sequelae. The most common sequelae of acute pneumonia are bronchiectasis (Fig. 3.31) and Swyer–James syndrome (Fig. 3.32). Bronchiectasis is enlargement of the diameter of the bronchi that is related to damage to the bronchial walls. It is best demonstrated by high-resolution CT (HRCT), on which the diagnostic finding is that the bronchus in question is larger in diameter than the adjacent pulmonary artery. Swyer–James syndrome is characterized by unilateral lung hyperlucency that is thought to be secondary to a virus-induced necrotizing bronchiolitis that leads to postinfectious obliterative bronchiolitis. Radiography shows a hyperlucent and enlarged or normal volume lung with a static lung volume. The pulmonary vessels are less prominent than on the normal side.

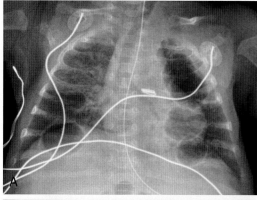

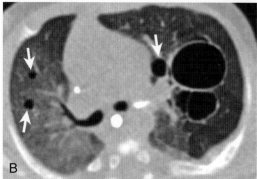

■ **FIGURE 3-28 Rapid development of necrosis and pneumatocele formation in an infant with multidrug-resistant *Staphylococcus aureus* pneumonia. A,** Radiograph obtained in the intensive care unit after intubation for respiratory failure shows several pneumatoceles in the left lung. Because the cysts are thin walled and without surrounding opacification, *pneumatocele* is acceptable terminology. **B,** Axial CT image taken a few weeks later shows additional smaller cysts (*arrows*), not well seen on conventional radiography.

Tuberculosis

The incidence of tuberculosis in children has been increasing. Children with primary tuberculosis can present with pulmonary consolidation within any lobe. It is often associated with ipsilateral hilar lymphadenopathy or pleural effusion. Therefore, when lung consolidation is seen with associated lymphadenopathy or effusion in a child who is not acutely ill, there should be a high suspicion for tuberculosis. Unilateral hilar lymphadenopathy (Fig. 3-33) is a common presentation for tuberculosis. Such cases should be considered tuberculosis until proven otherwise.

■ COMMON CHRONIC OR RECURRENT PULMONARY PROBLEMS IN SPECIAL POPULATIONS

In children with certain underlying conditions, the clinical scenarios and differential diagnoses differ greatly from those seen in the general population. Commonly encountered scenarios include the evaluation of pneumonia in immunocompromised children, acute chest syndrome in children with sickle cell anemia, and pulmonary complications in children with cystic fibrosis.

Pneumonia in Immunodeficient Children

Children can be immunocompromised for a variety of reasons, including cancer therapy, bone marrow transplantation, solid organ transplantation, primary immunodeficiency, and acquired immunodeficiency syndrome (AIDS). This is a population that continues to increase. Acute pulmonary processes are a common cause of morbidity and mortality in these patients. As with immunocompetent children, radiography is the primary modality used to confirm or exclude pneumonia. However, because many of the chest radiographs obtained in these children are portable and because of the consequences of missing an infection, CT plays a greater role in evaluating for an acute pulmonary process when chest radiographs are noncontributory. In large children's healthcare systems, the number of chest CTs obtained in immunocompromised children is potentially greater than the number of those obtained in immunocompetent children.

In immunocompetent children, the main question is whether a pulmonary process is viral or bacterial. In immunocompromised children, there are many more possible causes of acute pulmonary processes. They include alveolar hemorrhage, pulmonary edema, drug reaction, idiopathic pneumonia, lymphoid interstitial pneumonitis, bronchiolitis obliterans, bronchiolitis obliterans with organizing pneumonia, and chronic graft-versus-host disease. The CT findings for many of these entities are overlapping and nonspecific. A clinical question often posed is this: Is there evidence of fungal infection? The hallmark CT finding indicating fungal infection is the presence of nodules (Figs. 3-34 and 3-35). Fungal infection often presents as clustered nodules and may exhibit poorly defined margins, cavitation, or a surrounding halo that has the opacity of ground glass. However, many of these findings are also nonspecific. In these cases, CT does aid in directing potential interventions, such as bronchoscopy or percutaneous lung biopsy, to high-yield areas.

Acute Chest Syndrome in Sickle Cell Disease

Children with sickle cell anemia can develop acute chest syndrome, which is manifested by

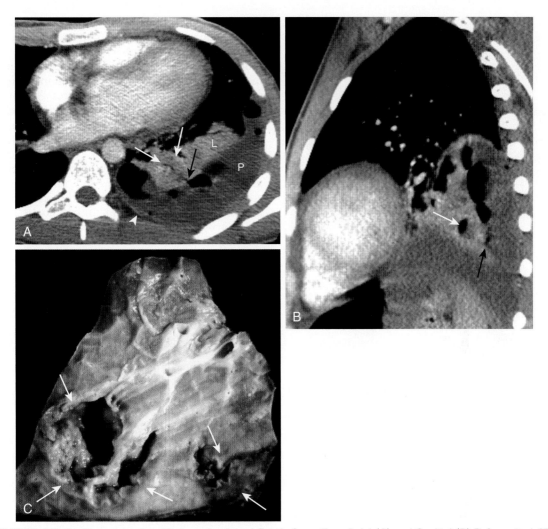

■ **FIGURE 3-29 Cavitary necrosis with bronchopleural fistula formation.** Axial (**A**) and Sagittal (**B**) Reformatted CT images show consolidation of the left lung. Portions of the lung demonstrate cavitary necrosis (*white arrows*). There are also areas of consolidated lung that enhance (*L*) and are not compromised. There is a pleural effusion (*P*) that contains both air and fluid. There are bubbles of gas in the pleural cavity (*black arrow*), consistent with a bronchopleural fistula. There is thickening and enhancement of the parietal pleura (*white arrowhead*). **C,** Photograph of surgical specimen (in different patient) shows consolidated lung (*tan area*) with areas of necrosis and cavity formation (*arrows*).

fever, chest pain, hypoxia, and pulmonary opacities on chest radiographs (Fig. 3-36). Acute chest syndrome is much more common in children than adults with sickle cell anemia. It occurs most commonly between 2 and 4 years of age and is the leading cause of death (25% of deaths) and the second most common cause of hospitalization in those affected with sickle cell disease. Although it is debated whether the cause of such episodes is more often related to infection or infarction, many believe the lung opacities are related to rib infarction, splinting, and subsequent areas of atelectasis. Other authors advocate

fat embolism, pulmonary infarctions, hypoventilation, and pulmonary or systemic infections as possible etiologies. Radiography often shows segmental to lobar pulmonary opacities but can also be normal. There can be an associated increase in cardiomegaly. Bone scans may show rib infarcts. The children are treated with oxygen, antibiotics, and pain control, and the pulmonary opacities are commonly monitored by radiography. Pneumonia occurs significantly more commonly in children with sickle cell disease, presumably related to impaired immune function and functional asplenia.

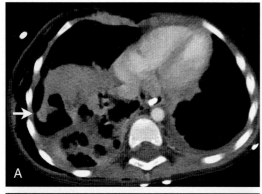

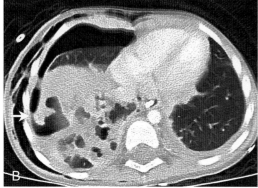

■ **FIGURE 3-30 Cavitary necrosis with bronchopleural fistula formation in a 5-year-old with a history of multidrug resistant *Staphylococcus aureus* pneumonia (MRSA).** Axial-enhanced CT images in soft tissue (**A**) and Lung (**B**) Windows show right lung cavitary necrosis. There is a right hydropneumothorax, which is in direct communication with the lung parenchyma via a bronchopulmonary fistula (*arrows*). The affected right lung parenchyma shows loss of the normal lung architecture, decreased parenchymal enhancement, and multiple thin-walled cavities containing air or fluid and lacking a distinct enhancing border. Notice associated subcutaneous emphysema.

Cystic Fibrosis

Cystic fibrosis is a genetic disease that most commonly affects the respiratory and gastrointestinal tracts. In the respiratory system, abnormally viscous mucus leads to airway obstruction and infection that causes bronchitis and bronchiectasis. Children may initially present with recurrent respiratory tract infections. Radiography may be normal at young ages but eventually demonstrates hyperinflation, increased peribronchial markings, mucus plugging, and bronchiectasis. The hilar areas can become prominent because of a combination of lymphadenopathy secondary to the chronic inflammation and enlarged central pulmonary arteries related to the development of pulmonary arterial hypertension. Chest radiography is used to monitor the disease and evaluate for complications during acute exacerbations. Such complications include focal pneumonia, pneumothorax, and pulmonary hemorrhage. To monitor the progression of disease, some institutions use low-dose CT with thin-section reconstruction, which demonstrates findings such as bronchiectasis and bronchial wall thickening in greater detail and earlier than does radiography (Fig. 3-37), often at similar radiation doses as a chest radiograph. Some authors advocate the use of MRI for follow-up imaging in patients with cystic fibrosis and other chronic conditions because it may allow the characterization of several different morphologic and functional imaging features without the use of ionizing radiation.

■ HIGH-RESOLUTION COMPUTED TOMOGRAPHY IN CHILDREN

High-Resolution Computed Tomography in Questioned Chronic Aspiration

A common indication for HRCT in the pediatric population is questioned chronic aspiration. Often this issue arises in children with neurologic abnormalities, such as cerebral palsy or chronic tracheotomy tubes, when decisions about methods of feeding are being entertained. HRCT findings of chronic aspiration include bronchiectasis, tree-in-bud opacities (Fig. 3-38), and increased interstitial linear opacities. Findings more often occur in lower lobes and dependent portions of the lungs.

Childhood Interstitial Lung Disease

Occasionally, neonates and infants present with pulmonary disorders characterized by extensive lung parenchymal abnormalities and impaired gas exchange primarily related to underlying developmental or genetic disorders constituting a heterogeneous group of diseases known as childhood interstitial lung diseases (chILDs). The chILDs classification recognizes four main categories: (1) diffuse developmental disorders, (2) alveolar growth abnormalities, which are the most common cause of chILDs and include conditions such as BPD and conditions associated with chromosomal abnormalities and congenital heart disease, (3) surfactant dysfunction disorders and related abnormalities, and (4) specific conditions of unknown or poorly understood etiology, including entities such as neuroendocrine cell hyperplasia of infancy (NEHI) (Fig. 3-39) and pulmonary interstitial glycogenosis (PIG).

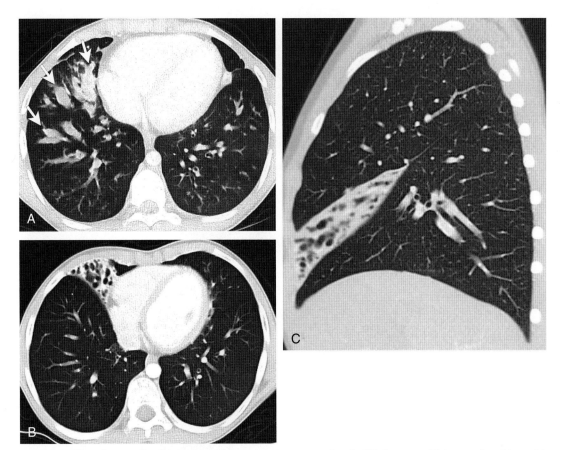

■ FIGURE 3-31 **Chronic complications related to recurrent pneumonias. A,** CT shows multiple round and branching, soft tissue density lesions in right middle and right and left lower lobes (*arrows*), consistent with bronchiectasis with mucus plugging, in a 14-year-old with cystic fibrosis. **B,** Axial and **C,** Sagittal reformatted CT images show marked bronchiectasis with volume loss in the right middle lobe in an 11-year-old boy with genetically proven primary cilia dyskinesia (DNAH11-associated PCD). The patient had multiple prior episodes of pneumonia, usually on the right side, documented radiographically.

On CT, NEHI is characterized by high lung volumes and geographic areas on ground-glass opacification in paramediastinal location, particularly in the right middle lobe and lingula (Fig. 3-39). Two forms of PIG have been described, the diffuse and the patchy forms, the latter being the more common form, which is typified by the presence of numerous cyst-like lucencies on the background of ground-glass opacification, septal thickening, and reticular changes.

The innumerable tiny (1−2 mm) subpleural cysts seen on Trisomy 21 (Fig. 3-40) are an example of a lung growth disorder associated with a genetic mutation. The prevalence of this abnormality in patients with Trisomy 21 ranges from 20% to 36%. Within the periphery of the lungs, the cysts may be seen with or without associated pleural thickening. The etiology and clinical relevance of this abnormality is not well understood; however, the presence of these characteristic cysts along the periphery, pleural reflections, or broncho-vascular bundles in this population should not be confused with other pathology.

Trauma

RIB FRACTURES AND LUNG CONTUSION

There is a greater component of cartilage than bone within the chest walls of children, so there is more compliance than there is in the chest walls of adults. Because of this increased compliance, the sequelae of trauma to the pediatric chest are unique in several ways. First, the incidence of rib fractures after high-speed motor vehicle accidents is lower in children than in adults. Second, the deceleration forces of high-speed collisions are more likely to be dispersed into the lung in children, resulting in lung contusion. Children with lung contusions have been shown to have higher morbidity and

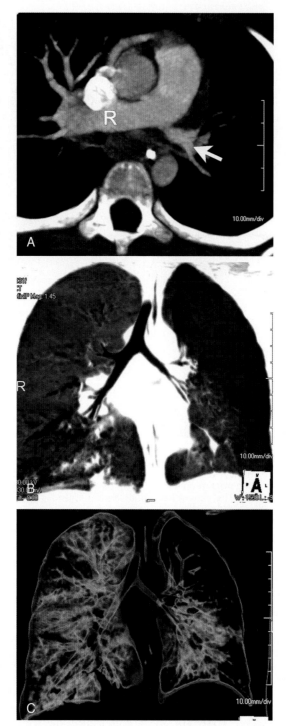

■ FIGURE 3-32 **Swyer–James syndrome in a 5-year-old with a remote history of adenovirus pneumonia. A,** Multiplanar reformatted CT image shows a small left main pulmonary artery (*arrow*), compared to the contralateral, normal right pulmonary artery (R). **B,** Coronal minimum intensity projection CT image shows relative normal size of the left lung, however, with diffuse hyperlucency. **C,** Coronal 3D volume-rendered CT image shows poor arborization of the left bronchial tree when compared to the right.

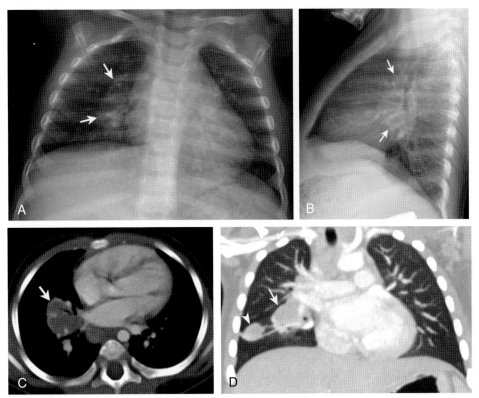

■ **FIGURE 3-33 Tuberculosis in a 14-month-old girl. A** and **B,** Frontal and Lateral radiographs of the chest demonstrate a right hilar mass (*arrows*) consistent with unilateral lymphadenopathy. **C,** Enhanced axial and **D,** Coronal reformatted CT images show unilateral, right hilar lymphadenopathy with a single right middle lobe pulmonary nodule (*arrowhead*). These findings are consistent with primary pulmonary tuberculosis (Ghon complex). Note that the enlarged lymph nodes show poor to no enhancement.

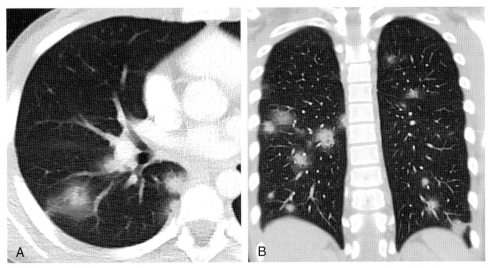

■ **FIGURE 3-34 Fungal pneumonia in a 15-year-old patient after bone marrow transplantation for acute lymphoblastic leukemia. A,** Axial and **B,** Coronal reformatted CT images show multiple poorly defined nodules and associated ground-glass opacity.

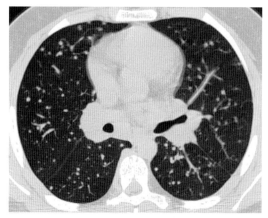

■ **FIGURE 3-35 Histoplasmosis infection**. CT shows multiple nodules bilaterally. Note bilateral hilar lymphadenopathy.

causes of lung opacification. The CT finding that classifies an opacified area as a lung laceration rather than a lung contusion is the presence of a blood- or air-filled cyst (traumatic hematocele or pneumatocele) or both within the opacified lung (Fig. 3-42). These cystic spaces result from torn lung.

Finally, the sites of rib fracture in children differ from those in adults. Rib fractures in young children in the absence of an obvious traumatic event are highly suspicious for child abuse (Figs. 3-43 and 3-44). Pediatric rib fractures are more likely to be posterior than lateral. In child abuse, as a result of squeezing an infant's thorax, the posterior ribs can be excessively levered at the costotransverse process articulation, causing posterior fracture at this site. In the

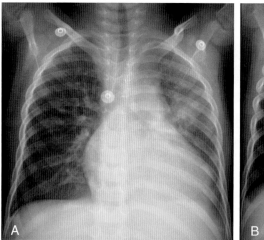
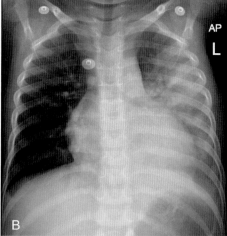

■ **FIGURE 3-36 Acute chest syndrome in a 4-year-old boy with sickle cell anemia. A,** Chest radiograph obtained at admission shows focal retrocardiac and faint left upper lobe airspace opacity. Notice moderate cardiomegaly. **B,** Chest radiograph obtained 1 day later shows consolidation of near the entire left lung.

mortality rates than those without lung contusions. Although chest CT is not commonly performed to evaluate for lung contusion, the lower lungs are often seen on CT when it is performed to evaluate for abdominal trauma. Characteristic findings in lung contusion on CT include nonlobar or nonsegmental distribution, posterior location, crescent shape, and mixed confluent and nodular characteristics (Fig. 3-41). In children with small lung contusions, the compliance of the chest wall can result in a rim of nonopacified lung between the consolidated contusion and the adjacent ribs seen on CT (Fig. 3-41). This *subpleural sparing* can be helpful in differentiating lung contusion from other

appropriately aged child, these findings are considered pathognomonic for child abuse.

MEDIASTINAL INJURY

The incidence of aortic injury is also much lower in children than in adults. This, in combination with the lower incidence of obesity in children as compared to adults, makes the "uncleared" mediastinum on a chest radiograph after trauma, a much less common scenario in children than in adults. Otherwise, the use of CT and angiography and the imaging findings of aortic injuries are no different from those encountered in adults.

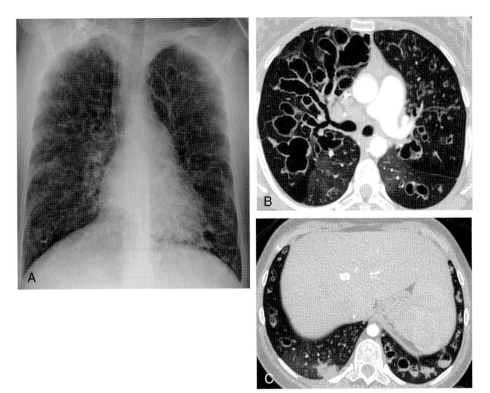

■ FIGURE 3-37 **Cystic fibrosis. A,** Radiograph shows areas of extensive bronchiectasis, most prominent in the upper lobes. Axial high-resolution **(B, C)** CT images show diffuse bronchiectasis and bronchial wall thickening, more pronounced within the right upper lobe. There are also multiple tree-in-bud opacities in the peripheral portions of the left lower lobe, which were not present on a prior study (not shown) and suggest superimposed infection. Notice air trapping throughout both lungs, although more pronounced in the right upper lobe.

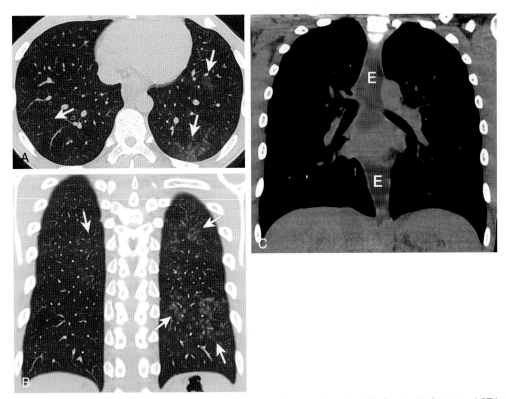

■ FIGURE 3-38 **Aspiration secondary to achalasia in a 14-year-old boy. A,** Axial and **B,** Coronal reformatted CT images show multiple ground-glass and tree-in-bud opacities in dependent portions of the lungs, left greater than right (*arrows*). **C,** Coronal reformatted CT image in soft tissue window shows significant fluid distention of the esophagus (*E*) in this patient with subsequently proven achalasia on upper GI study. Aspirative cellular bronchiolitis is a common complication of achalasia.

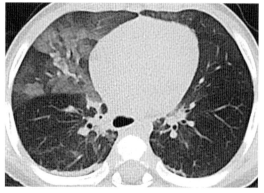

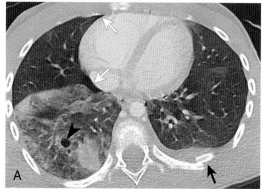

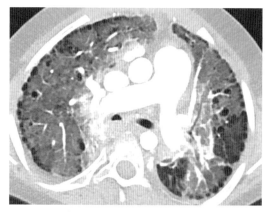

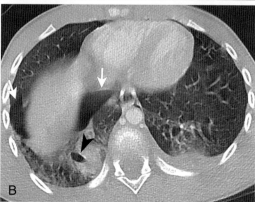

■ FIGURE 3-39 **Neuroendocrine cell hyperplasia of infancy in a 10-month-old**. HRCT images shows central predominant ground-glass opacities in the right middle lobe and to a lesser extent in the lingula, with air trapping in the lower lobes.

■ FIGURE 3-40 **Lung growth disorder in a 7-year-old with Trisomy 21**. Axial CT image shows innumerable, tiny, characteristic, peripheral subpleural cysts with mild pleural thickening on the right.

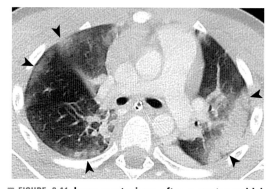

■ FIGURE 3-41 **Lung contusions after a motor vehicle accident in a 5-year-old**. CT shows characteristic findings of contusion on the left, including posterior location, crescent shape, nonsegmental distribution, and subpleural sparing (*arrowheads*). Milder contusions are seen anteriorly on the periphery of the right hemithorax.

■ FIGURE 3-42 **Lung contusions and lacerations with traumatic pneumatocele formation and pneumothorax in a 10-year-old following motor vehicle accident. A, B,** Axial CT images show a patchy area of opacity in the periphery of the right lung base with subpleural sparing consistent with lung contusion. No rib fractures present on the right. Notice a displaced left rib fracture (*black arrow*) with associated pleural effusion on the left. There are several air-filled cavities (*arrowheads*) consistent with lung laceration, and there is a small associated right pneumothorax (*white arrows*).

HYDROCARBON INGESTION

The aspiration of the hydrocarbons in gasoline, furniture polish, kerosene, or lighter fluid when young children get into and drink such liquids can cause a combination of chemical pneumonitis and atelectasis secondary to surfactant destruction. Radiographic findings may not manifest for up to 12 h after ingestion. However, a normal radiograph at 24 h after suspected ingestion excludes significant aspiration. The lung opacities tend to be in the lung bases (Fig. 3-45) and may persist for weeks after clinical improvement. Pneumatoceles are not uncommon sequelae.

■ MEDIASTINAL MASSES

The mediastinum is the most common location of primary thoracic masses in children. In

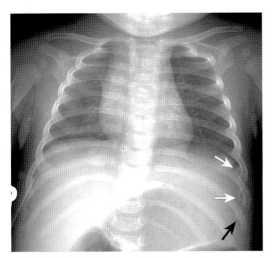

■ FIGURE 3-43 **Child abuse.** Radiograph shows healing rib fractures of the left seventh, eighth (*white arrows*), and ninth ribs. The fractures occurred at apparent different times. The ninth rib fracture appears more acute (*black arrow*). There is also callus formation involving the posteromedial right seventh and ninth ribs.

addition, the majority of mediastinal masses occur in children rather than in adults. As in adults, characterizing the location of the mass as anterior, middle, or posterior mediastinal can focus the differential diagnosis of mediastinal masses (Table 3-4).

Anterior Mediastinum

By far, the most commonly encountered issues in the anterior mediastinum are the normal thymus (when mistaken as a mass) and lymphoma. There are a large number of other potential but much less common causes of anterior mediastinal masses in children. They include teratoma (and other germ cell tumors), thymoma, multilocular thymic cysts seen in association with AIDS, and thymus enlargement and heterogeneity (often with calcifications or cysts) in Langerhans cell histiocytosis (Fig. 3-46).

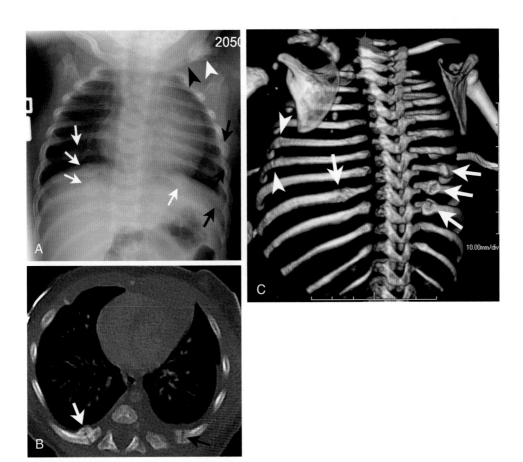

■ FIGURE 3-44 **Child abuse. A,** Radiograph shows multiple fractures that occurred at different times. There are multiple subacute healing rib fractures (*white arrows*) with callus formation and multiple more acute left-sided rib fractures (*black arrows*) without callus formation. The left clavicle shows an acute fracture involving the mid diaphyseal portion (*white arrowhead*) and a subacute, healing fracture (*black arrowhead*) more distally. **B,** Axial CT image shows callus around a healing right posterior rib fracture (*white arrow*). A characteristic acute fracture of the posterior rib (*black arrow*) is seen on the left. **C,** Coronal 3D volume-rendered CT image shows to better advantage left acute (*arrowheads*) and right subacute (*white arrows*), healing rib fractures.

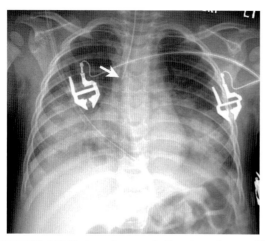

■ **FIGURE 3-45 Hydrocarbon aspiration in a 2-year-old boy who accidentally drank gasoline from an orange juice container.** Chest radiograph shows bibasilar lung consolidation. Note tip of the endotracheal tube in right mainstem bronchus (*arrow*).

✴ **TABLE 3-4** Common Mediastinal Masses by Location		
Anterior	**Middle**	**Posterior**
Normal thymus	Lymphadenopathy	Neuroblastoma
Lymphoma	Duplication cyst	
Teratoma (germ cell tumor)	Bronchogenic cyst	

NORMAL THYMUS

One of the most common areas of confusion in the imaging of children is related to differentiating the normal thymus from pathologic processes. This confusion led to thymic radiation therapy in the first half of the 20th century, when children with a normal, prominent thymus on chest radiography were radiated because of the erroneous belief that a big thymus compressed the airway and predisposed to death. Interestingly, it was the fallout around the unnecessary irradiation of thousands of children related to the misinterpretation of the large thymic shadow on chest radiographs that led to the recognition that children were not just "small adults" and gave rise to the first radiology subspecialty training fellowships—which were in pediatric radiology.

Distinguishing the normal thymus from disease continues to cause diagnostic problems today, particularly for those who do not often image children. In children, the thymus has a variable appearance in both size and shape. In children less than 5 years of age, and particularly in infants, the thymus can appear to be very large (Fig. 3-47). Large thymuses are said to be more common in boys but can also be seen in girls. The thymus also has variable configurations. A number of names have become associated with normal variations in the thymus, such as the sail sign (Fig. 3-48), which refers to a triangular extension of the thymus, most commonly to the right, on frontal chest radiography. It resembles a sail. This should not be confused with the spinnaker sail sign (Fig. 3-49), which is an indication of pneumomediastinum, in which the abnormally located air lifts the thymus up so it looks like the sail on the front of a racing boat. Typically, it is the left lobe that is lifted by the pneumomediastinum. If both lobes are lifted, the appearance is called angel's wing sign (Fig. 3-49).

Between 5 and 10 years of age, the thymus becomes less prominent radiographically because of the disproportionately decreased growth of the thymus in relationship to the growth of the rest of the body. During a child's second decade, the thymus should not be visualized as a discrete anterior mediastinal mass on chest radiography.

Abnormality of the thymus (or anterior mediastinum) is suspected when the thymic silhouette has an abnormal shape or an abnormal size in relationship to the patient's age. Displacement or compression of the airway or other structures is suspicious for abnormality. CT, US, MRI, and fluoroscopy can be used to help to differentiate the normal thymus from an abnormal mass, but CT is probably used most commonly. When CT is performed to evaluate suspicious cases, the normal thymus should appear homogeneous in attenuation, typically is quadrilateral in shape in young children (Fig. 3-50) and triangular in teenagers (Fig. 3-50), and may have slightly convex margins. US may be also used to evaluate the thymus. The normal infantile thymus has a characteristic sonographic appearance; it is relatively hypoechoic to the adjacent musculature and shows thin, echogenic strands and punctate bright foci. These findings allow for a confident diagnosis of normal thymus, when an abnormality is questioned on chest radiographs (Fig. 3-50).

Heterogeneity, calcification, and displacement or compression of the airway or vascular structures indicate an abnormality (Fig. 3-51; and see Fig. 3-46). True pathologic masses of the thymus are actually quite rare in children.

Thymic rebound is another source of confusion concerning normal thymic tissue. After a

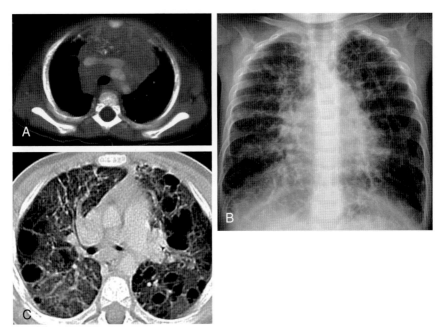

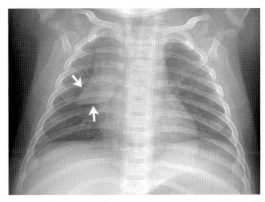

■ FIGURE 3-46 **Langerhans cell histiocytosis. A,** Thymus is enlarged and shows several punctate calcifications. Notice bilateral axillary lymphadenopathy. Chest radiograph (**B**) and Axial high-resolution CT image (**C**) Of pulmonary Langerhans cell histiocytosis in another child show numerous cysts and coarsening of the pulmonary interstitium throughout both lungs.

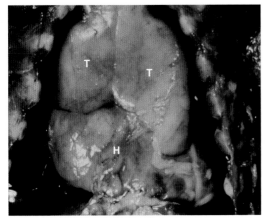

■ FIGURE 3-47 **Normal, prominent size of the thymus.** Photograph from autopsy of an infant who died of sudden infant death syndrome shows frontal view of thymus (*T*) after thoracotomy. Note the prominent size of the thymus in relation to the heart (*H*). The thymus is bilobed. In this patient, the left lobe is larger than the right. *Image courtesy Janet L. Strife, MD, Cincinnati, OH.*

■ FIGURE 3-48 **Normal, prominent thymus with "sail" sign.** Radiograph shows prominent but normal thymus with rightward triangular extension (*arrows*). This appearance should not be confused with right upper lobe pneumonia.

patient has ceased receiving chemotherapy for a malignancy, it is normal for the thymus to grow back, as seen in serial CT examinations. Thymic volume has been shown to vary cyclically by as much as 40% during rounds of chemotherapy. Thymic rebound may also occur in children recovering from a recent stress event such as pneumonia, treatment with steroids, surgery, or burns (Fig. 3.52). This intervallic increase in soft tissue attenuation in the anterior mediastinum should not be considered abnormal when encountered on conventional radiography or cross-sectional imaging.

LYMPHOMA

Lymphoma is the third most common tumor in children, exceeded only by leukemia and brain tumors. It is by far the most common abnormal anterior mediastinal mass in children,

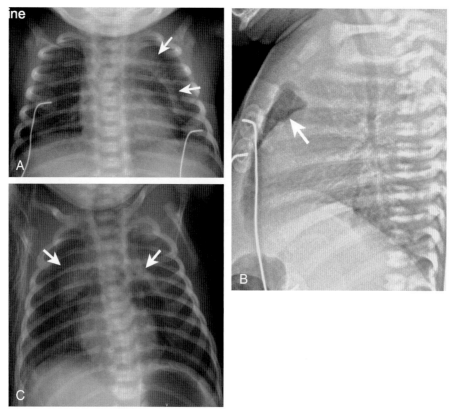

■ **FIGURE 3-49 Pneumomediastinum. A,** Frontal chest radiograph of a young infant shows thymus (*arrows*) lifted off of mediastinum by air in mediastinum—the "spinnaker sail sign." **B,** Notice the pneumomediastinum in retrosternal projection (*arrow*). **C,** Pneumomediastinum in a 36-week gestational age newborn with mild respiratory distress. Air is lifting both lobes of the thymus (*arrows*) resulting in an "angel's wing" pattern.

particularly in older children and teenagers. Therefore, lymphoma is the working diagnosis for newly diagnosed anterior mediastinal masses in children. Age is helpful in differentiating a normal thymus from lymphoma because a normal thymus is most common in small children and lymphoma is most common in teenagers. The most problematic case is the slightly prominent anterior mediastinum in an approximately 10-year-old child. One helpful clinical clue in identifying lymphoma is that mediastinal lymphoma is commonly associated with cervical lymphadenopathy.

The most common types of lymphoma that involve the mediastinum include Hodgkin lymphoma and the lymphoblastic type of non-Hodgkin lymphoma. Both lesions can appear as discrete lymph nodes or as a conglomerate mass of lymph nodes, most commonly within the anterior mediastinum (Fig. 3-51). Lung involvement, when present, is usually contiguous with mediastinal and hilar disease. Calcifications are rare in untreated lymphoma and when present should raise the possibility of other diagnoses,

such as teratoma (Fig. 3-53), a form of germ cell tumor.

Most mediastinal masses are initially identified on chest radiography and then further evaluated by CT, which confirms the presence of an anterior mediastinal mass, evaluates the extent of disease, and evaluates for potential complications. The potential complications related to mediastinal lymphoma include airway compression, compressive obstruction of venous structures (superior vena cava, pulmonary veins) (Fig. 3.51), and pericardial effusion (Fig. 3-54). Airway compression is especially important because it may influence decisions concerning surgical biopsy with general anesthesia versus US-guided percutaneous biopsy with local anesthesia. If a patient cannot lie recumbent for CT imaging because of airway compression, the images can usually be obtained with the patient positioned prone because the anterior mediastinal mass falls away from the airway. Compression of the airway by more than 50% from the expected round shape has been shown to be associated with a high risk for complications related to anesthesia.

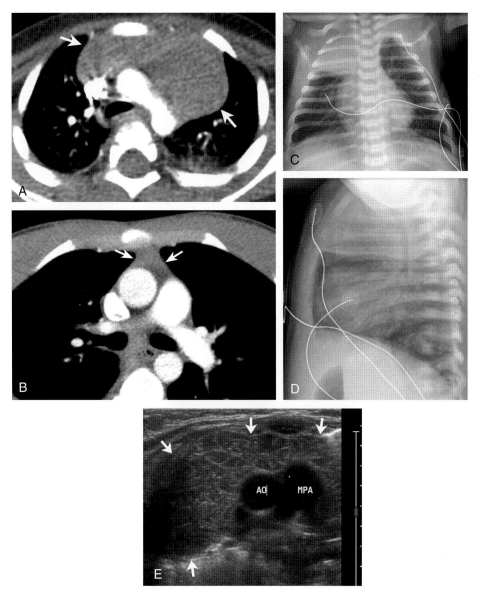

■ FIGURE 3-50 **Normal thymus on cross-sectional imaging. A,** CT in a young child shows thymus (*arrows*) to be quadrilateral in shape, have convex margins, and be of homogeneous attenuation. There is no compression of the trachea or superior vena cava. **B,** CT in a 17-year-old, note the typical triangular shape of the thymus. **C,** Frontal and **D,** Lateral chest radiographs obtained in a young infant at an outside institution raised concern for a mediastinal mass. On further review, it was suspected to be normal thymus. **E,** Transverse US scan through the mid right upper chest performed in same child as in (**C**) and (**D**) reveals normal thymic parenchyma with a relatively prominent right lobe of the thymus (*arrows*) and no abnormal mass. US in this case obviated the need of CT. *AO,* aorta; *MPA,* main pulmonary artery.

Middle Mediastinal Masses

Middle mediastinal masses are less common than anterior or posterior mediastinal masses and are usually related to lymphadenopathy or foregut duplication cysts. Lymphadenopathy can be inflammatory, most often secondary to granulomatous disease, such as tuberculosis or fungal infection, or to neoplastic growth secondary to metastatic disease or lymphoma. Foregut duplication cysts can be bronchogenic, enteric, or neurenteric. Foregut duplication cysts are well-defined masses that appear cystic on cross-sectional imaging. Neurenteric cysts, by definition, have associated vertebral anomalies. Pathologic processes related to the esophagus can also cause middle mediastinal abnormalities. Chronic foreign bodies can erode through the esophagus and cause a middle mediastinal mass, typically in the cervical esophagus at the level of

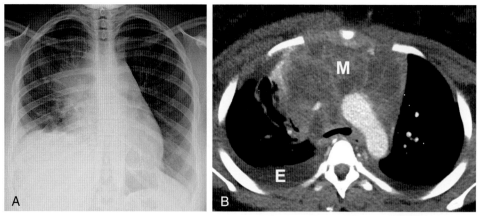

■ **FIGURE 3-51 Lymphoma. A,** Frontal radiograph shows enlargement of the superior mediastinum and associated large, right pleural, subpulmonic effusion, evidenced by elevation of the right hemidiaphragm. Axial (**B**) CT image shows a large, heterogeneous anterior mediastinal mass (*M*) with compression of the trachea at the level of the carina and superior vena cava, which is markedly narrowed. Notice the right pleural effusion (*E*).

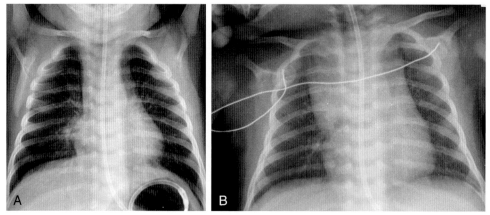

■ **FIGURE 3-52 Thymic rebound in a young infant poststress. A,** Frontal radiograph taken during a viral illness shows little thymic tissue. **B,** Radiograph taken several weeks later shows regrowth of the thymus. This should not be mistaken for a mediastinal mass.

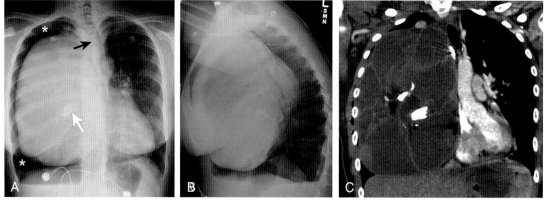

■ **FIGURE 3-53 Teratoma in a 15-year-old with dyspnea and chest pain. A,** Frontal and **B,** Lateral chest radiographs show a moderate right pneumothorax (*) and a large space occupying lesion resulting in tracheal displacement (*black arrow*) and mediastinal shift to the left. Notice a cluster of amorphous calcific densities (*white arrow*). **C,** Coronal CT shows a very large anterior mediastinal mass with fatty, cystic, and calcific components resulting in mediastinal shift.

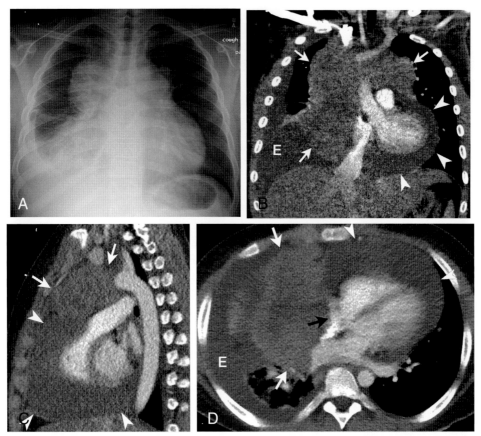

■ **FIGURE 3-54** **Lymphoma with pericardial effusion in a 14-year-old. A,** Chest radiograph shows a markedly enlarged superior mediastinum and associated right pleural effusion. **B,** Coronal and **C,** Sagittal reformatted CT images show a large anterior mediastinal mass (*white arrows*) resulting in mediastinal shift to the left on **B.** Note adjacent, massive pericardial effusion (*arrowheads*) encircling the heart. There is also a small-to-moderate pleural effusion (*E*). **D,** Axial CT image shows significant right atrial compression (*black arrow*).

the thoracic inlet (Fig. 3-55). A dilated esophagus resulting from achalasia or a hiatal hernia may also appear as a middle mediastinal mass on chest radiography.

Posterior Mediastinal Masses

There are a number of causes of posterior mediastinal masses in children. They include neural crest tumors, neurofibromas, lateral meningoceles, diskitis, hematoma, and extramedullary hematopoiesis. However, just as anterior mediastinal masses in older children are considered to be lymphoma, the working diagnosis for posterior mediastinal masses in young children is neuroblastoma until proven otherwise.

NEUROBLASTOMA

Neurogenic tumors (neuroblastoma, ganglioneuroblastoma, ganglioneuroma) are the most common posterior mediastinal masses in childhood. Neuroblastoma is discussed in detail in the genitourinary section. Approximately 15% of neuroblastomas occur in the posterior mediastinum, most occurring before a child is 2 years of age.

Most neuroblastomas are visible on frontal radiographs of the chest as a posterior opacity (Fig. 3-56). The soft tissue mass is often surprisingly poorly visualized on the lateral view. There is frequently erosion, destruction, or splaying of the adjacent posterior ribs. These findings may be subtle; so whenever a posterior chest opacity is identified, an effort should be made to look for rib erosion. The neuroforamina may appear enlarged on the lateral view, secondary to intraspinal extension of the tumor. Calcifications are reported to be visible on chest radiography in as many as 25% of cases, although in the author's experience it is less than that. Cross-sectional imaging with CT or MRI confirms the presence of the tumor and evaluates

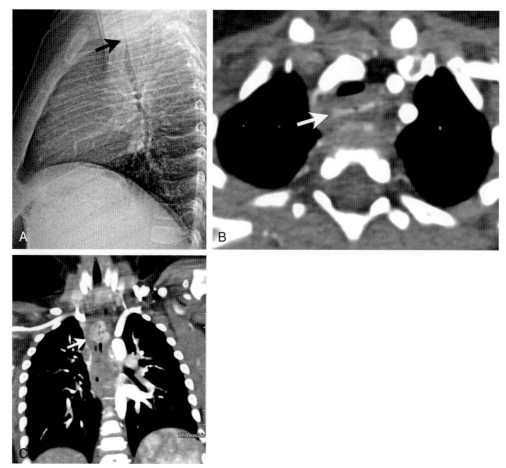

■ **FIGURE 3-55 Chronic esophageal foreign body presenting as stridor and worsening respiratory symptoms in a young child. A,** Lateral view of the chest shows focal airway, smooth narrowing at the thoracic inlet (*black arrow*). **B,** Axial CT image shows a distended upper esophagus with an internal radiodensity (*white arrow*) suspicious for a chronic foreign body within the upper esophagus with adjacent inflammatory changes. **C,** Coronal oblique reformatted CT image shows a heart-shaped foreign body (*arrow*) lodged in the upper esophagus.

extent of disease, particularly whether there is intraspinal extension. Thoracic neuroblastomas have better prognosis than abdominal neuroblastomas.

■ PEDIATRIC CHEST WALL MASSES

A number of primary malignant processes can arise in the chest walls of children. They include Ewing sarcoma, peripheral primitive neuroectodermal tumor of the chest wall (Askin tumor) (Fig. 3-57), and other sarcomas. Most of these lesions present with painful enlargement of the chest wall. Metastatic involvement by neuroblastoma, lymphoma, or leukemia is actually more common than are primary tumors. On imaging, all of these malignancies typically appear as nonspecific aggressive lesions with poorly defined margins that include or not bony destruction and pleural involvement. However, one must consider that as much as one third of children have variations in the configuration of the anterior chest wall, including asymmetric findings, such as tilted sternum, prominent convexity of anterior rib or costal cartilage (Fig. 3-58), prominent asymmetric costal cartilage, parachondral nodules, or mild degrees of pectus excavatum or carinatum. It is common for these asymmetric variants to be palpated by the pediatrician, parent, or patient, and because of the fear of malignancy, cross-sectional imaging is requested. In a previous study that reviewed cross-sectional examinations performed to evaluate children with suspected chest wall masses, all of the palpable lesions that were

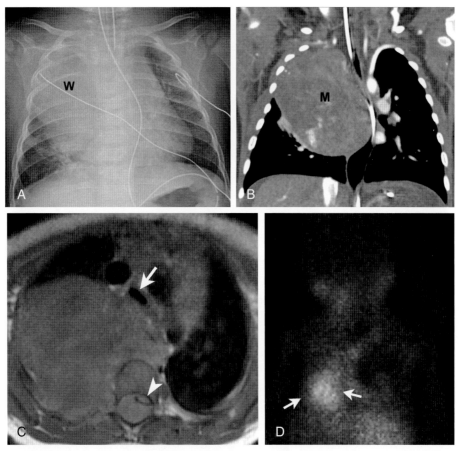

■ **FIGURE 3-56 Neuroblastoma in a 10-month-old girl. A,** Frontal chest radiograph shows a large mass in the right upper hemithorax. There is widening (*W*) between the fourth and fifth ribs and erosion of these ribs. **B,** CT shows a large posterior mediastinal mass (*M*) with speckled calcifications resulting in airway displacement and compression. **C,** Axial T1-weighted MR image shows extension into the spinal canal. The cord is displaced and compressed (*arrowhead*). Notice tracheal compression (*arrow*) **D,** Metaiodobenzylguanidine (MIBG) scan shows avid uptake of radiotracer within the mass (*arrows*), consistent with a neural crest tumor.

asymptomatic were related to normal anatomic variations. Knowledge that such variations are common should be communicated to referring physicians and parents when imaging is being contemplated in a child with an asymptomatic chest wall "lump." US is the initial imaging test of choice to demonstrate these anterior chest wall variations (Fig. 3.58) and exclude more concerning masses.

One of the most common abnormalities in chest wall configuration is pectus excavatum. Although the majority of associated problems due to this deformity are cosmetic, pectus deformities can cause chest pain, fatigue, dyspnea on exertion, palpitations, and restrictive lung disease. When the deformities are severe,

surgical repair can be performed. Pectus excavatum is commonly treated by the minimally invasive Nuss procedure. Before performing a Nuss procedure, surgeons commonly request CT or MR examination to document the Haller index, which quantifies the severity of the pectus deformity (Fig. 3-59). To calculate the Haller index, cross-sectional images are obtained through the level of the greatest degree of pectus deformity. The Haller index is equal to the transverse left-to-right diameter of the chest divided by the anterior-to-posterior diameter. The greater the Haller index, the more severe the pectus. A patient with a Haller index greater than 3.25 is considered a surgical candidate.

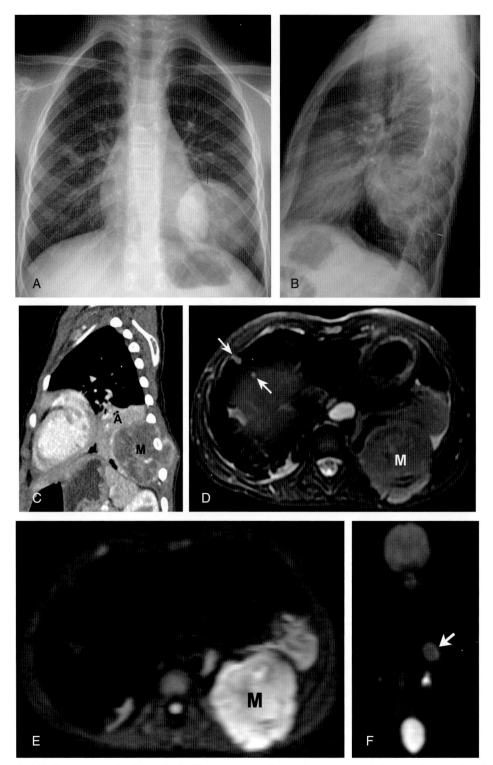

■ FIGURE 3-57 **Ewing sarcoma/peripheral primitive neuroectodermal tumor of the left posterior chest wall in a 5-year-old girl. A,** Frontal and **B,** Lateral chest radiographs show a large mass in the left hemithorax. **C,** Sagittal-enhanced CT image shows a heterogeneously enhancing large mass (*M*) involving the posterolateral left chest wall. Note adjacent atelectasis of the left lung (*A*). No rib abnormalities could be appreciated on bone windows (not shown). **D,** On axial T2-weighted MR image, the mass (*M*) shows intermediate signal. Notice two lung nodules in the contralateral lung (*arrows*); these were consistent with metastasis on CT. **E,** On axial diffusion–weighted MR image, the mass (*M*) shows restricted diffusion consistent with hypercellularity. **F,** The lesion (*arrow*) shows heterogeneous FDG activity (SUV 4.3) on F-18 FDG PET scan.

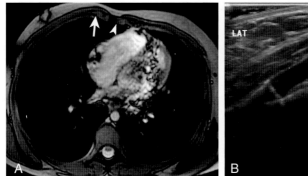 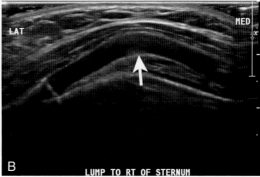

■ FIGURE 3-58 **Tilted sternum with prominent costal cartilage presenting as a palpable mass on physical exam. A,** Axial T2-weighted MR image shows the sternum (*arrowhead*) to be tilted with respect to the horizontal right-to-left axis of the body. The right margin of the sternum is more anterior than the right. The associated anterior position of the right costal cartilage (*white arrow*), a normal variant, caused the palpable finding on physical exam. **B,** Transverse US image over the palpable abnormality shows an exaggerated convexity (*arrow*) of the cartilaginous portion of one of the right lower ribs. *LAT*, lateral; *MED*, medial.

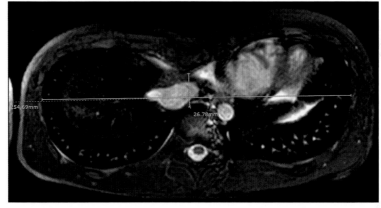

■ FIGURE 3-59 **Pectus excavatum.** Axial MR image shows severe pectus deformity of the anterior chest wall. Measurement lines are the anterior-to-posterior and left-to-right diameters of the chest. These are measured to calculate the Haller index, a quantitative measure of pectus severity. The Haller index in this patient was 9.5. Corrective surgery is considered for a Haller index of $\geq$3.25. Note the degree of cardiac displacement and compression.

SUGGESTED READING

Agrons GA, Courtney SE, Stocker JT, Markowitz RI: From the archives of the AFIP: lung disease in premature neonates: radiologic-pathologic correlation, *Radiographics* 25(4):1047–1073, 2005.

Bramson RT, Griscom NT, Cleveland RH: Interpretation of chest radiographs in infants with cough and fever, *Radiology* 236(1):22–29, 2005.

Cox M, Soudack M, Podberesky DJ, Epelman M: Pediatric chest ultrasound: a practical approach, *Pediatr Radiol* 47(9):1058–1068, August, 2017.

Donnelly LF: Maximizing the usefulness of imaging in children with community-acquired pneumonia, *AJR* 172:505–512, 1999.

Donnelly LF: Imaging issues in CT of blunt trauma to the chest and abdomen, *Pediatr Radiol* 39(Suppl 3):406–413, 2009.

Donnelly LF, Frush DP: Abnormalities of the chest wall in pediatric patients, *AJR* 173:1595–1601, 1999a.

Donnelly LF, Frush DP: Localized lucent chest lesions in neonates: causes and differentiation, *AJR* 172:1651–1658, 1999b.

Epelman M, Kreiger PA, Servaes S, et al.: Current imaging of prenatally diagnosed congenital lung lesions, *Semin Ultrasound CT MR* 31(2):141–157, 2010.

Erasmus JJ, McAdams HP, Donnelly LF, Spritzer CE: MR imaging of mediastinal masses, *Magn Reson Imag Clin N Am* 8(1):59–89, 2000.

Eslamy HK, Newman B: Pneumonia in normal and immunocompromised children: an overview and update, *Radiol Clin North Am* 49(5):895–920, 2011.

Griscom NT: Respiratory problems of early life now allowing survival into adulthood: concepts for radiologists, *AJR* 158:1–8, 1992.

Griscom NT, Wohl MB, Kirkpatrick JA: Lower respiratory infections: how infants differ from adults, *Radiol Clin North Am* 16:367–387, 1978.

Liang T, Vargas SO, Lee EY: Childhood interstitial (diffuse) lung disease: pattern recognition approach to diagnosis in infants, *AJR Am J Roentgenol*, March 5, 2019:1−10, March 5, 2019.

Liszewski MC, Stanescu AL, Phillips GS, Lee EY: Respiratory distress in neonates: underlying causes and current imaging assessment, *Radiol Clin North Am* 55(4):629−644, July, 2017.

Marcovici PA, LoSasso BE, Kruk P, Dwek JR: MRI for the evaluation of pectus excavatum, *Pediatr Radiol* 41(6):757−758, 2011.

Ranganath SH, Lee EY, Restrepo R, Eisenberg RL: Mediastinal masses in children, *AJR* 198(3):W197−W216, 2012.

Swischuk KE, John SD: Immature lung problems: can our nomenclature be more specific? *AJR* 166:917−918, 1996.

Thacker PG, Mahani MG, Heider A, Lee EY: Imaging evaluation of mediastinal masses in children and adults: practical diagnostic approach based on a new classification system, *J Thorac Imag* 30(4):247−267, 2015.

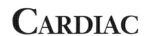

CHAPTER 4

CARDIAC

Evan J. Zucker

■ IMAGING MODALITIES IN CONGENITAL HEART DISEASE

Multiple imaging modalities are used to define the morphology, vascular connections, and function of the heart in children with congenital heart disease (CHD). Such modalities include radiography, echocardiography, nuclear scintigraphy, computed tomography (CT), magnetic resonance imaging (MRI), and catheter angiography.

Multiple insults can occur in utero that can lead to CHD. In many cases, a specific insult results in a single type of anatomic lesion, such as ventricular septal defect (VSD) or coarctation of the aorta. However, insults can result in a variety of anatomic abnormalities or "complex" CHD. Historically, chest radiography and clinical symptoms played a larger role in narrowing the differential diagnosis of the types of CHD that may be present in a particular patient. With technologic advances and increased use of other imaging modalities, the dependency on chest radiography findings to diagnose the specific type of CHD has decreased, although it remains important in the identification of the possible presence of CHD.

Diagnosing a specific type of CHD by radiography is difficult. The role of radiography in making the diagnosis of CHD has probably been overemphasized in education. This is particularly true nowadays because most of the classically described radiographic findings of specific CHD do not manifest until after the neonatal period, and most patients in developed nations are diagnosed with CHD and are treated surgically during the neonatal period (and often prenatally identified). However, in some cases, the radiologist may be the first person to recognize that the radiographic findings in a newborn suggest that CHD rather than a pulmonary disorder is the cause of respiratory distress. Therefore, it is important to get some understanding of the radiographic findings and role of radiography in relation to the other imaging modalities in the management of CHD.

Echocardiography

Echocardiography is the mainstay of CHD identification and diagnosis. This is particularly true during the fetal and neonatal periods. Most of the highly detailed anatomic and functional information needed for the medical and surgical management of patients with CHD can be obtained by ultrasound. Color Doppler can be used to identify areas of stenosis or regurgitation. However, there are populations of patients in whom echocardiography is less easily obtained and more prone to inaccuracy. These populations include older children, adults, and postsurgical patients. In these patients, the acoustic window is decreased and echocardiography is more difficult. It is in these circumstances that echocardiography may not provide the necessary information needed for care, so CT and MRI play a role. It is important to keep in perspective the current relatively small (albeit growing) role of CT and MRI in cardiac imaging as compared with that of ultrasound.

Computed Tomography

The role of CT, with angiographic technique, in the evaluation of CHD has rapidly increased as a result of the advent of multidetector CT technology, improved temporal resolution, and decreased ionizing radiation doses. The rapid speed of acquisition, ability to acquire volumetric data that may even be used to create three-dimensional (3D) printed models, and ability to obtain thin collimation have made CT very useful in patients with CHD. CT is beneficial in depicting those anatomic structures that are not easily seen on echocardiography, such as the pulmonary arteries, aorta, pulmonary veins, right-sided chambers, and vascular conduits. CT also enables a more global assessment of the airway and pulmonary parenchyma, which may also be abnormal in patients with CHD. CT is often used to depict complex CHD preoperatively and to evaluate the postoperative patient (Fig. 4-1) for potential complications, such as stenoses, occlusions, and pseudoaneurysms. It is

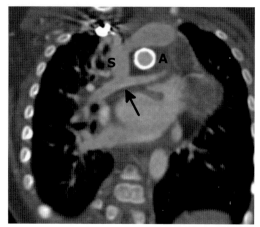

■ FIGURE 4-1 Oblique coronal reformatted image from a CT angiogram performed to evaluate patency of a Glenn shunt. The image shows a widely patent Glenn shunt (direct connection between the superior vena cava (*S*) and the pulmonary arteries [*arrow*]). An aortic stent (*A*) is also present.

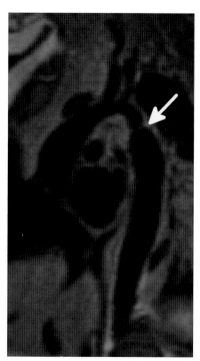

■ FIGURE 4-2 Double inversion recovery, T1-weighted, black-blood, oblique sagittal ("candy cane") image shows a focal narrowing of the aortic isthmus (*arrow*) consistent with coarctation.

useful in evaluating the pulmonary veins, such as in suspected anomalous pulmonary venous return. CT is also useful in patients in whom pacemakers may preclude the use of MRI, including functional assessment. Evaluation of metal stents is often less hampered by artifact in CT than in MRI, especially with new metal reduction algorithms and dual-energy/spectral techniques available on modern CT scanners. Although ionizing radiation exposure remains of paramount concern in medical imaging of children, the advent of newer technologies, such as iterative reconstruction, volume acquisition, and high-pitch capable dual-source scanners, has resulted in dramatic decreases in radiation exposure, improvement in temporal resolution associated with cardiac CT, and a resultant renewal of interest in CT's role in CHD evaluation.

Magnetic Resonance Imaging

MRI has become a mainstay in the evaluation of certain types of CHD. MRI studies offer both anatomic and functional information. Cardiac-gated spin echo imaging and double inversion recovery imaging, also known as "black-blood" imaging (Fig. 4-2), have traditionally been used to demonstrate anatomic detail and spatial relationships between adjacent structures. These sequences allow for precise measurement of anatomic structures.

Cardiac-gated cine MRI, or "bright-blood" imaging, can be obtained with a number of sequences. Predominantly, a balanced steady-state free precession sequence is used (e.g., FIESTA,

TRUFISP, bFFE; Fig. 4-3), but a T2* GRE sequence (e.g., FLASH, SPGR) can also be used for "bright-blood" imaging. Data from these sequences can be processed to provide functional

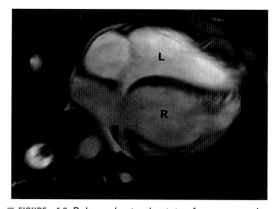

■ FIGURE 4-3 Balanced steady-state free precession (bSSFP) bright-blood four-chamber image in a child with congenitally corrected (L-) transposition of the great arteries (L-TGA) shows the morphologic left ventricle (*L*) anterior and to the right of the morphologic right ventricle (*R*). Such images through the heart can be obtained in cine mode and are used to evaluate cardiac motion and functional parameters, such as ventricular ejection fraction.

information, such as ventricular ejection fractions, and can also be used to demonstrate dynamic findings, such as turbulent blood flow related to stenosis or regurgitation. Phase-contrast imaging can be used to evaluate flow dynamics within vasculature structures. Magnetic resonance (MR) angiography using gadolinium or ferumoxytol as an off-label blood agent and maximum intensity projection or shaded surface 3D reconstructions is also useful in demonstrating complex anatomic relationships. While long, technically challenging exams with extensive breath-holding requirements historically prohibited the greater use of cardiac MRI; newer acquisition methods such as 3D time-resolved phase contrast or four-dimensional (4D) flow, combined with novel acceleration techniques (e.g., compressed sensing, deep learning) now permit complete evaluation of anatomy, function, and flow on the order of minutes in a single volumetric acquisition. Moreover, promising techniques such as ultrashort echo time imaging may facilitate simultaneous assessment of lungs and airways on par with CT.

Computed Tomography Versus Magnetic Resonance Imaging

With both CT and MRI becoming increasingly useful in the evaluation of patients with CHD, there is frequent debate regarding which examination is better for specific clinical indications. Although there are no clear-cut answers, there are advantages and disadvantages of both examinations. The benefits of CT include rapid acquisition time, avoiding the need for sedation in many cases, greater access for critically ill infants, less artifact resulting from metal stents and other structures, lack of pacemaker safety issues, and visualizing the airway and lungs. The major disadvantage of CT is radiation exposure. Techniques used in adults, including cardiac gating, overlapping imaging acquisition, and acquiring multiple sets of images, result in very high radiation doses relative to other CT examinations. Because of the radiosensitivity of children, many of these techniques may not be appropriate when imaging children. Other disadvantages of CT include dependence on intravenous contrast bolus and relative lack of functional information compared to MRI. The primary advantages of MRI include lack of ionizing radiation, ability to show more detailed anatomy in some circumstances, and greater depiction of functional and flow information. A disadvantage of MRI is the usually greater requirement for sedation or anesthesia in younger children who may otherwise be able to undergo a CT without the need for sedation or anesthesia. However, with increasingly faster MR techniques, requirements for sedation and particularly deep anesthesia continue to decrease.

Catheter Angiography

The use of diagnostic angiography in cases in which percutaneous intervention is not performed is dramatically decreasing because of improvements in noninvasive imaging tools, such as echocardiography, MRI, and CT. At the same time, that the role of diagnostic angiography in the evaluation of CHD is decreasing, percutaneous interventional procedures, such as ductus arteriosus, atrial septal defect (ASD), and VSD closure device deployment, are increasing in number. Diagnostic angiography is commonly performed as part of these interventional procedures to define the anatomy of these abnormalities and provide procedure guidance, as well as physiologic data such as pressure measurements.

Approach to the Chest Radiograph in Congenital Heart Disease

It is important to have a basic understanding of the radiographic findings of CHD because the radiologist may be the first to recognize that respiratory symptoms are secondary to cardiac rather than respiratory disease. In addition, understanding the radiographic findings provides a framework for understanding the pathophysiology behind CHD. When evaluating a chest radiograph in a patient with potential CHD, it is important to evaluate pulmonary vascularity, cardiac size, situs, and the position of the aortic arch.

PULMONARY VASCULARITY

An important radiographic feature for determining the appropriate differential diagnosis in CHD is the pulmonary vascularity. Unfortunately, it is probably also the most difficult radiographic finding to evaluate and one that can be altered iatrogenically by the administration of fluids or diuretics to a patient. In addition, the appearance of pulmonary vascular prominence can be increased by low lung volumes and portable radiographic technique. The pulmonary vascularity can be normal or can reflect increased pulmonary arterial flow, increased pulmonary venous flow, or decreased pulmonary flow.

In cases of increased pulmonary arterial flow, the pulmonary arteries appear too prominent both in size and in the number of visualized

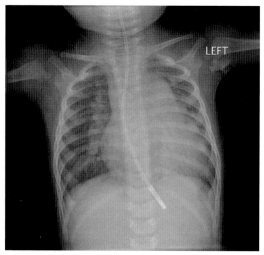

■ FIGURE 4-4 Frontal chest radiograph in a child with a perimembranous ventricular septal defect shows shunt vascularity with increased number and size of visible pulmonary arteries. Cardiomegaly is present as well.

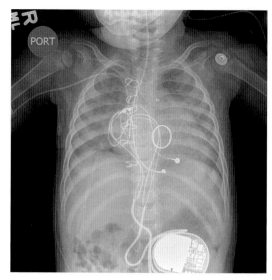

■ FIGURE 4-5 Increased pulmonary venous flow/pulmonary edema in a neonate posttricuspid valve repair and mitral valve replacement. Note the prominent but indistinct pulmonary vascularity.

pulmonary arterial structures (Fig. 4-4). A helpful rule is that if the right interlobar pulmonary artery is larger in diameter than the trachea, one should consider increased pulmonary arterial flow to be present. The prominent vascular structures seen in increased pulmonary arterial flow are very distinct and have well-defined borders. It can at times be difficult to differentiate increased pulmonary arterial flow from the increased peribronchial markings seen with reactive airway disease or viral pneumonia.

In cases with increased pulmonary venous flow, although the pulmonary vascular structures appear prominent in size and distribution, they are very indistinct and poorly defined (Fig. 4-5). Increased pulmonary venous flow is akin to pulmonary venous congestion or mild pulmonary edema. In many cases, such as in left-to-right shunts, there is both increased pulmonary arterial flow resulting from left-to-right shunting and increased pulmonary venous flow due to congestive heart failure. If any of the pulmonary arteries in a particular case appear very well defined, it is important to consider at least a component of increased pulmonary arterial flow to be present.

In decreased pulmonary arterial flow, there is a paucity of visualized arterial structures throughout the lung (Fig. 4-6).

CARDIAC SIZE

Cardiac size may be normal or enlarged. In older children and adults, there may be findings that suggest specific chamber enlargement. However,

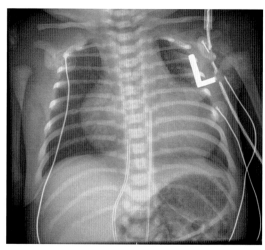

■ FIGURE 4-6 Critical pulmonic stenosis on frontal chest radiograph. Note the decrease in identifiable pulmonary markings consistent with decreased pulmonary flow. The heart is also enlarged.

specific chamber enlargement may be difficult to ascertain in infants because they usually undergo an anteroposterior radiographic technique and have large thymus glands. It is for this same reason that measuring the transverse diameter of the cardiac silhouette and comparing it with the transverse diameter of half the thoracic base may overestimate cardiac size. In these infants, the lateral view commonly offers greater insight into whether cardiomegaly is truly present than does the frontal view (Figs. 4-7A and B, and 4-8A and B). On the lateral view, if the posterior aspect of

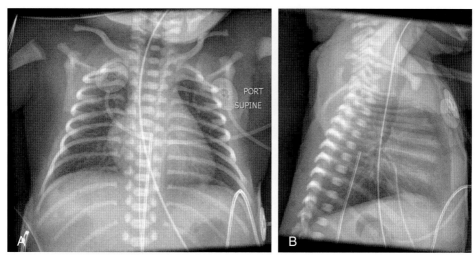

■ FIGURE 4-7 **Normal size heart on radiography. A,** Frontal chest radiograph shows that the transverse diameter of the cardiac silhouette is less than 50% of the diameter of the chest. **B,** Lateral radiograph demonstrates the posterior border of the heart to be normally positioned and not to extend posteriorly beyond the spine. No cardiomegaly is present.

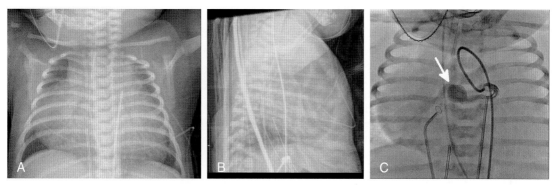

■ FIGURE 4-8 **Coronary-atrial fistula causing severe cardiomegaly. A,** Frontal chest radiograph demonstrates a markedly enlarged cardiac silhouette. **B,** Lateral radiograph confirms cardiomegaly. Note that the posterior aspect of the cardiac silhouette extends to the anterior border of the spine. **C,** Coronal projection of the chest during catheter angiography shows an abnormal fistulous communication between the left main coronary artery and atria with associated aneurysm (*aneurysm*), the underlying cause of cardiac dysfunction and resultant cardiomegaly.

the cardiac silhouette extends over the vertebral bodies, cardiomegaly should be considered present.

Cardiac axis is the term given to the configuration of the apex of the heart; it indicates whether the apex points superiorly or inferiorly. If the cardiac apex is oriented superiorly, right-sided cardiac enlargement is suggested, and if the cardiac axis or apex is oriented inferiorly, left-sided cardiac enlargement is suggested.

SITUS

Situs is defined as the relationship of asymmetric organs to the midline. Identifying disturbances in normal situs (the presence of heterotaxy syndromes) is important because they are associated with the presence of CHD. Situs should not be confused with the actual location of the heart within the thoracic cavity. Levoposition describes a heart mainly located in the left chest, whereas dextroposition describes a heart located primarily within the right chest. The term *mesoposition* is used to describe a heart located in the midline. The term *dextrocardia* strictly refers to a heart located in the right hemithorax with the base–apex relationship tilted rightward.

The important structures when evaluating situs on chest radiography are the cardiac apex, stomach bubble, and position of the liver. When

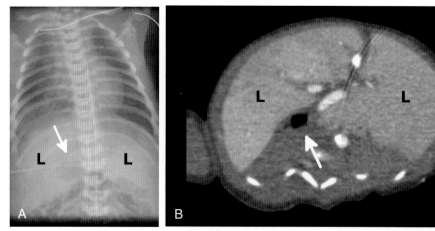

■ **FIGURE 4-9 Asplenia. A,** Frontal chest radiograph in child with complex congenital heart disease shows a normal left-sided cardiac apex left-sided aortic arch. The stomach (*arrow*) is on the right, and the liver shadow (*L*) extends across midline. No splenic shadow is seen. **B,** Axial contrast-enhanced CT image in the same patient shows a midline liver (*L*), a right-sided stomach (*arrow*), and absence of the spleen.

the cardiac apex and gastric bubble appear on the same side, left or right, there is a much lower incidence of CHD than in cases in which the cardiac apex is on the opposite side of gastric bubble. When there is discordance between the side of the cardiac apex and gastric bubble, there is a near 100% incidence of CHD. Situs solitus is the name given to the normal configuration; it is associated with a 0.6% incidence of CHD. Situs inversus is the mirror image of normal and is associated with a 3%−5% incidence of CHD. With situs ambiguous, there is no clear, straightforward left- or right-sidedness. The major types of situs ambiguous include asplenia (bilateral right-sidedness) and polysplenia (bilateral left-sidedness). Definitive determination of situs requires identifying the relationship between the atrial chambers and adjacent organs, which is not possible radiographically.

Asplenia (Fig. 4-9A and B) is associated with complex, cyanotic CHD. Patients are susceptible to infections by encapsulated bacteria because of the lack of a spleen. Other abnormalities that may be present include malrotation, microgastria, and midline gallbladder. Radiographic findings include a midline liver, bilateral right-sided appearing bronchi, decreased pulmonary arterial flow, azygous continuation of the inferior vena cava (IVC), and other findings reflecting the specific type of cyanotic heart disease.

Polysplenia (Fig. 4-10) is typically associated with less complex acyanotic heart disease, usually left-to-right shunts. Other associations include azygous continuation of the IVC, bilateral superior vena cava (SVC), malrotation, and absent

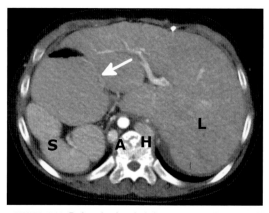

■ **FIGURE 4-10 Polysplenia.** Axial contrast-enhanced CT image shows multiple spleens (*S*) in the right upper quadrant, a predominantly left-sided liver (*L*), a right-sided stomach (*arrow*), and prominent azygous (*A*) and hemiazygous (*H*) veins.

gallbladder. Radiographic findings include absence of the IVC shadow, prominent azygous vein, midline liver, and increased pulmonary arterial flow.

POSITION OF AORTIC ARCH

The identification of a right-sided aortic arch should increase suspicion for the presence of CHD. The most common congenital heart lesions that have an associated right-sided aortic arch are tetralogy of Fallot, truncus arteriosus, tricuspid atresia, and transposition of the great arteries. When the aortic knob can be identified, as in most cases in adults and older children, it is obvious which side the aortic arch is on. However, in infants, the aortic knob is often not easily identified. In such cases, secondary findings for the presence of the aortic arch must be used. Such findings include the position of the descending aorta (though this does not universally correspond with the side of the arch), tracheal displacement, and tracheal indentation. In a normal left-sided aortic arch, the trachea is displaced slightly toward the right as it moves inferiorly. Also, in such cases, there is an indentation on the left aortic border of the trachea as visualized on the frontal view of the chest. If the trachea deviates slightly leftward as it moves inferiorly or if there is a soft tissue indentation on the right aortic border of the trachea, a right-sided aortic arch should be suspected. A double aortic arch may manifest on a chest radiograph simply as a midline trachea with no indentation.

■ CATEGORIZATION OF CONGENITAL HEART DISEASE

In the traditional classification of CHD, two of the major features that place the disease into a particular diagnostic category include (1) whether or not the patient is cyanotic (blue) and (2) whether the pulmonary arterial flow is decreased, normal, or increased (Table 4-1). Once these two major features have been identified, other radiographic findings will help to limit the differential diagnosis.

Another important factor to consider is the frequency of occurrence of the various types of CHD (Table 4-2). Approximately 50% of cases of CHD are left-to-right shunts. Many of the types of CHD discussed here are highlighted because of striking anatomic findings but are actually quite rare. It is also important to remember that there are other systems for classifying CHD that are used by cardiac imagers, most commonly the segmental approach described by Van Praagh (see Suggested Readings). The following discussion serves as a basic introduction to the classification of congenital heart teaching from a traditional radiography approach.

Blue, Decreased Pulmonary Arterial Flow, Mild Cardiomegaly

The differential diagnosis of patients who are cyanotic and demonstrate decreased pulmonary arterial flow on chest radiograph can be narrowed according to whether the patient has mild or massive cardiomegaly. In the cases in which

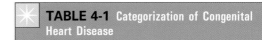

TABLE 4-1 Categorization of Congenital Heart Disease

Blue

  Decreased flow
    Normal heart size
      Tetralogy of Fallot
    Giant heart size
      Ebstein anomaly
      Pulmonary atresia with intact ventricular septum
  Increased flow
    Truncus arteriosus
    Total anomalous pulmonary venous return
  Variable flow
    D-TGA
    Tricuspid atresia

Pink

  Increased pulmonary arterial flow and left-to-right shunt (VSD, ASD, AVC, PDA)
  Increased pulmonary venous flow
    Congestive heart failure in the newborn
  Normal pulmonary flow
    Obstructive lesions
      Coarctation of the aorta
      Aortic stenosis
      Pulmonary artery stenosis
    Postsurgery

ASD, Atrial septal defect; *AVC*, atrioventricular canal; *D-TGA*, D-transposition of the great arteries; *PDA*, patent ductus arteriosus; *VSD*, ventricular septal defect.

TABLE 4-2 Incidence of More Common Types of Congenital Heart Disease

Diagnosis	% Congenital Heart Disease
Left-to-right shunts (VSD, ASD, atrioventricular canal, persistent PDA)	50 (VSD, 28)
Pulmonic stenosis	9.3
Aortic stenosis—bicuspid aortic valve	7.7
Tetralogy of Fallot	7.5
Coarctation of the aorta	3.8
Single ventricle	2.7
Hypoplastic left heart syndrome	1.8
D-TGA	1.8
Tricuspid atresia	1.6
Total anomalous pulmonary venous return	1.4
Truncus arteriosus, L-transposition of great arteries, pulmonary atresia, Ebstein anomaly	Each ≤1

ASD, Atrial septal defect; *D-TGA*, D-transposition of the great arteries; *PDA*, patent ductus arteriosus; *VSD*, ventricular septal defect.

the heart size is normal or there is only mild cardiomegaly, the differential diagnosis includes tetralogy of Fallot and pulmonary atresia with an associated VSD. These two entities are essentially different spectrums of the same disease.

TETRALOGY OF FALLOT

Tetralogy of Fallot is the most common type of cyanotic CHD in children. It is usually diagnosed by 3 months of age. There are four classic anatomic components of tetralogy of Fallot: (1) right ventricular outflow tract obstruction, (2) VSD, (3) overriding aorta, and (4) right ventricular hypertrophy. Radiographic features include a normal-sized to slightly enlarged cardiac silhouette with uplifting of the ventricular apex (a superiorly oriented cardiac axis) secondary to right ventricular hypertrophy The main pulmonary artery segment is concave because of the small associated pulmonary arteries. The combination of the deficient main pulmonary artery and the upturned cardiac apex makes the configuration of the cardiac silhouette appear to be "boot shaped." The pulmonary vascularity is generally decreased. In tetralogy of Fallot, the central pulmonary arteries may be confluent or nonconfluent. This is often difficult to evaluate with echocardiography, so MRI or CT can be used to evaluate the status of the pulmonary arteries in patients with tetralogy of Fallot. A right aortic arch is present in approximately 25% of tetralogy of Fallot patients (see Fig. 4-11). Pulmonary atresia with a VSD is considered to be the most severe form of tetralogy of Fallot. It is synonymous with pseudotruncus or truncus arteriosus type 4 because of the larger bronchial arteries, or collaterals, arising from the aorta and supplying the lungs.

Blue, Decreased Pulmonary Arterial Flow, Massive Cardiomegaly

In patients who are cyanotic and demonstrate decreased pulmonary flow but have massive cardiomegaly, the first two entities that should be considered are Ebstein anomaly and pulmonary atresia with an intact ventricular septum. With these two entities, the degree of cardiomegaly may be the most massive encountered on radiography. The right atrium can dilate to massive size, rather like a balloon; therefore, when massive cardiomegaly is encountered, abnormalities that lead to marked enlargement of the right atrium should be considered.

EBSTEIN ANOMALY

In Ebstein anomaly, there is redundancy of the tricuspid valve, which is displaced into the right ventricle, causing atrialization of part of the right ventricle. There is functional obstruction at the level of the tricuspid valve that results in massive dilatation of the right atrium and the atrialized portion of the right ventricle. The age of presentation is variable. When the anomaly is severe, infants present with severe cyanosis. On radiography, massive cardiomegaly and decreased pulmonary arterial flow are seen (Figs. 4-12 and 4-13). Ebstein anomaly is a rare entity.

PULMONARY ATRESIA WITH INTACT VENTRICULAR SEPTUM

Unlike cases of pulmonary atresia with VSD (tetralogy of Fallot), patients with pulmonary atresia and an intact septum have no forward flow from the right heart. This leads to massive

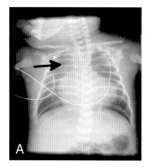
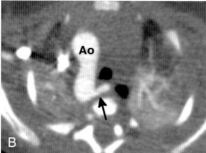
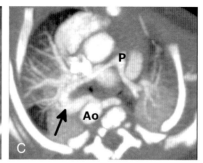

■ **FIGURE 4-11 Tetralogy of Fallot. A,** Frontal chest radiograph shows cardiomegaly with an upturned cardiac apex and a right-sided aortic arch (*arrow*). **B,** Axial contrast-enhanced CTA image shows a right-sided aortic arch (*Ao*) with an aberrant subclavian artery (*arrow*). **C,** Axial MIP-reformatted image from the same CTA shows small, confluent pulmonary arteries (*P*), with the right pulmonary artery partially supplied by a major aortopulmonary collateral (*arrow*), arising from the descending aorta (*Ao*).

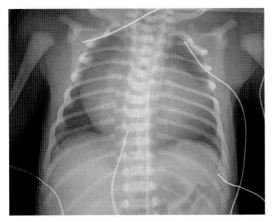

■ **FIGURE 4-12 Ebstein Anomaly.** Frontal chest radiograph in a newborn shows massive cardiomegaly and relatively decreased pulmonary blood flow.

dilatation of the right atrium and, to a lesser degree, the right ventricle. Such patients present with marked cyanosis in infancy. The radiographic appearance (Fig. 4-14) may be indistinguishable from that of Ebstein anomaly.

Note that there are many other abnormalities that may cause the appearance of a massive cardiopericardial silhouette on the chest radiograph of a newborn. They include cardiac tumors (Fig. 4-15A and B), such as rhabdomyoma, noncardiac mediastinal masses, congenital diaphragmatic hernia before aeration of the herniated bowel, and peripheral arterial venous fistulas with associated high output failure. However, when massive cardiomegaly is encountered in the presence of decreased pulmonary flow, Ebstein anomaly and pulmonary atresia with intact septum should be the primary considerations.

Blue, Increased Flow

Patients who are cyanotic and have increased pulmonary arterial flow have admixture lesions, in which the systemic and pulmonary circulations are mixed. In infancy, the two entities that should be considered most likely are truncus arteriosus and total anomalous pulmonary venous return (TAPVR).

TRUNCUS ARTERIOSUS

In truncus arteriosus, there is failure of the normal division of the primitive truncus arteriosus into an aorta and a pulmonary artery. Therefore, one single vessel arises from the heart and gives rise to the coronary, systemic, and pulmonary circulations. There is always an associated VSD. The types of truncus arteriosus are classified according to how the pulmonary arteries arise from the primitive truncus. It is an uncommon lesion and usually presents with cyanosis early in infancy.

On chest radiography, there is increased pulmonary arterial flow. A right aortic arch is present in approximately one third of patients. The identification of a right aortic arch in the presence of increased pulmonary arterial flow in a cyanotic child is highly suggestive of the diagnosis (Fig. 4-16). There is usually moderate cardiomegaly, as well as superimposed pulmonary venous congestion.

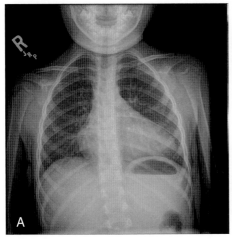
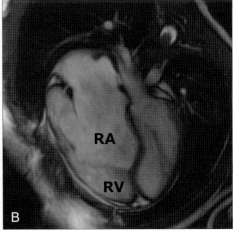

■ **FIGURE 4-13 Ebstein anomaly with marked cardiomegaly. A,** Frontal radiograph shows significant cardiac enlargement. **B,** Four-chamber bright-blood bSSFP image shows marked enlargement of the right atrium (*RA*) and atrialization of a portion of the right ventricle (*RV*), a hallmark of Ebstein anomaly.

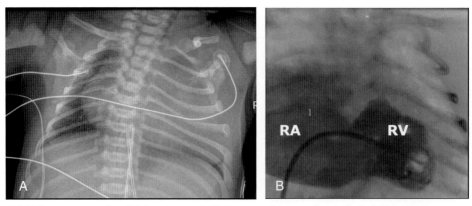

■ FIGURE 4-14 **Pulmonary atresia with intact ventricular septum in a newborn. A,** Radiograph shows massive cardiomegaly filling the entire chest. **B,** Contrast injection of the right ventricle shows massive dilatation of the right atrium (*RA*) as well as dilation of the right ventricle (*RV*).

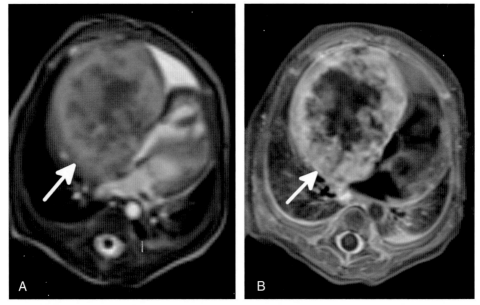

■ FIGURE 4-15 **Cardiac sarcoma.** Axial **A,** bright-blood bSSFP and **B,** T1-weighted, fat-saturated post-contrast MR images show a large, heterogeneous, infiltrative right-sided cardiac mass (*arrows*) with associated mass effect on the left heart and a small pericardial effusion. Final pathology demonstrated a rare, spindle-cell sarcoma.

TOTAL ANOMALOUS PULMONARY VENOUS RETURN

In TAPVR, the pulmonary venous return does not connect to the left atrium but instead connects to the SVC, IVC, right atrium, or portal vein. TAPVR can be divided into supracardiac, cardiac, or infracardiac subtypes. Supracardiac is the most common form; in this form, the pulmonary veins converge and form a left vertical vein that runs superiorly and connects into the innominate vein. With infracardiac TAPVR, the returning veins penetrate the diaphragm and connect to the IVC or portal veins below the level of diaphragm. These veins may become obstructed, and the patient may present with a pulmonary edema pattern on chest radiography (Fig. 4-17). If the veins are not obstructed, the lesion may appear with cardiomegaly and increased pulmonary arterial flow, similar to other left-to-right shunts (Fig. 4-18).

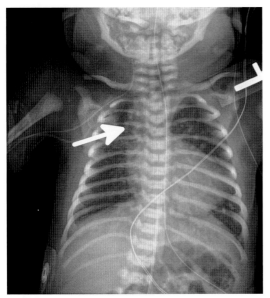

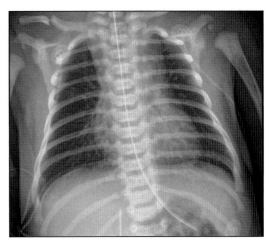

■ FIGURE 4-18 **TAPVR, cardiac type, without venous obstruction in a newborn.** Frontal chest radiograph shows only mild cardiomegaly and increased pulmonary arterial flow in a child with unobstructed cardiac TAPVR to the coronary sinus.

■ FIGURE 4-16 **Truncus arteriosus.** Frontal chest radiograph shows increased pulmonary arterial flow, cardiomegaly, and right-sided aortic arch (*arrow*).

Supracardiac TAPVR classically demonstrates a "snowman" appearance, in which the dilated left vertical vein and dilated SVC form the superior portion of the snowman and the cardiac silhouette forms the inferior portion (Fig. 4-19). This classic appearance does not develop until later in

life and is not often seen now because these lesions are repaired during infancy.

Blue, Variable Pulmonary Arterial Flow

Both D-transposition of the great arteries (D-TGA) and tricuspid atresia can present with variable flow, depending on the anatomy associated with the lesion, as well as the age of the patient.

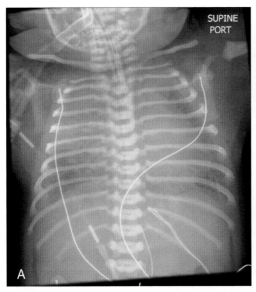

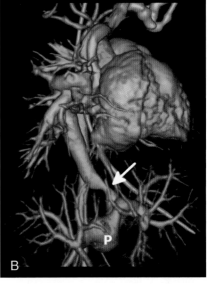

■ FIGURE 4-17 **TAPVR with venous obstruction. A,** Frontal chest radiograph demonstrates cardiomegaly, diffuse pulmonary opacity with indistinctness of the pulmonary vascularity consistent with pulmonary edema, and bilateral pleural effusions in a newborn with obstructed supracardiac TAPVR. **B,** Three-dimensional reformatted CTA image in a different newborn shows an anomalous narrowed (*arrow*) connection between the pulmonary veins and dilated portal vein (*P*), consistent with obstructed infracardiac TAPVR.

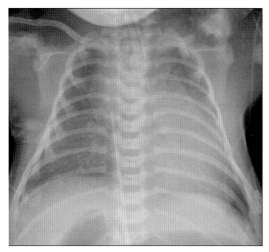

■ FIGURE 4-19 **TAPVR, unobstructed supracardiac type.** Frontal chest radiograph shows the classic "snowman" appearance of the cardiomediastinum. There is enlargement of the superior mediastinum secondary to the dilated left vertical vein and SVC.

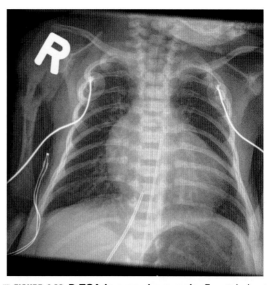

■ FIGURE 4-20 **D-TGA in a newborn male.** Frontal chest radiograph shows classic "egg-on-a-string" appearance of the heart and mediastinum. This is a relatively rarely encountered appearance for TGA. More commonly the chest radiograph is normal in these patients.

D-TRANSPOSITION OF THE GREAT ARTERIES

D-TGA is the most common CHD presenting with cyanosis during the first 24 h of life. With this abnormality, the aorta and pulmonary arteries are transposed. The ascending aorta arises from the right ventricle, and the pulmonary artery arises from the left ventricle. Therefore, blood flow runs in two parallel circuits, systemic and pulmonary. Survival depends on communication between these two circuits via a patent foramen ovale, ASD, VSD, or patent ductus arteriosus (PDA). Historically, D-TGA was categorized as a cardiac lesion associated with increased pulmonary arterial flow. However, in areas with developed healthcare systems, pulmonary arterial switch procedures are performed during the first week of life; therefore, increased pulmonary flow, which is seen in older children with transposition, is now rarely seen. The most common chest radiographic appearance of a newborn child with D-TGA is normal. Classically described radiographic findings include narrowing of the superior mediastinum due to decreased thymic tissue and abnormal relationships of the great vessels and to increased pulmonary arterial flow, as previously mentioned. The appearance of such a mediastinum has been likened to that of an "egg-on-a-string" (Fig. 4-20).

TRICUSPID ATRESIA

In tricuspid atresia, the classic description is that the right atrium is markedly enlarged, causing marked cardiomegaly associated with decreased pulmonary flow. However, this classic appearance is seen only in a minority of patients. The radiograph can vary greatly in cases of tricuspid atresia, making radiographic diagnosis a humbling experience (Fig. 4-21A and B).

Pink, Increased Pulmonary Arterial Flow

Children who are acyanotic and demonstrate increased pulmonary arterial flow on chest radiography have left-to-right shunts. Potential shunts include ASD, VSD (Fig. 4-4), PDA (Fig. 4-22A and B), atrioventricular canal, partial anomalous pulmonary venous return, and aortopulmonary window. The particular cardiac chamber enlargement is a clue to which type of shunt is present. In ASD, the right atrium and right ventricle are enlarged. In VSD, the right ventricle, left atrium, and left ventricle are enlarged. In PDA, the left atrium, left ventricle, and aorta are enlarged. However, as previously mentioned, determining chamber enlargement on chest radiographs is next to impossible in infants. Perhaps a more practical way of predicting which type of shunt is present is by determining the age at presentation. Patients with very large shunts, such as VSDs or atrioventricular canals, present in infancy. ASDs typically present later in childhood or in early adulthood. PDAs occur most commonly in

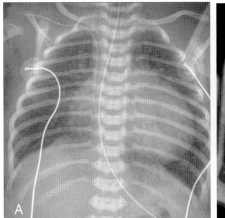
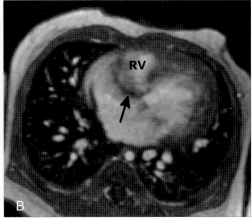

■ **FIGURE 4-21 Tricuspid atresia in a 3-day-old girl. A,** Frontal chest radiograph shows a prominent heart with increased pulmonary vascularity. **B,** Axial ferumoxytol-enhanced T1-weighted ultrashort echo time MR image shows a small, hypertrophied right ventricle (*RV*) with an atretic tricuspid valve (*arrow*).

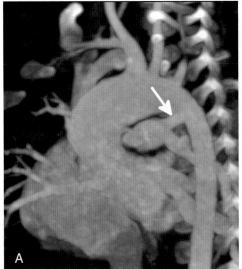
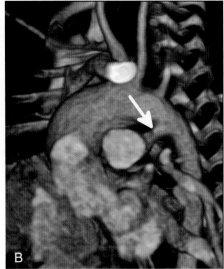

■ **FIGURE 4-22 PDA. A,** MIP and **B,** 3D reformatted images from a chest CTA show a connection (*arrows*) between the descending and main pulmonary artery, consistent with a PDA.

premature infants. Atrioventricular canals occur with increased prevalence in patients with Down syndrome.

On chest radiography, neonates with left-to-right shunts demonstrate increased pulmonary arterial flow, a variable amount of associated increased pulmonary venous flow (pulmonary edema), and cardiomegaly (see Fig. 4-4). It is common for infants with large left-to-right shunts also to have marked hyperinflation on chest radiography. This hyperinflation is thought to be secondary to air trapping due to the peribronchial edema. Therefore, the presence of

marked hyperinflation should not dissuade one from the diagnosis of a left-to-right shunt in favor of viral small airway disease.

Pink (or Dusky) With Increased Pulmonary Venous Flow

An acyanotic patient with increased pulmonary venous flow is essentially a patient with congestive heart failure. In the neonate, the differential diagnosis of congestive heart failure is quite extensive and somewhat different from that seen in older children and adults. Radiology trainees

TABLE 4-3 Differential Diagnosis for Congestive Heart Failure in the Newborn

Anatomic

  Coarctation

  Aortic stenosis

  Left ventricular dysfunction and
    Anomalous origin of the left coronary artery

    Myocarditis

    Shock myocardium (birth asphyxia)

    Glycogen storage disease

    Infant of diabetic mother
  Hypoplastic left heart

  Mitral stenosis

  Cor triatriatum

  Pulmonary venous atresia or stenosis

Systemic

  Anemia–polycythemia

  Hypoglycemia and hyperglycemia

  Hypothyroidism and hyperthyroidism

  Sepsis

  Peripheral arteriovenous malformation
    Vein of Galen malformation

    Hepatic hemangioendothelioma

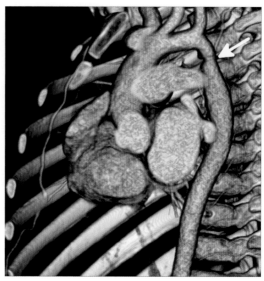

■ FIGURE 4-23 **Coarctation of the aorta.** Three-dimensional reformation of a CT angiogram demonstrates a focal coarctation at the aortic isthmus (*arrow*).

often have difficulty providing a reasonable differential diagnosis of congestive heart failure in a newborn. An easy way to approach the differential diagnosis is to consider two large categories of disease. The first category is anatomic left-sided obstruction (Table 4-3). Anything that obstructs the left side of the heart can cause congestive heart failure. If one works his or her way proximally, starting at the level of the aorta, one will not forget to mention any of the likely candidates. In the aorta, both coarctation of the aorta (Fig. 4-23) and critical aortic stenosis can cause left-sided obstruction. Anything that causes the left ventricle to be dysfunctional also can cause left-sided heart obstruction. The list of possibilities is long and includes cardiomyopathy, glycogen storage disease, anomalous origin of the left coronary artery with associated cardiac ischemia (see Fig. 4-8), birth asphyxia (shock myocardium), infants of diabetic mothers, myocarditis, and hypoplastic left heart syndrome (Fig. 4-24). Within the region of the left atrium, both mitral valve stenosis and cor triatriatum can cause left-sided heart failure. Cor triatriatum is defined as the presence of a membrane dividing the left atrium into two separate chambers. The membrane has a pin-like hole centrally that is the only route for forward blood flow and causes

relative obstruction. Pulmonary venous atresia can also cause left-sided heart failure. The most commonly encountered of these abnormalities include hypoplastic left heart syndrome and coarctation of the aorta.

The second large category of entities that can cause left-sided heart failure includes systemic causes of failure, such as anemia and polycythemia, sepsis, or high output failure resulting from a peripheral arteriovenous malformation.

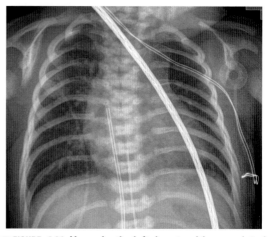

■ FIGURE 4-24 **Hypoplastic left heart with associated mild congestive heart failure in a newborn.** Frontal chest radiograph shows cardiomegaly and indistinct pulmonary vasculature. Note that patients with hypoplastic left heart do not necessarily have hearts that appear to be small.

HYPOPLASTIC LEFT HEART SYNDROME

Hypoplastic left heart syndrome refers to a combination of hypoplasia or aplasia of the ascending aorta, aortic valve, left ventricle, and mitral valve. Children present with congestive heart failure at birth. The lesion is dependent on a PDA. Systemic flow goes from the main pulmonary artery to the descending aorta via the PDA. Flow to the coronary and cranial areas is retrograde via the hypoplastic ascending aorta. On radiography, there is cardiomegaly and increased pulmonary venous flow (pulmonary edema; see Fig. 4-24). Treatment is typically the Norwood procedure or variant thereof (Table 4-4).

Pink, Normal Pulmonary Arterial Flow

The three main categories of CHD that are associated with cyanosis and normal pulmonary arterial flow include obstructive lesions, extrinsic airway compression, and CHD with increased or decreased pulmonary arterial flow that has been surgically corrected (Extrinsic airway compression was discussed in Chapter 2).

TABLE 4-4 Common Surgical Procedures for Congenital Heart Disease		
Procedure	**Indication**	**Connection**
Fontan	Tricuspid atresia Single ventricle Hypoplastic right ventricle Complex congenital heart disease	IVC-to-PA conduit or anastomosis
Glenn	Tricuspid atresia Hypoplastic RV Pulmonary atresia	SVC-to-right PA anastomosis (bidirectional provides flow to both pulmonary arteries)
Rastelli	Pulmonary atresia	RV-to-PA conduit
Mustard–Senning (intraatrial baffle)	TGA	Atrial rerouting of venous blood flow. Mustard uses pericardium to create baffle and Senning uses atrial wall
Arterial switch procedure (Jatene)	TGA	Switch of aorta and PA with reanastomosis of coronary arteries
Norwood	Hypoplastic left heart syndrome	First stage: use of main PA as ascending aorta, enlargement of aortic arch, systemic or right ventricle shunt to PA
		Second stage: Glenn
		Third stage: Fontan
Blalock–Taussig shunt	Palliative shunt for obstruction of pulmonary blood flow (TOF, pulmonary atresia, tricuspid atresia)	Subclavian artery-to-PA graft
Sano shunt	Palliative shunt for obstruction of pulmonary blood flow (TOF, pulmonary atresia, tricuspid atresia)	Right ventricle-to-PA graft
Closure device deployment	Left-to-right shunts (ASD, PDA)	Percutaneous catheter placement of "plugging" closure device across left-to-right shunt
Waterston–Cooley	Palliative shunt for obstruction of pulmonary blood flow	Ascending aorta-to-right PA anastomosis
Potts	Palliative shunt for obstruction of pulmonary blood flow	Descending aorta-to-left PA anastomosis
PA banding	Left-to-right shunting	Band around main PA

ASD, Atrial septal defect; *PA*, pulmonary artery; *PDA*, patent ductus arteriosus; *IVC*, inferior vena cava; *RV*, right ventricle; *SVC*, superior vena cava; *TGA*, transposition of the great arteries; *TOF*, tetralogy of Fallot.

OBSTRUCTIVE LESIONS

Obstructive lesions of the great arteries include aortic stenosis, pulmonic stenosis, and coarctation of the aorta. These lesions can have subtle findings on chest radiography, so when there is a scenario that suggests CHD but one's initial impression is that the chest radiograph is normal, a second glance for subtle mediastinal contour abnormalities may prove fruitful.

AORTIC STENOSIS

Aortic stenosis may occur secondary to a bicuspid aortic valve or previous rheumatic disease. With aortic valvular stenosis, there may be dilatation of the ascending aorta secondary to the "jet" effect through the stenotic valve (Fig. 4-25A and B). The ascending aorta should never be identified in a normal child on frontal radiography. If the rightward border of the ascending aorta is visualized, a dilated aorta should be suspected (see Fig. 4-25). In addition to aortic stenosis, another cause of a dilated ascending aorta is an aneurysm secondary to a disorder such as Marfan syndrome. Another supporting sign for aortic stenosis is left ventricular enlargement secondary to hypertrophy. Aortic stenosis can also be supravalvular in location. Williams syndrome is associated with supravalvular stenosis, peripheral pulmonary artery stenosis, and other symptoms, including intellectual disability.

PULMONIC STENOSIS

In pulmonary valvular stenosis, there may be dilation of the main pulmonary artery secondary to the jet effect (Fig. 4-26). On frontal chest radiography, this appears as a prominent main pulmonary arterial segment (Fig. 4-27).

COARCTATION OF THE AORTA

Coarctation is defined as a congenital narrowing of the aorta. This narrowing can be either diffuse or localized. The localized type, which is more common, is typically located just beyond the left subclavian artery origin in the vicinity of the level of ductus arteriosus. The clinical presentation is determined by the severity of the narrowing. Severe narrowing presents in infancy with congestive heart failure. Coarctation can be an isolated lesion or can appear as part of more complex anatomic anomalies (see Figs. 4-2, 4-23, 4-28, and 4-29). Less severe narrowing may present later in childhood with upper extremity hypertension. On chest radiography, the appearance of the leftward border of the superior mediastinum has been likened to the numeral 3 in coarctation (Fig. 4-29A–C), particularly in older children. The superior portion of the 3 is caused by the prestenotic dilation of the aorta above the coarctation. The middle or narrow part of the 3 is caused by the coarctation itself, and the inferior part of the 3 is caused by the

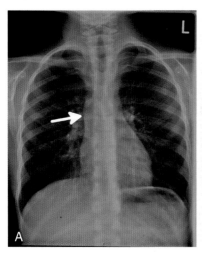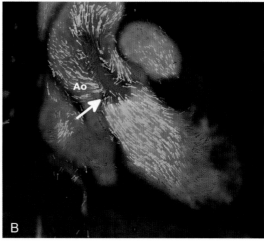

■ FIGURE 4-25 **Aortic stenosis with poststenotic dilatation. A,** Frontal chest radiograph shows visualization and prominence of the shadow of the ascending aorta (*arrow*). Normally, the shadow of the ascending aorta is not seen in children. **B,** Coronal, ferumoxytol-enhanced 4D flow MR image in the same patient shows a dilated ascending aorta (*Ao*) resulting from a flow jet (*white arrow*) through the stenotic aortic valve. The small color-coded vectors illustrate the direction, magnitude, and velocity of flow.

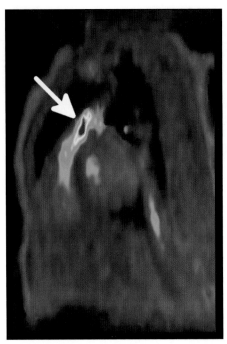

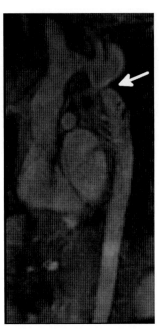

■ FIGURE 4-28 **Coarctation of the aorta.** Noncontrast, three-dimensional SSFP candy cane reformatted MR image demonstrates coarctation at the aortic isthmus (*arrow*).

■ FIGURE 4-26 **Pulmonic stenosis in a 1.5-month-old boy.** Gadolinium-enhanced 4D flow MR image in the oblique sagittal/right ventricular outflow tract plane shows flow acceleration (*arrow*) across the pulmonic valve, indicating stenosis.

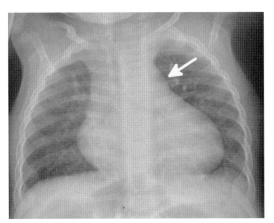

■ FIGURE 4-27 **Pulmonic stenosis in a 5-month-old girl.** Frontal chest radiograph shows prominence of the main pulmonary artery (*arrow*).

poststenotic, dilated portion of the descending aorta. Inferior rib notching may be present secondary to pressure from dilated intercostal arteries (see Fig. 4-29); it most commonly occurs at the level of the fourth through eighth ribs. In

patients with coarctation of the aorta, there is increased association with bicuspid aortic valve, which can present later in life with resultant aortic stenosis. Treatment involves balloon dilation and stent placement or surgical resection (see Fig. 4-29). In cases of coarctation, CT and MRI can be used for diagnosis and presurgical planning (site, length, severity, relationship to left subclavian artery, and extent of collateralization), as well as for postsurgical follow-up in the evaluation of restenosis, stent patency (if applicable), aneurysm, or left ventricular hypertrophy.

■ ABNORMALITIES OF CONOTRUNCAL ROTATION

Several types of CHD can result from abnormalities of conotruncal rotation. There is often confusion concerning this group of diseases. The primitive truncus is an anterior midline structure during fetal development. Normally, the

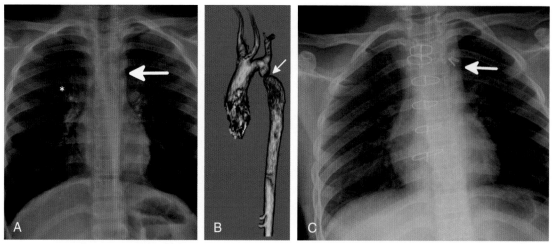

■ **FIGURE 4-29 Coarctation of the aorta treated with surgery. A,** Frontal chest radiograph shows a three-shaped appearance of the left superior mediastinal border made up of dilated aorta above the coarctation, coarctation (*arrow*), and poststenotic dilation of the descending aorta inferior to the coarctation. Also note subtle rib notching (*asterisk—example*). **B,** Three-dimensional reconstruction from a gadolinium-enhanced MR angiogram confirms the coarctation (*arrow*). **C,** Post surgery, the coarctation has been resolved, with a now normal appearance of the aortic knob (*arrow*).

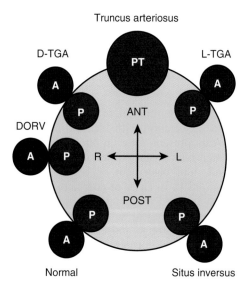

■ **FIGURE 4-30 Conotruncal rotation.** Diagram shows relationship of the great arteries at the level of the semilunar valves as depicted by axial cross-sectional CT or MRI. During embryologic development, the primitive truncus is an anterior midline structure. With normal development, the primitive truncus divides into the aorta and the pulmonary artery, which then rotate 150 degrees clockwise. The pulmonary artery then lies anterior to and left of the aorta. Variations in this rotation are characteristic of various conotruncal abnormalities. *A,* Aorta; *DORV,* double outlet right ventricle; *P,* pulmonary artery; *PT,* primitive truncus; *TGA,* transposition of the great arteries.

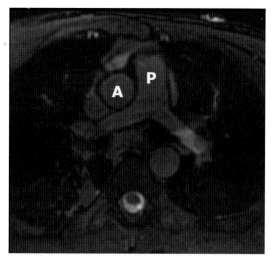

■ **FIGURE 4-31** Normal conotruncal position on axial reformatted image from a 3D SSFP MR acquisition. The main pulmonary artery (*P*) is anterior and leftward in relationship to the aorta (*A*).

primitive truncus divides into the aorta and pulmonary artery, which rotate clockwise 150 degrees (Figs. 4-30 and 4-31). As a result, the pulmonary artery ends up anterior and to the left of the aorta. Abnormal division or rotation of this primitive truncus may result in a number of diseases, including L-transposition of the great arteries (L-TGA; Figs. 4-3 and 4-32); D-TGA (Figs. 4-20, 4-33, and 4-34); truncus arteriosus; double-outlet right ventricle; and situs inversus. The anatomic relationship between the aorta and pulmonary artery as viewed in cross-section at the level of the semilunar valves is characteristic of these abnormalities. With truncus arteriosus, there is a failure of division of the primitive truncus into a separate aorta and pulmonary

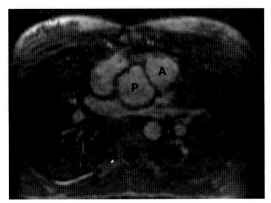

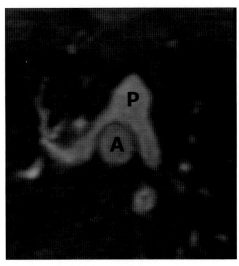

■ **FIGURE 4-32** L-transposition of the great vessels shown on axial reformatted image from a ferumoxytol-enhanced, T1-weighted, 3D-spoiled gradient echo MRA acquisition. The aorta (A) is to the left of and anterior to the pulmonary artery (P).

■ **FIGURE 4-34** Axial reformatted image from a gadolinium-enhanced, 3D-spoiled gradient echo MRA acquisition shows D-transposition of the great vessels following an arterial switch (Jatene) procedure with LeCompte maneuver, with typical postswitch anatomy. The pulmonary artery (P) is now anterior to and draped over the more posteriorly positioned ascending aorta (A).

artery. Therefore, a single large vessel gives rise to the coronary, systemic, and pulmonary arterial circulation. Truncus arteriosus was discussed previously.

In L-TGA or congenitally corrected transposition of the great arteries, the ventricles and atrioventricular valves are inverted such that there are both atrioventricular and ventriculoarterial discordance. Therefore, the morphologic right ventricle is in the position of and serves as the anatomic left ventricle. L-TGA is often associated with complex CHD but may occur as an isolated lesion. With L-TGA, there is a 30-degree clockwise rotation of the primitive truncus, which causes the aorta to be anterior and leftward as compared with the pulmonary artery (see Figs. 4-30 and 4-32).

In contrast, with D-TGA or complete transposition of the great arteries, there is ventricular great vessel discordance, in which the aorta arises from the right ventricle and the pulmonary

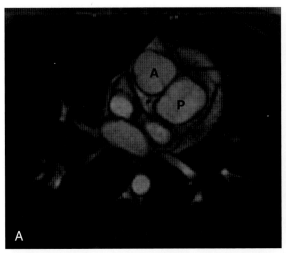

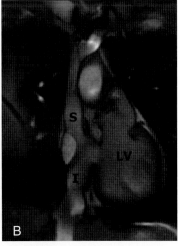

■ **FIGURE 4-33 D-transposition of the great vessels. A,** Axial bright-blood bSSFP MR image shows the aorta (A) is anterior and rightward in relationship to the pulmonary artery (P). **B,** Oblique coronal bSSFP MR image after Mustard intraatrial baffle demonstrates baffling of the SVC (S) and IVC (I) toward the left atrium and left ventricle (LV) instead of the right atrium and right ventricle. Thus, deoxygenated blood is directed toward the left side of the heart, which pumps to the pulmonary artery to the lungs.

artery arises from the left ventricle. With D-TGA, there is a 30-degree counterclockwise rotation of the primitive truncus, which means that the aorta is rightward and anterior to the pulmonary artery (see Figs. 4-30, 4-33, and 4-34).

In the case of a double-outlet right ventricle, more than half of the origins of the great arteries arise from the morphologic right ventricle. The only outlet for the left ventricle is a VSD. This lesion is commonly associated with other complex CHD. During development, there is a 45-degree counterclockwise rotation of the primitive truncus, which causes the aorta and pulmonary artery to be side by side with the aorta on the right (see Fig. 4-30).

In situs inversus, the rotation of the aorta and pulmonary artery is completely opposite of that which would be considered normal (see Fig. 4-30).

■ SURGERIES FOR CONGENITAL HEART DISEASE

To understand the imaging appearances on chest radiography and cross-sectional studies of patients who have undergone surgery or interventional procedures for CHD, basic knowledge of the types of procedures performed is required. Table 4-4 lists the names, indications, and flow alterations of commonly performed cardiac procedures. The imaging findings related to a number of procedures are also illustrated: aortic stenting (see Fig. 4-1) as may be performed for coarctation of the aorta, intraatrial baffle (see Fig. 4-33), arterial switch procedure (see Fig. 4-34), Amplatzer occlusion devices (Fig. 4-35A–D), Glenn shunt (see Fig. 4-1), and Fontan procedure (Fig. 4-36).

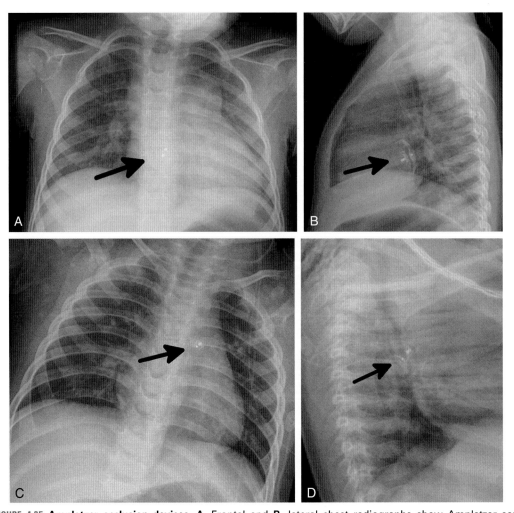

■ FIGURE 4-35 **Amplatzer occlusion devices. A,** Frontal and **B,** lateral chest radiographs show Amplatzer septal occluder device (*arrows*) in the location of an ASD. Note the two disk-shaped portions, each one resting on one or the other side of the defect, holding the device in place and blocking flow. **C,** Frontal and **D,** lateral chest radiographs show an Amplatzer duct occluder device (*arrows*) closing a PDA.

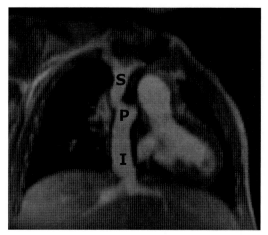

■ FIGURE 4-36 **Fontan procedure.** Coronal magnitude image from a ferumoxytol-enhanced 4D flow MR acquisition shows anatomy of the Fontan procedure. The SVC (*S*) and IVC (*S*) are connected directly to the pulmonary arteries (*P*).

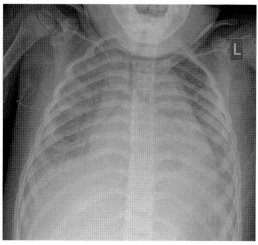

■ FIGURE 4-37 **Kawasaki disease in a 4-year-old child resulting in acute myocarditis and associated heart failure.** Chest radiograph shows cardiomegaly, bilateral pleural effusions, and indistinct, prominent pulmonary vasculature consistent with venous congestion.

Acquired Heart Disease

In addition to CHD, there are multiple types of acquired heart disease that can occur during childhood. Many of these, such as cardiomyopathy and rheumatic heart disease, have features in common with those found in adult disease. One of the unusual types of acquired heart disease that can occur in children is Kawasaki disease.

KAWASAKI DISEASE

Kawasaki disease (mucocutaneous lymph node syndrome) is an inflammatory disease of unknown cause. Characteristic findings include fever, rash, conjunctivitis, erythema of the lips and oral cavity, and cervical lymphadenopathy. There is an associated generalized vasculitis. Cardiac involvement includes an acute myocarditis, which can lead to congestive heart failure (Fig. 4-37). Delayed cardiac complications include the development of coronary artery aneurysms (Fig. 4-38), as well as coronary artery stenoses. Chest radiographs can show findings of congestive heart failure when the myocarditis is severe. Rarely, the coronary artery aneurysms can calcify. Gallbladder hydrops, as seen on ultrasound, has also been described as a finding. However, this is not included as one of the criteria in making the diagnosis, and ultrasound of the upper abdomen is rarely useful in diagnosing the disease. Treatment with gamma globulin and aspirin can decrease the severity of

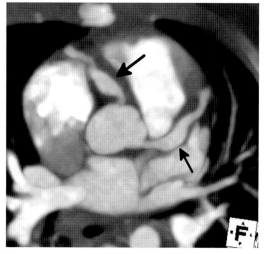

■ FIGURE 4-38 **Kawasaki disease with coronary artery aneurysms.** Axial MIP reformation from a CT angiogram shows multiple coronary aneurysms (*arrows*).

the illness and can decrease the likelihood of delayed complications such as coronary aneurysms. Of note, the novel severe acute respiratory syndrome coronavirus 2 causing COVID-19 has been associated with a pediatric Kawasaki-like illness, termed multisystem inflammatory syndrome in children (MIS-C), with potential overlapping cardiac features including myocarditis and coronary dilation.

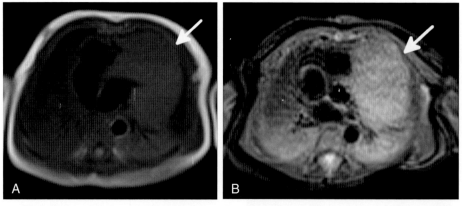

■ FIGURE 4-39 **Rhabdomyoma in a girl with tuberous sclerosis. A,** Axial T1-weighted black-blood and **B,** axial T2-weighted, fat-saturated MR images show a large cardiac mass (*arrows*) blending with the myocardium.

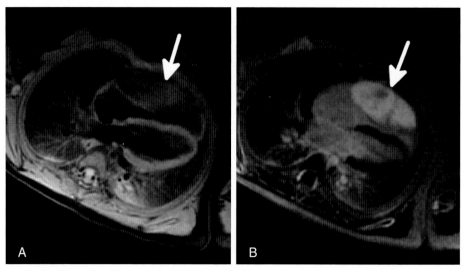

■ FIGURE 4-40 **Pediatric cardiac fibroma.** Four-chamber **A,** T2-weighted triple inversion recovery and **B,** delayed gadolinium enhancement MR images show a large circumscribed solid mass within the anterior aspect of the heart (*arrows*).

CARDIAC MASSES

There are a number of causes of cardiac masses in children. The majority of pediatric cardiac masses are present during the newborn period. By far, the most common type of congenital heart mass is rhabdomyoma (Fig. 4-39A and B). This lesion is most commonly seen in patients with tuberous sclerosis. Rhabdomyomas typically involute over time and are usually treated conservatively. Other potential cardiac masses include sarcoma (Fig. 4-15), particularly angio-sarcoma, fibroma (Fig. 4-40), teratoma, and hemangioma. The most common cause of cardiac tumor associated with pericardial effusion is a hemangioma. These cases are often initially diagnosed on in utero or postnatal sonography and then further characterized by MRI.

SUGGESTED READING

Applegate KE, Goske MJ, Pierce G, Murphy D: Situs revisited: imaging of the heterotaxy syndrome, *Radiographics* 19:837−852, 1999.

Chan FP, Hanneman K: Computed tomography and magnetic resonance imaging in neonates with congenital cardiovascular disease, *Semin Ultrasound CT MR* 36:146−160, 2015.

Coussement AM, Gooding CA: Objective radiographic assessment of pulmonary vascularity in children, *Radiology* 109:649−654, 1973.

Donnelly LF, Gelfand KJ, Schwartz DC, et al.: The wall to wall heart: differential diagnosis for massively large cardiothymic silhouette in newborns, *Appl Radiol* 26:23−28, 1997.

Donnelly LF, Higgins CB: MR imaging of conotruncal abnormalities, *AJR* 166:925−928, 1996.

Ferguson EC, Krishnamurthy R, Oldham SA: Classic imaging signs of congenital cardiovascular abnormalities, *Radiographics* 27:1323–1334, 2007.

Frank L, Dillman JR, Parish V, et al.: Cardiovascular MR imaging of conotruncal anomalies, *Radiographics* 30:1069–1094, 2010.

Gaca AM, Jaggers JJ, Dudley LT, Bisset GS: Repair of congenital heart disease: a primer Part 1, *Radiology* 247:617–631, 2008.

Gaca AM, Jaggers JJ, Dudley LT, Bisset GS: Repair of congenital heart disease: a primer Part 2, *Radiology* 248:44–60, 2008.

Goo HW: State-of-the-art CT imaging techniques for congenital heart disease, *Korean J Radiol* 11:4–18, 2010.

Kellenberger CF, Yoo SJ, Valsangiacomo Büchel ER: Cardiovascular MR imaging in neonates and infants with congenital heart disease, *Radiographics* 27:5–18, 2007.

Leschka S, Oechslin E, Husman L, et al.: Pre- and postoperative evaluation of congenital heart disease in children and adults with 64-section CT, *Radiographics* 27:829–846, 2007.

Ntisnjana HN, Hughes ML, Taylor AM: The role of cardiovascular magnetic resonance in pediatric congenital heart disease, *J Cardiovasc Magn Reson* 13:51, 2011.

Pouletty M, Borocco C, Ouldali N, et al.: Paediatric multisystem inflammatory syndrome temporally associated with SARS-CoV-2 mimicking Kawasaki disease (Kawa-COVID-19): a multicentre cohort, *Ann Rheum Dis* 79:999–1006, 2020.

Pushparajah K, Duong P, Mathur S, Babu-Narayan S: EDUCATIONAL SERIES IN CONGENITAL HEART DISEASE: cardiovascular MRI and CT in congenital heart disease, *Echo Res Pract* 6:R121–R138, 2019.

Schallert EK, Danton GH, Kardon R, Young DA: Describing congenital heart disease by using three-part segmental notation, *Radiographics* 33:E33–E46, 2013.

Schicchi N, Fogante M, Esposto Pirani P, et al.: Third-generation dual-source dual-energy CT in pediatric congenital heart disease patients: state-of-the-art, *Radiol Med* 124:1238–1252, 2019.

Schweigmann G, Gassner I, Maurer K: Imaging the neonatal heart–essentials for the radiologist, *Eur J Radiol* 60:159–170, 2006.

Siripornpitak S, Pornkul R, Khowsathit P, et al.: Cardiac CT angiography in children with congenital heart disease, *Eur J Radiol* 82:1067–1082, 2013.

Strife JS, Sze RW: Radiographic evaluation of the neonate with congenital heart disease, *Radiol Clin North Am* 37:1093–1107, 1999.

Swischuk LE, Stansberry SD: Pulmonary vascularity in pediatric heart disease, *J Thorac Imag* 4:1–6, 1989.

van der Hulst AE, Roest AA, Westenberg JJ, et al.: Cardiac MRI in postoperative congenital heart disease patients, *J Magn Reson Imag* 36:511–528, 2012.

Vasanawala SS, Hanneman K, Alley MT, Hsiao A: Congenital heart disease assessment with 4D flow MRI, *J Magn Reson Imag* 42:870–886, 2015.

Winer-Muram HT, Tonkin IL: The spectrum of heterotaxic syndromes, *Radiol Clin North Am* 27(6):1147–1170, 1989.

Zucker EJ, Koning JL, Lee EY: Cyanotic congenital heart disease: essential primer for the practicing radiologist, *Radiol Clin North Am* 55:693–716, 2017.

CHAPTER 5

GASTROINTESTINAL

Michael P. Nasser

■ NEONATAL

Necrotizing Enterocolitis

Necrotizing enterocolitis (NEC) is an idiopathic enterocolitis that predominantly involves the gastrointestinal (GI) tract of premature infants. The majority of cases occur in low birth weight infants (BW < 1500 g) and those born less than 32 weeks gestation. Mortality rates can be as high as 30% and are inversely correlated to birth weight and gestational age. Term infants who develop NEC typically have a preexisting condition, including congenital heart disease or sepsis.

NEC is suspected to occur from a combination of ischemia and infection. Infants who develop NEC usually present with sudden feeding intolerance. This can also include abdominal distention, increased residuals via nasogastric (NG) tube, emesis (often bilious), and bloody stools. The onset of symptoms is also found to be inversely related to gestational age.

Management of NEC includes making the patient NPO, decompression with an NG tube, and the administration of brood spectrum antibiotics. Surgical intervention is usually reserved for patients with perforation or those with a declining clinical state. Patients with NEC have historically been monitored with serial abdominal radiographs. This includes a supine abdominal X-ray with either a left decubitus or supine cross-table lateral view to look for free air.

Radiographic findings suspicious for NEC include focally dilated bowel or generalized bowel distention. The dilated bowel often has a featureless appearance with separation of bowel loops suggesting bowel wall thickening. An abnormal bowel gas pattern that remains unchanged on multiple subsequent images increases the specificity for NEC. A diagnostic finding of NEC is the presence of pneumatosis (gas in the bowel wall). Pneumatosis may appear as multiple bubble-like or curvilinear lucencies overlying bowel (Fig. 5-1). The bubble-like lucencies may be confused with meconium or stool. Pneumatosis will remain relatively stable or progress in degree on subsequent images. Meconium and stool will change with time. Portal venous gas is

another finding associated with NEC. This will appear as linear or branching lucencies overlying the liver (Fig. 5-1).

Free intraperitoneal air is an indication for surgical intervention. When present, free air results in a generalized lucent appearance to the abdomen. In a supine patient, free air will layer in the most nondependent portion of the anterior abdomen, often the proximal abdomen (Fig. 5-2). Free air may outline the falciform ligament on the supine view (football sign). Free air can also result in the visualization of both sides of the bowel wall, the classic Rigler sign (Fig. 5-2). On the cross-table lateral view, free air will layer anterior to the liver or bowel (Fig. 5-3). On the left decubitus view, free air may collect along the lateral border of the liver (Fig. 5-4) or bowel. An acute change from an abdomen with multiple distended bowel loops to a gasless abdomen is highly suspicious for perforation.

Ultrasound has an increasing role for the diagnosis of NEC. This modality has several advantages over radiographs, including real-time visualization of the bowel wall, assessment of bowel perfusion via Doppler and detecting signs of early perforation. It is particularly useful in children with a relatively gasless abdomen on radiographs.

Initial signs of NEC include dilated, fluid-filled, and aperistaltic bowel. The bowel wall may be thickened, measuring more than 2–3 mm thick in the transverse diameter. In later stages of NEC, with the development of ischemia and necrosis, the bowel wall may become thinned. Ultrasound may even detect a focal mural defect. The modality of ultrasound is unique in its ability to assess bowel wall perfusion with color Doppler. Initially, those suspected of having NEC will demonstrate increased bowel wall perfusion. With the development of ischemia and necrosis, bowel perfusion will be diminished. Other signs of NEC include generalized increased bowel wall echogenicity (Fig. 5-5). Focal areas of pneumatosis will present as punctate echogenic foci within the bowel wall (Fig. 5-6).

Signs of perforation include free peritoneal air and peritoneal fluid. Free air will appear as linear

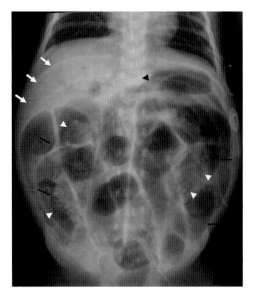

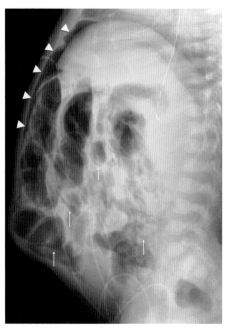

■ FIGURE 5-1 NEC in a premature infant. Supine abdominal radiograph demonstrates multiple dilated bowel loops throughout the abdomen. There are both curvilinear (*small black arrows*) and bubbly (*white arrowheads*) lucencies associated with bowel, consistent with pneumatosis. Branching lucencies over the liver are consistent with portal venous gas (*large white arrows*). Incidental note is made of a malpositioned NG tube in the distal esophagus (*black arrowhead*).

■ FIGURE 5-3 Free peritoneal air in a premature infant with NEC. Cross-table lateral view demonstrates multiple dilated bowel loops with pneumatosis (*small white arrows*). There is free air layering along the nondependent abdomen, anterior to the liver and bowel (*white arrowheads*).

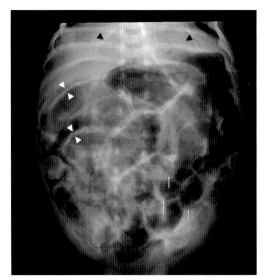

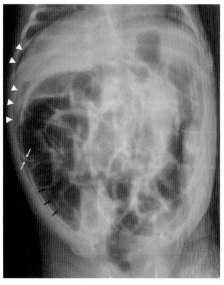

■ FIGURE 5-2 Complications of NEC in a premature infant. Supine radiograph demonstrates multiple dilated bowel loops with curvilinear lucencies (*small white arrows*) representing pneumatosis. There is a large rounded lucency in the upper mid abdomen (*black arrowheads*) representing free intraperitoneal air. Several examples of Rigler (*double wall*) sign are present in the right hemiabdomen (*white arrowheads*).

■ FIGURE 5-4 Free peritoneal air in a premature infant with NEC. A left decubitus radiograph demonstrates dilated bowel with pneumatosis (*small black arrows*). There is free air layering along the nondependent right abdomen, lateral to the liver and bowel (*white arrowheads*). Another example of Rigler (*double wall*) sign (*small white arrows*).

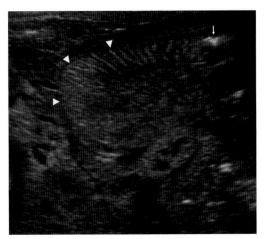

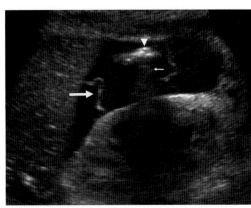

■ FIGURE 5-7 Perforation on abdominal ultrasound of a premature infant. Transverse ultrasonographic image demonstrates echogenic free air in the nondependent anterior abdomen (*white arrowhead*). Reverberation artifact is also present (*small white arrow*). There is complex free fluid present with septations (*large white arrow*).

■ FIGURE 5-5 Ultrasound of NEC in a premature infant. Transverse ultrasonographic image demonstrates a moderate length segment of echogenic small bowel (*white arrow heads*). There are also localized punctate echogenicities (*small white arrow*) representing pneumatosis.

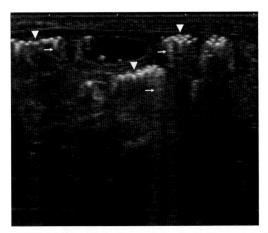

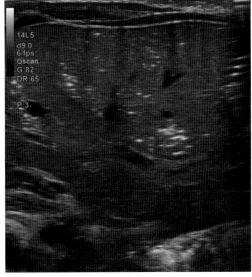

■ FIGURE 5-6 Pneumatosis on abdominal ultrasound of a premature infant. Transverse ultrasonographic image demonstrates several loops of small bowel with punctate echogenic foci consistent with pneumatosis (*white arrowheads*). Note the reverberation artifact posterior to the echogenic foci (*small white arrows*).

■ FIGURE 5-8 Portal venous gas on abdominal ultrasound. Portal venous gas in a premature infant with NEC. There are multiple punctate echogenic foci throughout the liver. These echogenic foci may be dynamic, changing location during real-time imaging.

or punctate echogenic foci outside of bowel, usually along the nondependent abdomen (Fig. 5-7). Free air may demonstrate reverberation artifact posterior to these echogenic foci (Fig. 5-7). Free peritoneal fluid may be simple (anechoic) or complex (mixed echogenicity). Free fluid may be localized or diffuse within the abdomen. Finally, ultrasound will help to directly visualize portal gas. Portal gas will appear as punctate or branching echogenic foci in the liver (Fig. 5-8).

A delayed complication in those that survive NEC may be bowel stricture. Strictures can involve both small and large bowel. Evaluation of bowel strictures can be conducted with a UGI/small bowel follow-through (SBFT) or a contrast enema (Fig. 5-9).

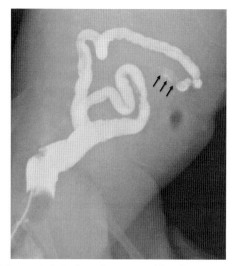

■ FIGURE 5-9 **Colonic stricture resulting from previous NEC.** Contrast enema demonstrates a stricture in the region of the hepatic flexure (*small black arrows*) from prior instance of NEC.

Intestinal Obstruction in Neonates

Neonates with suspected intestinal obstruction can present with emesis (bilious or nonbilious), feeding intolerance, abdominal distention, failure to pass meconium, or clinical deterioration. Abdominal radiographs are usually the first imaging exam performed for evaluation. The visualized obstruction can be divided into a proximal versus a distal etiology.

Neonates with a proximal intestinal obstruction usually present with early emesis in contrast to those with a more distal process. Radiographs may show distension of the stomach, duodenum, proximal jejunum, or all three, depending on the level of the obstruction. There are fewer distended bowel loops in a proximal obstruction in contrast to a more distal obstruction (Fig. 5-10A and B). The most common causes of a proximal intestinal obstruction in neonates include duodenal atresia or stenosis, duodenal web, annular pancreas, malrotation with midgut volvulus or LADD bands, and jejunal atresia. The most common causes of a distal intestinal obstruction in neonates include Hirschsprung disease, Meconium plug syndrome (small left colon syndrome), ileal atresia, meconium ileus, and anal atresia/anorectal malformations (Table 5-1).

PROXIMAL INTESTINAL OBSTRUCTION IN NEONATES

Duodenal Atresia, Stenosis, and Web

A congenital obstruction of the duodenum can be intrinsic or secondary to an extrinsic etiology. The intrinsic etiologies include duodenal atresia, stenosis, and web. The extrinsic causes include malrotation with midgut volvulus, malrotation with LADD bands, and an annular pancreas. Congenital duodenal obstruction is the most common form of congenital bowel obstruction. More than half are premature and there is an

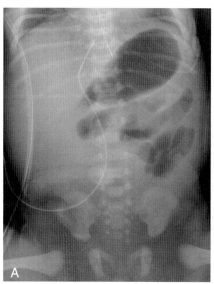
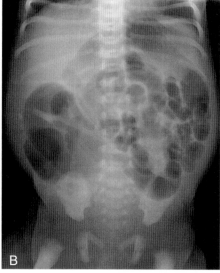

■ FIGURE 5-10 **Proximal versus distal intestinal obstruction in a neonate. A,** Supine abdominal radiographs demonstrate distention of the stomach, duodenum, and a few proximal jejunal bowel loops, concerning for a proximal obstructive process. **B,** Supine abdominal radiographs demonstrate multiple distended bowel loops throughout the abdomen (jejunal and ileal), concerning for a distal obstructive process.

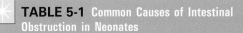

TABLE 5-1 Common Causes of Intestinal Obstruction in Neonates

Proximal

- Duodenal atresia or stenosis
- Duodenal web
- Malrotation with midgut volvulus or LADD bands
- Annular pancreas
- Jejunal atresia

Distal

- Ileal atresia
- Meconium ileus
- Hirschsprung disease
- Meconium plug syndrome (small left colon syndrome)
- Anal atresia and anorectal malformations

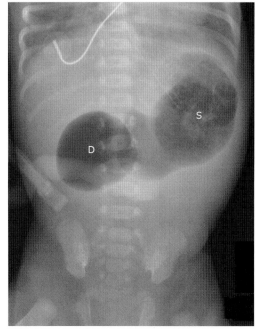

■ **FIGURE 5-11 Duodenal atresia.** Supine abdominal radiograph demonstrates a dilated stomach (S) and duodenal bulb (D) constituting the double bubble sign. It is important to note that there is no distal bowel gas.

association with cardiac defects, renal anomalies, tracheoesophageal fistulas (TEFs), biliary anomalies, Trisomy 21, and VATER. Approximately 30% of cases with duodenal atresia are associated with Down syndrome. Up to 5% of those with congenital duodenal obstruction may also have a second more distal site of obstruction.

Duodenal atresia is the most common congenital duodenum obstruction. Duodenal atresia most often occurs in the second portion of the duodenum, just past the ampulla of Vater. This location has several ramifications. The first is that the neonate will present with bilious emesis, usually after the very first feeding. The location of the atresia also results in the classic double bubble configuration on radiographs (Fig. 5-11). The double buddle is composed of the dilated stomach and duodenal bulb. The dilatation of the duodenal bulb signifies that the process is chronic instead of acute (such as a midgut volvulus). With a true duodenal atresia, there should be no air in distal bowel. A double buddle sign and the absence of air in distal bowel is pathognomonic for duodenal atresia. Further imaging with UGI is not indicated.

Duodenal stenosis and web are in the same spectrum as an atresia. They result from failure of recanalization of the duodenum during embryological development. There is also a strong correlation between annular pancreas and duodenal stenosis. The degree of stenosis may vary but the location is also often found in the second portion of the duodenum, just past the ampulla of Vater. Duodenal stenosis can present with either bilious or nonbilious emesis, usually with a latter presentation than a true atresia. The abdominal radiograph will present with distension of the

stomach and duodenal bulb, with varying degrees of distal bowel gas (Fig. 5-12).

Duodenal web is an incomplete or partial obstruction. It presents with an intraluminal membrane that has a tiny central fenestration. The size of the opening within the intraluminal membrane dictates the degree of proximal dilatation and the timing in presentation of clinical symptoms such as emesis. The duodenal web will occur in the second or third portion of the duodenum, past the ampulla of Vater. The abdominal radiographs will demonstrate distention of the stomach and duodenum with varying degrees of air in distal bowel, similar to duodenal stenosis (Fig. 5-12). During the UGI, the web may stretch downstream, forming a windsock configuration (Fig. 5-13).

Malrotation and Midgut Volvulus

Malrotation with a midgut volvulus is a surgical emergency. Any radiologist taking general call should have a basic understanding of the pathology and be able to perform an emergent UGI. A delay in the diagnosis of midgut volvulus can result in ischemic necrosis of bowel and possibly death.

During normal embryological development, herniated midgut will rotate 270 degrees in a counterclockwise fashion around the superior

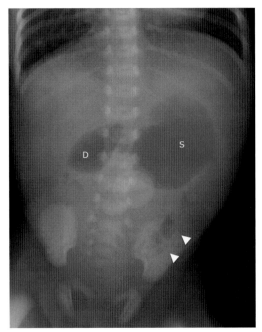

■ FIGURE 5-12 **Duodenal stenosis and web**. Supine abdominal radiograph demonstrates a distended stomach (S) and duodenal bulb (D), slightly less that a true atresia. There is also air (*white arrowheads*) in distal bowel, making duodenal atresia unlikely.

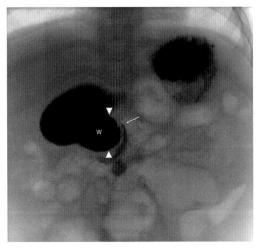

■ FIGURE 5-13 **Duodenal web in a neonate with emesis**. Single view from a UGI demonstrates distention of the proximal duodenum. There is a rounded windsock configuration (W) of the duodenum at the level of the obstructing membrane (*white arrow heads*). A small amount of contrast can be seen extruding through the small central fenestration (*small white arrow*).

mesenteric artery (SMA) prior to returning to the abdomen. In a normally rotated patient, there are two points of fixation. The duodenojejunal junction (DJJ) is fixed in the left upper quadrant of the abdomen and the cecum (ileocecal junction) will attach in the right lower quadrant of the abdomen. This will result in

small bowel having a long mesenteric attachment extending between these two points. The long fixed base keeps the small bowel mesentery from twisting upon itself. A malrotated patient will have abnormal fixation of one or both of these attachment points. As a result, the mesenteric base of the small bowel may be short and predispose the bowel to twist upon itself, resulting in a midgut volvulus. With malrotation, one can also have obstruction of the duodenum secondary to crossing LADD bands.

For clarification, note the following definitions:

- *Malrotation:* Embryologic abnormality of rotation that results in abnormal fixation of the small bowel mesentery and results in a short mesenteric base.
- *Midgut volvulus:* Abnormal twisting of the small bowel around the axis of the SMA. Volvulus can result in bowel obstruction, ischemia, or infarction.
- *Ligament of Treitz:* Also referred to as the DJJ (duodenojejunal junction). This is the anatomic location where the duodenum passes through the transverse mesocolon and becomes jejunum. It is also where the bowel changes from retroperitoneal (duodenum) to intraperitoneal (jejunum). This anatomic location is not visualized but is inferred on UGI.
- *Ladd bands:* Abnormal fibrous peritoneal bands that can occur in patients with malrotation. They are a potential causes of duodenal obstruction, in addition to volvulus.

The diagnosis of malrotation has traditionally been made on a UGI. The UGI determines that the duodenum is retroperitoneal (right lateral view) and that the DJJ is normally positioned (frontal view). On a frontal view, the DJJ is considered normally positioned when it is located to the left of the spine and at the same level as the duodenal bulb (Fig. 5-14C). On the right lateral view, the duodenum is considered retroperitoneal, when contrast exiting the stomach initially moves in a posterior and caudal direction (Fig. 5-14A). The contrast column will then move in a cranial and anterior direction (Fig. 5-14B). The two limbs of the visualized duodenum should overlap on the lateral view. The portion that starts to move in an anterior direction is the DJJ and should be at the same level as the duodenal bulb. It is important to evaluate the position of the DJJ on the first pass of contrast through the duodenum and proximal jejunum. Once the contrast column enters the proximal jejunum, it may obscure any further detailed evaluation of the duodenal sweep.

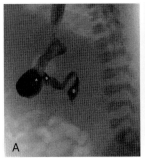
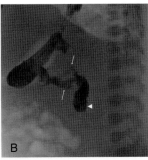
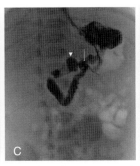
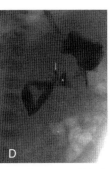

■ **FIGURE 5-14 Normal duodenal sweep on UGI. A,** The right lateral view demonstrates the gastric antrum (A), the duodenal bulb (B), and the retroperitoneal proximal duodenum (D). Initially, the contrast column will move in a posterior and then caudal direction. **B,** The contrast column will then move in a cranial (*white arrowhead*) and then anterior fashion. The two limbs of the retroperitoneal duodenum should overlap on the lateral view (*small white arrows*). **C,** The frontal view demonstrates the positioning of the duodenal bulb (*white arrowhead*) relative to the DJJ (*small white arrow*). The normal DJJ is positioned to the left of the spine and at the same level as the duodenal bulb. **D,** The left oblique view confirms the normal positioning of the DJJ. The DJJ overlaps the duodenal bulb (*small white arrow*).

Most cases of malrotation are grossly obvious. The duodenal sweep will not be completely retroperitoneal on the lateral view (5-15A), the duodenum and proximal jejunum may be in the right hemiabdomen, never crossing midline (Fig. 5-15C), the DJJ may be positioned below the level of the duodenal bulb (Fig. 5-15B), or the cecum may be high riding (Fig. 5-15D). However, when performing UGIs in children, there may be instances where the positioning of the DJJ is borderline. The criteria for a normal DJJ are not quite met but are very close. In these cases, it is good practice to continue with a SBFT. Follow the contrast column to the level of the cecum and document its exact position. If the borderline DJJ and jejunum are in the left upper quadrant and the ileum and cecum are in the right lower quadrant, the patient most likely has a long mesenteric attachment. This suggests a low risk for volvulus.

The DJJ is a mobile structure in children and can "factitiously" be moved into an abnormal position by a space-occupying lesion, such as a mass, dilated stomach or distended bowel. In addition, the presence of a nasojejunal tube or a gastrojejunal tube may alter the apparent position of the DJJ.

In patients who are malrotated, midgut volvulus may happen at any age; however, the majority are present during first 3 months of life. Midgut volvulus can be seen on a UGI as an abrupt duodenal obstruction (Fig. 5-16A and B) or a corkscrew appearance of the duodenum and proximal jejunum (Fig. 5-16C and D). The presence of bilious emesis and findings of malrotation on a UGI, with or without findings of midgut volvulus, is considered a surgical emergency.

Those with malrotation may also have LADD bands. They are fibrous peritoneal bands that

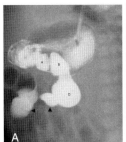
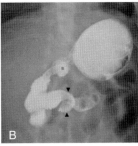
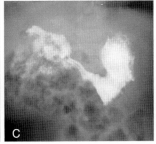
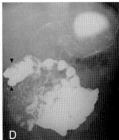

■ **FIGURE 5-15 Malrotation on a UGI and SBFT. A,** The right lateral view demonstrates the gastric antrum (A), the duodenal bulb (B), and the proximal limb of the duodenal sweep (D). The distal limb of the sweep moves in an anterior fashion (*black arrowheads*) instead of a cranial fashion. The distal limb does not ascend to the level of the duodenal bulb. This indicates that the duodenal sweep is not completely retroperitoneal. **B,** The frontal view demonstrates a midline and low lying DJJ (*black arrowheads*). The DJJ is below the level of the duodenal bulb (B). **C,** The delayed frontal view of the abdomen demonstrates contrast-filled duodenum and multiple jejunal loops in the right upper abdomen. No proximal bowel crosses midline or is positioned in the left upper abdomen. **D,** The image from an SBFT demonstrates the cecum (*black arrowheads*) to be positioned in the right mid abdomen, slightly medial, instead of the right lower abdomen.

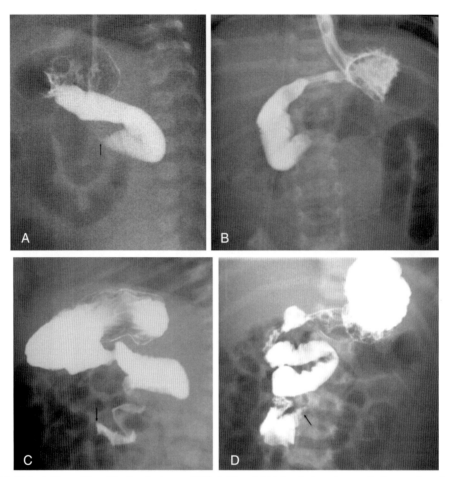

■ FIGURE 5-16 **Malrotation with midgut volvulus on UGI. A,** The right lateral view demonstrates an abrupt obstruction within the distal duodenum. There is a bird beak configuration at the site of the volvulus (*small black arrow*). **B,** The abrupt obstruction is remonstrated on the frontal view. Note distal bowel gas is present. This suggests that the volvulus was an acute process. **C,** The right lateral view demonstrates a corkscrew configuration of the duodenum and proximal jejunum. The bird beak configuration indicates the site of the volvulus (*small black arrow*). **D,** The frontal view offers another view of the corkscrew configuration of proximal small bowel, and the bird beak configuration indicates the site of the volvulus (*small black arrow*). The small bowel never reaches the left abdomen.

extend from the cecum to the liver or posterior abdominal wall. They can cross the second or third portion of the duodenum resulting in an obstruction.

Even though an UGI is still considered the gold standard for the documentation of malrotation and midgut volvulus, these entities may also be depicted with ultrasound or abdominal computed tomography (CT). Most often these exams will show a swirling pattern of bowel about the superior mesenteric vessels. These imaging studies may be ordered to evaluate abdominal pain or emesis, particularly in older children, in whom malrotation is not initially suspected. There are those that advocate ultrasound as an alternative to the UGI for the documentation of malrotation and midgut volvulus. It has been my experience that the surgical service will request an UGI to confirm

any abnormal findings on ultrasound or CT, prior to surgery, if the patient is clinically stable.

If you are performing an ultrasound on a neonate to assess for malrotation with/without volvulus, there are three main findings to document. The first is the orientation of the superior mesenteric artery (SMA) and the superior mesenteric vein (SMV). Normally the SMV is larger in caliber, positioned to the right and slightly anterior in position. The SMA is smaller in caliber, positioned to the left, with an echogenic rim (Fig. 5-17A). The majority of neonates suspected of having malrotation have an abnormal SMA/SMA orientation on ultrasound (Fig. 5-17B). Secondly, those with malrotation and midgut volvulus may demonstrate a swirling pattern (whirlpool sign) of bowel and mesenteric vessels about the SMA (Fig. 5-18). The third finding is the retroperitoneal position of the duodenum,

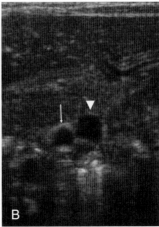
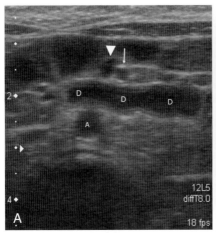

■ **FIGURE 5-17 Orientation of the SMA/SMV on abdominal ultrasound. A,** Transverse image of the superior mesenteric vessels. The SMV (*white arrowhead*) is slightly larger in caliber and positioned to the right. The SMA (*small white arrow*) is slightly smaller in caliber and positioned to the left. Note the thin echogenic rim that identifies the SMA. The third portion of the retroperitoneal duodenum (D) courses between the SMA and the aorta (A). **B,** Transverse image from a malrotated patient. The SMV (*white arrowhead*) is positioned to the left of the SMA (*small white arrow*).

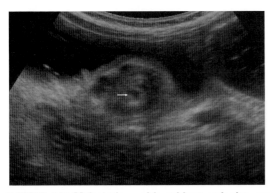

■ **FIGURE 5-18 Malrotation with midgut volvulus on abdominal ultrasound.** Transverse image demonstrates the swirling of bowel and vessels (*whirlpool sign*) about the SMA (*small white arrow*).

specifically segment three (D3). The third segment of the duodenum should course between the SMA and the aorta (Fig. 5-17A). In neonates with malrotation, the third portion of the duodenum will not pass between these structures.

Performing an Upper Gastrointestinal Series in an Infant

There are various ways to perform a UGI in an infant, and there is much debate by pediatric radiologists about the details. In my personal experience, I have found that the radiologist requires the assistance of both the radiology technologist and the parent/parents/caretaker to help hold the patient and to administer the contrast. In the event of an emergent UGI at night, the ordering ER physician or nurse can also help. In an ideal situation, the radiologist will stand by the fluoroscopic tower to obtain the necessary images, the radiology technologist will be on the opposite side of the table holding the patient in the necessary positions for imaging, and the caretaker(s) will be at the head of the table to administer the contrast. There are multiple variations on this theme, but I encourage you to always ask for more help than you think you will need. The key is to have enough help to make the exam move quickly and for you to get the necessary images, specifically the duodenal sweep. The radiologist should also spend a few minutes of time prior to the exam, instructing each member of the team on their exact role. The time spent preparing everyone will result in less surprises during the exam.

The most common questions I receive pertaining to pediatric fluoroscopy relates to the type of contrast required for each exam. The majority of UGI exams are performed using barium. It is readily available, cheap, and safe. A low-osmolality water-soluble contrast can be substituted if the patient is acutely ill or if there is a high suspicion for complications such as a perforation. Barium can be administered using a bottle with nipple or may by syringed into the side of the patient's mouth in small amounts (30 or 60 cc slip tip syringe). When performing an emergent UGI, the patient may already have an NG tube in place. Once you confirm that the tip of the NG tube is in the stomach (including any side holes), then this is the ideal method of contrast delivery.

The first step of any fluoroscopic procedure is to obtain a scout view of the abdomen. If the patient is small enough, then a fluorographic supine view of the abdomen can be obtained with the fluoro tower. If the patient is older/larger, then a radiographic supine view of the abdomen should be obtained. Check the scout for any complication, such as free air, prior to the study.

In a routine UGI, the patient will be placed in a left lateral decubitus position. The esophagus will be imaged while the patient is drinking contrast. Collimation should be tailored to image the contrast-filled and well-distended esophagus in its entirety. The patient is then placed in a supine position and imaging of the esophagus is performed in the frontal projection, including the GE junction. Note the contour and motility of the esophagus.

The next step is one of the most critical, particularly in an emergent patient. The patient is placed in the right lateral decubitus position. Once contrast starts emptying from the stomach, the radiologist must document that the duodenum is entirely retroperitoneal. The contrast column will initially move in a posterior then caudal direction (Fig. 5-14A). The contrast will then ascend in a cranial and then anterior fashion (Fig. 5-14B). The two limbs of the duodenum on the lateral view should overlap (Fig. 5-14B). The segment that moves in an anterior fashion is the DJJ and it should be at the same level as the duodenal bulb.

Once the contrast column starts to move in a cranial fashion and reaches the same level as the duodenal bulb, the patient should **immediately** be paced in a supine position. The supine position should document the exact location of the DJJ. The normal DJJ should be positioned to the left of the spine and at the same level as the duodenal bulb (Fig. 5-14C). If the infant is turned supine too early and not enough contrast is in the duodenum, the contrast will not pass leftward over the spine. You can always put the child back into the right-side-down position and get more contrast in the duodenum. If the child is turned supine too late (the worst-case scenario), the contrast will have passed into more distal loops of jejunum and may obscure visualization of the DJJ.

The final image of a UGI is a delayed (5−10 min) supine view of the abdomen. This delayed image should demonstrate several contrast-filled jejunal loops in the left upper abdomen.

Obtaining the appropriate images of the duodenal sweep is a source of much anxiety for radiologists, particularly those who do not routinely perform pediatric fluoroscopic exams. The timing and comfort in performing an UGI improves with experience, so it is imperative to perform as many as possible during your training. Furthermore, I encourage those who are not as experienced to use the last image hold button on the fluoroscopic tower to obtain the necessary images of the duodenal sweep or to use cine clips if this function is available.

If the patient has an NG tube in place, I strongly recommend using it once you have confirmed appropriate positioning of the tip. The use of the NG tube will expedite the exam and decrease the number of images necessary. After you obtain the scout image, place the patient in the right lateral decubitus position. Inject contrast under fluoroscopic visualization. One can also use an air-filled syringe to gently encourage contrast to empty from the stomach. Once the whole duodenum is filled with contrast, **immediately** turn the patient supine and document the position of the DJJ. It is good practice to drain the stomach of contrast and any fluid at the end of the study to decrease the chances of emesis and/or aspiration in an obstructed patient.

One image that I add to all UGIs is a left oblique view of the duodenal sweep (Fig. 5-14D). This view is very helpful in documenting the contour of the duodenum from a different projection. It is also a good view to confirm that the DJJ is at the same level at the duodenal bulb. This projection will be very helpful if you have placed too much contrast into the stomach and have obscured the duodenum on the supine views. The oblique positioning with help to displace the contrast-filled stomach and visualize the duodenal sweep.

Distal Intestinal Obstruction in Neonates

When abdominal radiographs demonstrate multiple distended bowel loops, a distal intestinal obstruction should be considered (Fig. 5-19A). Patients may present with failure to pass meconium, abdominal distension, or emesis (bilious vs. nonbilious). The only proximal bowel process that may be associated with multiple dilatated loops of bowel is midgut volvulus, when bowel dilates secondary to ischemia or infarction. These infants are very ill as compared to patients with a distal bowel obstruction.

In such patients, abdominal radiographs show multiple dilatated loops of bowel. They are otherwise clinically stable and will be evaluated with a contrast enema. Common causes of distal intestinal obstruction in neonates include ileal atresia, meconium ileus, Hirschsprung disease, meconium plug syndrome (small left colon), and anal atresia/anorectal malformation (Fig. 5-24).

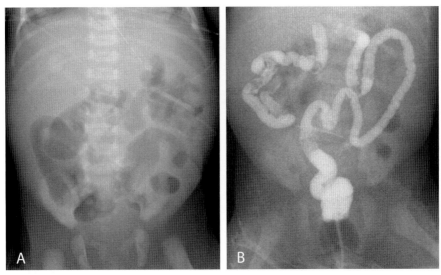

■ FIGURE 5-19 **Microcolon in a neonate that presents with emesis and failure to pass meconium. A,** Supine abdominal radiograph demonstrates multiple distended bowel loops concerning for a distal obstructive process. **B,** Diagnostic contrast enema demonstrates a microcolon, secondary to disuse. The patient was eventually diagnosed with meconium ileus.

Diagnostic enemas are most often performed using low-osmolality, water-soluble contrast agents. The most common contrast used for enemas is Cysto-Conray. Barium is not typically used because it can make the evacuation of meconium plugs in meconium ileus more difficult, whereas water-soluble enemas can be therapeutic. The best method of delivery is a Foley catheter (8-10F) with the balloon deflated and manual compression of the buttocks. Alternatively, the Foley balloon can be inflated **externally** and held against the anus to create a tight seal. As always, with pediatric fluoroscopy, I encourage you to have extra help to perform these exams. Holding the Foley catheter in place, positioning the patient, and imaging is not a one-person job.

ILEAL ATRESIA AND MECONIUM ILEUS

A microcolon is a narrow-caliber colon that results secondary to disuse (Fig. 5-19B). A distal ileal pathology is the likely cause of a microcolon. During a diagnostic contrast enema, if contrast is refluxed into a collapsed terminal ileum and the more proximal noncontrast-filled bowel is disproportionately dilatated, the diagnosis is likely to be ileal atresia (Fig. 5-20B). If the terminal ileum is distended and has multiple filling defects, the diagnosis is most likely meconium ileus (Fig. 5-21D).

Meconium ileus occurs secondary to obstruction of the distal ileum due to accumulation of abnormally tenacious meconium. It occurs exclusively in patients with cystic fibrosis

(CF). It may be complicated by perforation, volvulus of the bowel, or meconium peritonitis with/without meconium pseudocyst. Radiographs show findings of distal obstruction, which may be associated with bubble-like lucencies secondary to the accumulated meconium or with calcification secondary to perforation (Fig. 5-21A and C). Serial water-soluble enemas are commonly used in an attempt to remove the obstruction nonsurgically. There is debate about the optimal contrast agent to use for these therapeutic enemas. At our institution, we perform a therapeutic enema on those with meconium ileus using a high-osmolality water-soluble contrast such as Gastrografin (usually dilated 2:1 or 3:1 with sterile water). Any use of a high-osmolality contrast in a neonate requires special considerations (such as increased intravenous (IV) hydration) as it can cause fluid shifts in neonates and potentially an unstable clinical scenario. I strongly suggest that therapeutic enemas using high-osmolality contrast be 2performed by experienced pediatric fluoroscopists with appropriate clinical support. Table 5-2 shows a summary of the meconium-related GI diseases.

HIRSCHSPRUNG DISEASE

When performing a diagnostic enema for the evaluation of a distal obstruction, if the proximal colon is distended, relative to the distal colon, the cause of the obstruction is colonic, secondary to Hirschsprung disease or meconium plug syndrome.

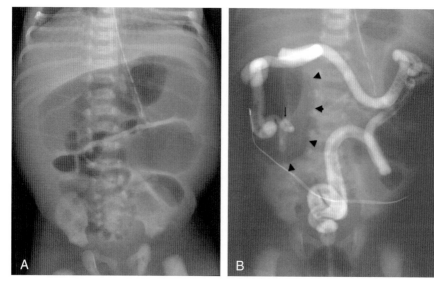

■ FIGURE 5-20 **Ileal atresia. A,** Supine abdominal radiograph demonstrates multiple dilated bowel loops concerning for a distal obstructive process. **B,** Image from a diagnostic contrast enema demonstrates a microcolon. Contrast could not be refluxed into the proximal dilated small bowel (*black arrow heads*). Note the contrast-filled appendix (*small black arrow*) that identifies the cecum.

Hirschsprung disease is related to the absence of ganglion cells that innervate the colon. The denervated colon spasms and causes a functional obstruction. Therefore, the affected portions of colon are small in caliber, and the more proximal, normally innervated colon is dilatated secondary to the obstruction (Fig. 5-22A and B). The rectum and a variable amount of more proximal colon are affected in a contiguous fashion; there are no skip lesions. Most patients with Hirschsprung disease present in the neonatal period with failure to pass meconium. However, patients can present later in life with problems related to chronic constipation. Hirschsprung disease is much more common in boys (4:1) and is associated with Down syndrome in 5% of cases.

When an enema is being performed to evaluate for possible Hirschsprung disease, it is essential to obtain early filling views, collimated to include the rectum and sigmoid colon, in both the lateral and frontal positions. Findings of Hirschsprung disease include a transition zone from an abnormally small rectum and distal colon to a dilated proximal colon (Fig. 5-22A and B). In a normal patient, the rectum has the largest luminal diameter of the left-sided colon. When the rectum is involved by Hirschsprung disease, the sigmoid colon is larger than the rectum. This is referred to as an abnormal rectosigmoid ratio. Another, but less common, finding is fasciculations or saw-toothed irregularity of the denervated colonic segment. If the entire colon is involved by Hirschsprung disease

(very rare), the entire colon may appear small in caliber and may mimic a microcolon.

Patients with Hirschsprung disease may present with associated colitis. Therefore, in patients who are suspected to have Hirschsprung disease and are acutely ill, contrast enemas should be avoided.

Definitive diagnosis is obtained by rectal biopsy, and patients are treated by surgical resection of the denervated segment. The transition zone depicted on enema does not always accurately predict where the transition from absent to present ganglion cells occurs histologically.

MECONIUM PLUG SYNDROME

Meconium plug syndrome, also referred to as *functional immaturity of the colon* or *small left colon* syndrome, is a common cause of distal neonatal obstruction. It is the most common encountered diagnosis in neonates who fail to pass meconium. It is thought to be related to functional immaturity of the ganglion cells. As in Hirschsprung disease, the distal colon does not have normal motility, which causes functional obstruction. Unlike Hirschsprung disease, it is a temporary phenomenon and resolves. Although most neonates with meconium plug syndrome are otherwise normal and have no abnormal associations, increased incidence occurs in patients who are infants of diabetic mothers or mothers who have received magnesium sulfate for eclampsia. In neonates with meconium plug syndrome, there is

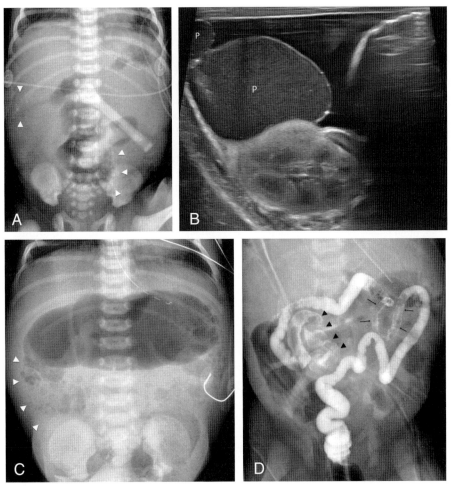

■ FIGURE 5-21 **Meconium ileus in a newborn with abdominal distention and failure to pass meconium. A,** The supine abdominal radiograph demonstrates clusters of small speckled calcifications (*white arrowheads*) in the right upper and left lower abdomen. This is seen with meconium peritonitis in a patient with an intrauterine perforation. **B,** Transverse image from an abdominal ultrasound demonstrates a complex bilobed cystic structure (P) consistent with a meconium pseudocyst. Note the tiny punctate peripheral echogenicities consistent with calcifications. There is also free ascites. **C,** Supine abdominal radiograph demonstrates a large dilated small bowel loop as well as a mottled appearance to bowel in the right hemiabdomen (*white arrowheads*). This is secondary to retained meconium in the distal ileum in a different patient with meconium ileus. **D,** Image from a diagnostic contrast enema in same patient as in C demonstrates a microcolon. There are multiple filling defects in the distal ileum (*black arrowheads*) and the transverse colon (*small black arrows*) consistent with meconium pellets. Note the noncontrast-filled dilated small bowel proximal to the meconium-filled distal ileum.

always concern about underlying Hirschsprung disease, so at many centers, all neonates who have findings of meconium plug syndrome undergo rectal biopsy. In contrast to meconium ileus, there is no significant relationship between meconium plug syndrome and CF.

On contrast enema, multiple filling defects (meconium plugs) are seen within the colon. The right and transverse colons may be more dilated than the left colon (small left colon syndrome), although these findings are variable (Fig. 5-23B). Microcolon does not occur. The rectum tends to be normal in luminal diameter, as compared with the rectums in infants with Hirschsprung disease.

The enema is often therapeutic; plugs of meconium are commonly passed during or shortly after the enema, and symptoms of obstruction often resolve within hours after the enema.

Esophageal Atresia and Tracheoesophageal Fistula

Esophageal atresia (EA) may present with or without a tracheoesophageal fistula (TEF). Patients present in two ways, the first are those with known EA on prenatal ultrasound or fetal magnetic resonance imaging (MRI). Findings include polyhydramnios, dilated blind-ending pharyngeal

---

TABLE 5-2 Summary of Meconium-Related Gastrointestinal Diseases

Meconium Ileus

- Occurs only in patients with cystic fibrosis
- Tenacious meconium causes obstruction of distal ileum
- Contrast enema: Microcolon, dilatated distal small bowel with filling defects (meconium pellets)

Meconium Plug Syndrome (Small Left Colon Syndrome)

- Not associated with cystic fibrosis
- Immaturity of colon; functional obstruction
- Self-limited, often relieved by contrast enema
- Contrast enema: Filling defects (meconium plugs) in colon, small-caliber left colon

Meconium Peritonitis

- Result of in utero perforation of bowel secondary to bowel atresia, in utero volvulus, or meconium ileus
- Imaging: bowel obstruction, peritoneal calcifications, meconium pseudocyst in peritoneal cavity

---

The atretic esophagus in EA is variable in length. The most common location is the junction between the proximal and middle third of the esophagus. EA can occur with or without a TEF. Of the five established types of fistulas, more than 80% involve a fistula between the trachea and the distal esophageal segment. Less common variations include a fistula between the trachea and the proximal or both the proximal and distal esophageal segments. Rarely, TEFs can occur in the absence of EA; this is called an H-type fistula.

Radiographs of the chest and abdomen are usually the first exam ordered in a neonate with suspected EA. Plain films may show a dilated pharyngeal pouch with or without a proximal coiled NG tube. If there is absence of bowel gas in the abdomen (Fig. 5-25A), then no TEF is suspected. If there is bowel gas present, then a TEF is suspected (Fig. 5-25B). Fluoroscopic imaging is rarely performed as surgical repair occurs within 1–2 days of birth. Surgery for EA is performed through a thoracotomy contralateral to the aortic arch. As a result, it is important to document the side of the aortic arch, which is usually confirmed by echocardiogram.

EA is usually associated with other congenital anomalies. The acronym VACTERL is used: vertebral anomalies, anal atresia, cardiac anomalies, TEF, renal anomalies, and limb anomalies. Chest radiographs in such patients should be scrutinized for vertebral and cardiac anomalies.

pouch, or the absence of a stomach bubble. The second group present shortly after birth with failure to ingest feeds, chronic drooling, regurgitation of feeds, and failed NG tube placement.

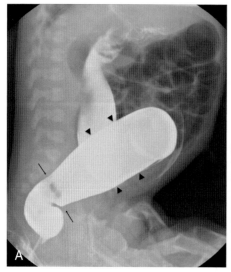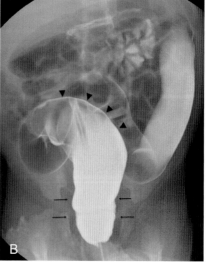

■ **FIGURE 5-22 Hirschsprung disease in a neonate with abdominal distention and failure to pass meconium. A,** Left lateral view from a diagnostic contrast enema demonstrates an abnormal rectosigmoid ration. The rectum (*small black arrows*) is smaller in caliber than the sigmoid colon (*black arrowheads*). Note the numerous distended small bowel loops throughout the abdomen suggesting a distal obstructive process. **B,** The frontal projection from the contrast enema further demonstrates a mildly serrated appearance to the narrowed rectum (*small black arrows*). The sigmoid colon (*black arrowheads*) remains larger in caliber than the rectum.

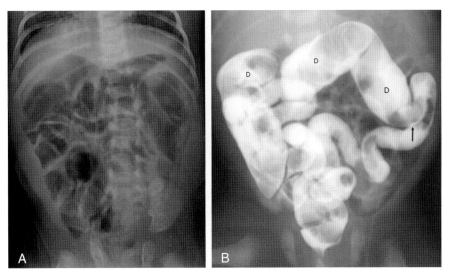

■ FIGURE 5-23 **Meconium plug syndrome (small left colon) in a neonate with distended abdomen and failure to pass meconium. A,** Abdominal radiograph demonstrates multiple distended bowel loops concerning for a distal obstruction. **B,** Diagnostic enema demonstrates a small left colon with a transition point at the splenic flexure (*small black arrow*). The colon proximal to the splenic flexure is distended (D). There are multiple filling defects throughout the colon consistent with meconium plugs.

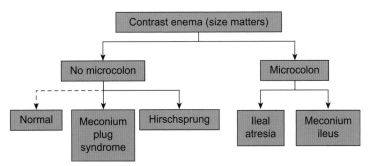

■ FIGURE 5-24 **Schematic representation for differential diagnosis of contrast enema findings in an infant with failure to pass meconium and distended abdomen.** In this scenario, there is a high incidence of pathology, and a normal study is uncommon. If the child has a microcolon, it indicates ileal pathology. If the child does not have a microcolon, the cause is probably colonic.

Children with an H-type fistula present with coughing or choking during feeds or with recurrent pneumonia. A UGI may be requested to exclude an H-type fistula. When performing a UGI for the evaluation of a TEF, it is important to obtain images with the patient in the prone or lateral projection. Supine positioning alone will often miss the fistula. The esophagus should be imaged fully distended with contrast, via the use of a bottle, syringe, or proximally placed NG tube.

Complications following repair of EA include postoperative leak, anastomotic stricture, recurrent fistula, esophageal dysmotility, and gastroesophageal reflux. A large extrapleural or paramediastinal opacity in a postsurgical patient is concerning for a leak.

Abnormalities of the Anterior Abdominal Wall

The closure of the anterior abdominal wall occurs early during fetal life. Failure of proper closure results in a number of abnormalities, including omphalocele, gastroschisis, and cloacal exstrophy. These abnormalities are diagnosed by prenatal ultrasound or fetal MRI. The location of the anterior wall defect (AWD) relative to the insertion of the umbilical cord is crucial for proper diagnosis.

Omphalocele is a midline AWD with herniation of the abdominal viscera into the base of the umbilical cord. The defect can vary in size and may contain both bowel and liver. The herniated viscera are covered by a membrane

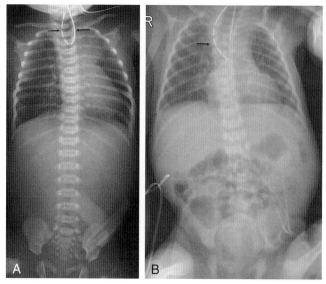

■ FIGURE 5-25 **Esophageal Atresia with and without TEF. A,** Supine view of the chest and abdomen demonstrate a coiled NG tube (*small black arrows*) in the distended pharyngeal pouch of the neck. Note there is no bowel gas in the abdomen, suggesting that a TEF is unlikely. **B,** Radiograph on a different patient demonstrates an NG tube (*small black arrow*) in a distended proximal esophageal pouch. There are multiple air-filled bowel loops in the abdomen suggesting the presence of a TEF.

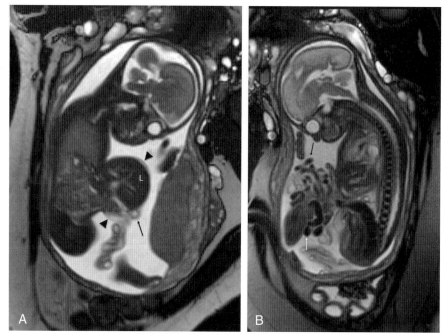

■ FIGURE 5-26 **Anterior abdominal wall defects on fetal MR. A,** Omphalocele: Sagittal view from a fetal MRI demonstrates a large omphalocele containing the liver (L). The black arrowheads delineate the membrane covering the herniated viscera. The umbilical cord attaches to the membranous sack (*small black arrow*). **B,** Gastroschisis: Sagittal view from a fetal MRI demonstrates gastroschisis with herniation of small (*small black arrow*) and large (*small white arrow*) bowel. Note there is no membrane covering the herniated viscera and it floats freely in the amniotic fluid.

creating a sac to which the umbilical cord attaches (Fig. 5-26A). More than two thirds of patients with an omphalocele have associated congenital anomalies that include cardiac, chromosomal, and urogenital. Omphalocele may also be a component of cloacal exstrophy.

Gastroschisis is an AWD that occurs lateral to the umbilical cord insertion, usually on the right

(Fig. 5-26B). The herniation most often involves bowel (small and large) and there is no covering membrane. Due to the absence of a covering membrane, the bowel is directly exposed to amniotic fluid, which is toxic to bowel. As a result, these patients will often develop bowel dysmotility and present with multiple episodes of pseudoobstruction. SBFTs are requested in an effort to differentiate pseudoobstruction from a true anatomic obstruction. These exams may take a full day or two to complete secondary to the degree of dysmotility. A final note on those with gastroschisis. They are rarely associated with other congenital anomalies, unlike omphaloceles. Cardiac anomalies are the most common if one does exist.

The cloaca is the common precursor to the intestinal, urinary, and genital tracts. Cloacal exstrophy is a severely low AWD in which there is exstrophy of the components of the cloaca. Findings may include an omphalocele, bladder exstrophy with diastasis of the pubic symphysis, imperforate anus, and spinal dysraphism. Hydrometrocolpos can be associated with cloacal exstrophy and cause renal failure if not identified due to compression and extrinsic obstruction of the distal ureters. There is a high association with renal abnormalities and dedicated renal ultrasound is usually part of the antenatal workup.

The Vomiting Infant

One of the most common exams performed in pediatric fluoroscopy is a UGI for excessive spitting up or chronic emesis in an infant. These clinical symptoms are most often associated with feeding and are usually nonbilious. The most common etiology is gastroesophageal reflux, which usually improves with age or with pharmaceutical treatment. The problem for pediatricians is that spitting up after feedings is a common and normal event. The degree of spitting up is also variable. How does a pediatrician differentiate prominent but normal regurgitation from emesis secondary to an obstruction or other pathologic etiologies? Associated problems such as failure to gain weight, failure to thrive, or respiratory symptoms suggest pathology. This difficult question often results in performing an UGI. Although such UGIs are often ordered to rule out reflux, they are actually performed to exclude an anatomic reason for excessive reflux, rather than to exclude reflux itself. There are a number of significant causes of excessive vomiting in infants. They include hypertrophic pyloric stenosis, gastroesophageal reflux, congenital stenosis, lactobezoar, and midgut volvulus. Although it is appropriate to document the presence and anatomic extent of gastroesophageal reflux when it occurs, it is not necessary to perform maneuvers to provoke reflux.

Hypertrophic Pyloric Stenosis

Hypertrophic pyloric stenosis is an idiopathic thickening of the muscle of the pylorus that results in a progressive gastric outlet obstruction. It usually occurs in infants between 1 week and 3 months of age who present with nonbilious, projectile emesis. It is much more common in males (5:1 ratio). On physical examination, the hypertrophied pylorus can be palpated as an olive-sized mass in the right upper quadrant. Hypertrophic pyloric stenosis is a diagnosis made by imaging and all children have imaging prior to surgery. It should be noted that imaging to confirm or exclude hypertrophic pyloric stenosis is not a medical emergency.

Ultrasound is the modality of choice to make a diagnosis of hypertrophic pyloric stenosis. Ultrasound allows direct visualization of the pyloric muscle and does not use radiation. The pylorus is anatomically located near the gallbladder, so an easy technique is to find the gallbladder and turn obliquely sagittal to the body in an attempt to visualize the pylorus longitudinally. The hypertrophied muscle is hypoechoic, and the central mucosa is hyperechoic. With hypertrophic pyloric stenosis, the pylorus does not open during real-time evaluation. The stomach is often distended with air and milk/formula. The pyloric muscle thickness (diameter of a single muscular wall on a transverse image) should normally be less than 3 mm. The length (longitudinal diameter) should not exceed 15 mm (Fig. 5-27B−D). Another good rule of thumb is that an easily visualized pylorus is likely to be abnormal. A normal pylorus is much more of a challenge to image (Fig. 5-27B).

Findings of hypertrophic pyloric stenosis can also be seen on an UGI. There will be delayed gastric emptying with hypertrophic pyloric stenosis. When some contrast does pass into the duodenum, the pylorus appears elongated with a narrow pyloric channel (string sign). The lumen may be puckered and have more than one apparent lumen (the double-track sign). The pylorus may indent the contrast-filled antrum (the shoulder sign) or the base of the duodenal bulb (the mushroom sign), and the entrance to the pylorus may be beak shaped (the beak sign). After the diagnosis is made, excess barium should be removed from the stomach by NG tube to avoid the risk for aspiration.

On abdominal radiographs, children with hypertrophic pyloric stenosis may show gastric distension, peristaltic waves (caterpillar sign), and mottled retained gastric content (Fig. 5-27A).

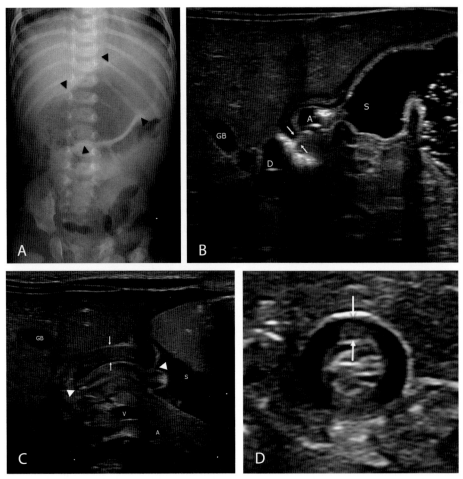

■ **FIGURE 5-27 Hypertrophic pyloric stenosis. A,** Supine abdominal radiograph demonstrates a distended stomach with lobulation (*black arrowheads*) due to hyperperistalsis. This appearance is known as the caterpillar sign. **B,** Longitudinal view of the normal pyloric channel (*small white arrows*). A normal pyloric channel may be difficult to visualize by a less experienced sonographer. The gastric antrum (A) is proximal to the channel and the duodenal bulb (D) is distal. **C,** Longitudinal view (in a different patient than in B) of the abnormal pyloric channel. With hypertrophic pyloric stenosis, the pyloric channel is elongated (*white arrowheads*), measuring 15 mm or more. The mucosa of the channel is echogenic. The individual muscular wall measures 3 mm or more (*small white arrows*). The hypertrophied pyloric musculature is hypoechoic. Note that the pyloric channel is adjacent to the gallbladder (GB). Note the normal orientation of the SMA (A) and SMV (V). **D,** A transverse view demonstrates the hypertrophied hypoechoic pyloric musculature (*small white arrows*). Again, the central mucosa is echogenic. Wall measurements are most accurately made on the transverse image.

■ INTESTINAL OBSTRUCTION IN CHILDREN

The key finding of bowel obstruction on abdominal radiographs is the presence of disproportionately dilated proximal bowel as compared to less dilated or decompressed distal small bowel or colon. With infants and small children, it may be difficult to differentiate small bowel from colon secondary to a lack of well-defined haustra and valvulae conniventes. The addition of a prone view to the standard two-view abdominal series (supine and either upright, cross-table lateral, or left decubitus view) can be helpful when differentiating between small and large bowel. On the prone view, air moves into the more posterior (nondependent) structures of the colon—the ascending and descending colon as well as the rectum. On supine views, air lies in the more anterior structures, the transverse and sigmoid colon. The position of air on this combination of views may help to localize air to the colon rather than in dilated small bowel. The presence or absence of air in the ascending colon may be of particular help when evaluating the potential existence of an ileocolic intussusception.

The most common causes of bowel obstruction in children are listed in Table 5-3. The mnemonic *take AAIIMM* against small bowel

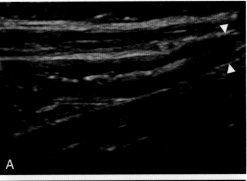

TABLE 5-3 Common Causes of Intestinal Obstruction in Older Children: Take AAIIMM

Adhesions

Appendicitis

Intussusception

Incarcerated inguinal hernia

Malrotation with volvulus

Meckel diverticulum

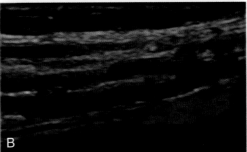

■ **FIGURE 5-28** **Normal appendix on ultrasound. A,** Longitudinal view demonstrates a blind-ending tubular structure (*white arrowheads*). The normal appendix will measure less than 6 mm in the largest transverse dimension. Notice the normal mucosa in the center of the appendix is echogenic and well delineated. **B,** Same longitudinal view with color Doppler demonstrates no hyperemia to suggest an acute inflammatory process. There are no surrounding inflammatory changes as well.

obstruction is helpful for recalling this list when under pressure. Each letter in AAIIMM represents a pertinent diagnosis. Appendicitis, intussusception, and Meckel diverticulum will be discussed in further detail.

Appendicitis

Appendicitis is the most common etiology for abdominal surgery in children. Obstruction of the appendiceal lumen results in distention of the appendix, superimposed infection, ischemia, and eventually perforation. In older children with nonperforated appendicitis, the classic symptoms include pain that begins in the periumbilical region and then migrates to the right lower quadrant. Patients may have tenderness over McBurney point, anorexia, nausea, vomiting, diarrhea, and fever. The clinical presentation is nonspecific in up to one third of patients. This is particularly true in young patients, whose diagnoses may be delayed due to limitations in communication, resulting in higher rates of perforation. Historically, the decision to operate has been made on physical examination and laboratory results; however, patients now undergo some form of imaging prior to surgery. The goal of imaging includes decreasing the negative laparotomy rates, increasing the speed of diagnosis to reduce the rate of perforation, and identifying any other alternative diagnoses.

There is much debate about the appropriate imaging algorithm for suspected appendicitis. In pediatric patients, the ideal modality is ultrasound due to its lack of radiation (Fig. 5-28A and B). However, the accuracy of ultrasound is operator dependent. Body habitus also limits the diagnostic value of ultrasound. This is why abdominal CT is still a mainstay for appendicitis workup at many medical facilities. Dedicated pediatric hospitals will advocate the primary use of ultrasound in their imaging protocols, with CT reserved for further evaluation of questionable cases. In a female patient, in whom ovarian pathology may be a cause of right lower quadrant pain (such as hemorrhagic cyst or torsion), ultrasound is usually the first exam performed. A pelvic ultrasound is usually ordered at the same time as the appendicitis study.

CT is the preferred modality in patients with suspected perforation, for visualization of a suspected abscess, in postoperative evaluations, and in obese patients. There is perpetual debate about the technical factors related to CT: IV contrast, oral contrast, rectal contrast, or noncontrast studies. In cases of uncomplicated acute appendicitis, specifically those with a short clinical presentation, IV contrast only is used to perform an abdominal CT. This will expedite the exam and any surgical intervention for an acutely ill patient.

Ultrasound evaluation of appendicitis uses graded compression of the right lower quadrant with a high-frequency transducer. Findings include a dilated blind-ending tubular structure measuring more than 6 mm, noncompressibility, echogenic shadowing appendicolith, increased flow within the walls of the appendix on color Doppler, and increased echogenicity in the surrounding mesentery (Fig. 5-29A and B). With perforation, findings include surrounding free fluid, phlegmon, or abscess in the right lower quadrant or pelvis (Fig. 5-30A).

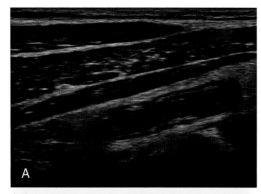

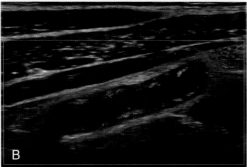

■ FIGURE 5-29 **Acute nonperforated appendicitis on ultrasound. A,** Longitudinal view demonstrates a noncompressible blind-ending tubular structure that measures more than 6 mm in the transverse dimension. There is increased echogenicity in the immediate surrounding mesentery. These findings all suggest an active inflammatory process. **B,** Longitudinal view with color Doppler demonstrates hyperemia within the wall of the inflamed appendix. Again note the increasing echogenicity in the surrounding mesentery, particularly at the tip.

CT findings include an increased appendiceal diameter (>6 mm), mural enhancement with IV contrast, induration of the surrounding mesenteric fat, appendicolith, focal ileus, and thickening of the terminal ileum and cecum. In cases of perforated appendicitis, there may also be surrounding free fluid, phlegmon, or abscess in the right lower quadrant or pelvis, as well as an evolving small bowel obstruction (Fig. 5-30B).

Radiographs no longer play a primary role in the diagnosis of patients with suspected appendicitis but may be the first imaging exam obtained for the evaluation of abdominal pain. Radiographs demonstrate an appendicolith in 5%–10% of patients with appendicitis (Fig. 5-31). Other findings may include air–fluid levels localized to the right lower quadrant, a dilated sentinel bowel loop in the right lower quadrant, splinting, and loss of the right psoas margin. With perforated appendicitis, there may be findings of small bowel obstruction, right lower quadrant extraluminal gas, and displacement of bowel loops from the right lower quadrant by a soft tissue mass. Free intraperitoneal gas is extremely uncommon secondary to appendicitis.

Noncontrast-enhanced MRI with rapid sequences has become an increasingly used tool in the diagnosis of appendicitis (Fig. 5-32A and B). The benefit of MRI is that there is no radiation and multiple studies have demonstrated its high sensitivity and specificity. There are several limitations that have prevented its full implementation, including the availability of staffing 24 hr a day as well as the potential need for sedation in younger pediatric patients.

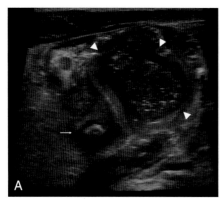

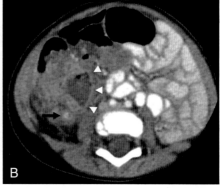

■ FIGURE 5-30 **Perforated appendicitis with abscess. A,** Transverse ultrasound through the right lower abdomen demonstrates a large loculated fluid collection (*white arrowheads*) consistent with an abscess secondary to perforation. Note the echogenic shadowing echogenicity consistent with an appendicolith adjacent to the abscess (*small white arrow*). **B,** Axial view from the abdominal CT that followed, demonstrating the same abscess (*white arrowheads*) with the adjacent appendicolith (*black arrow*). Note the diffuse mesenteric induration lateral to the abscess representing phlegmon.

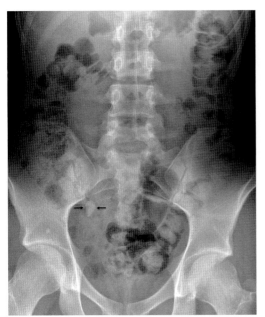

■ FIGURE 5-31 **Appendicolith on abdominal radiograph.** Supine abdominal radiograph demonstrates a calcified appendicolith in the right lower abdomen (*small black arrows*).

Intussusception

Intussusception occurs when a segment of proximal bowel (the intussusceptum) invaginates into the lumen of distal bowel (the intussuscipiens) in a telescopic manner. This process results in an obstruction, which left untreated, may develop ischemia, necrosis, and bowel perforation. The predominant types of intussusception include idiopathic ileocolic intussusception, intussusception secondary to a pathologic lead point, and incidentally noted small bowel–small bowel intussusception.

The most common form of intussusception in children is the idiopathic ileocolic type. The mechanism is thought to be due to lymphoid hypertrophy in the terminal ileum secondary to a viral illness. The terminal ileum then acts as the intussusceptum, invaginating into the proximal colon (intussuscipiens). Cases of intussusception are more prevalent in the viral months of winter and spring. The majority of patients with idiopathic ileocolic intussusception present between the ages of 3 months and 3 years. If the child is less than 3 months or older than 3 years of age, a pathologic lead point should be considered. Examples of a pathologic lead point include an inflamed appendix, Meckel diverticulum, duplication cyst, intraluminal polyps, HSP, or lymphoma. Presenting symptoms of intussusception include crampy abdominal pain, bloody (currant jelly) stools, emesis, and palpable right-sided abdominal mass.

Ultrasound is the primary imaging modality for the evaluation of children with suspected intussusception. The benefits include a lack of radiation and high sensitivity and specificity. Intussusception appears as a mass with alternating rings of hypoechogenicity and hyperechogenicity (Fig. 5-33A and B). In the transverse plane, the mass has been described as a target or donut sign and in the longitudinal plane as a pseudokidney. Ileocolic intussusception will usually measure larger than 2.5 cm in the transverse dimension. This will help to differentiate it from a small bowel–small bowel intussusception, which usually measures less than 2 cm in the transverse dimension (Fig. 5-34). When using ultrasound to evaluate for suspected intussusception, it is important to image all four quadrants of the abdomen. The intussusception can travel the entire length of the colon and

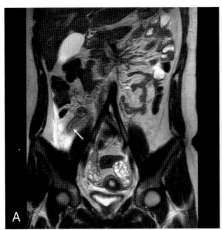
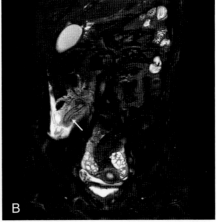

■ FIGURE 5-32 **Acute appendicitis on MRI. A,** Coronal T2 image demonstrates a dilated tubular structure in the right lower abdomen (*small white arrow*). There is free fluid lateral and inferior to the inflamed appendix. **B,** Coronal T2 image with fat saturation further accentuates the inflammatory changes about the inflamed appendix (*white arrow*). Note the normal-appearing left and right ovaries.

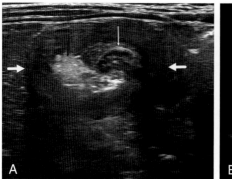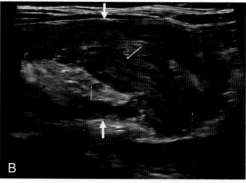

■ **FIGURE 5-33 Ileocolic intussusception on ultrasound. A,** Transverse view of an intussusception demonstrates the intussusceptum (*small white arrow*) and the intussuscipiens (*large white arrows*). There is also echogenic mesenteric fat present (*small black arrow*). The appearance of an ileocolic intussusception in the transverse plain has been likened to a target or donut sign. **B,** Longitudinal view of an ileocolic intussusception demonstrates the intussusceptum (*small white arrow*) and the intussuscipiens (*large white arrows*). There is also echogenic mesenteric fat present (*small black arrow*). The appearance of an ileocolic intussusception in the longitudinal plain has been likened to a psuedokidney.

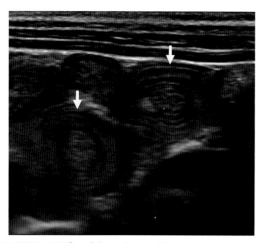

■ **FIGURE 5-34 Small bowel–small bowel intussusception on ultrasound.** Transverse view demonstrates two adjacent small bowel–small bowel intussusceptions (*white arrows*). They also demonstrate similar concentric ring pattern of varying echogenicity. The transverse dimensions of both measure smaller (<2 cm) than the ileocolic type (>2.5 cm). Small bowel–small bowel intussusceptions are predominantly transient and will usually spontaneously reduce. They are often encountered as incidental findings on abdominal ultrasound or CT.

therefore may be located in any quadrant of the abdomen.

There are associated findings on ultrasound that signify an intussusception may be difficult to reduce (higher rate of failure) or that there is a higher risk of perforation with an air reduction. Diminished or nonexistent flow within the intussusception on color Doppler indicates the presence of ischemia or necrosis. Free intraperitoneal fluid, fluid trapped within the layers of the intussusception, and the presence of a small bowel obstruction also indicated the potential for

a difficult reduction or higher chance of perforation (Fig. 5-35A and B). I would strongly suggest a discussion with the covering surgical service prior to any reduction in a child with these associated findings on ultrasound. Having representation from the emergency department or pediatric surgery on hand to help manage any potential complications is a good idea.

Abdominal radiographs are generally insensitive in the identification of an intussusception even when viewed in retrospect. However, radiographs are rarely completely normal in positive cases. Abnormal findings include a paucity of gas within the right hemiabdomen, the absence of an air-filled cecum or proximal colon, a meniscus of a soft tissue mass within the ascending or transverse colon (Fig. 5-36), and small bowel obstruction. A left decubitus or prone view may help to fill the cecum and proximal colon with air, making the presence of an ileocolic intussusception less likely. Even with these abnormal findings, an ultrasound is the appropriate exam to document the presence or absence of an ileocolic intussusception. The primary use for abdominal radiographs is to exclude free air prior to performing an air reduction in a confirmed case of intussusception.

CT plays no role in the workup of suspected intussusception. An ileocolic intussusception may be seen on CT when it is obtained for nonspecific abdominal pain, particularly in older children. When encountered on CT, ileocolic intussusception appears as a mass in the cecum or ascending colon with alternating rings of low and high attenuation (Fig. 5-37A). It is more common to see an incidental small bowel–small bowel intussusceptions on abdominal CT (or ultrasound) for the evaluation of abdominal

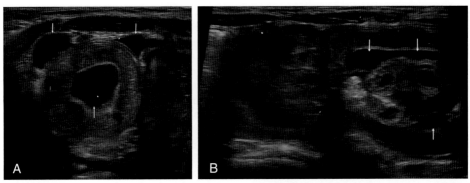

■ FIGURE 5·35 **Findings on ultrasound that suggest poor reducibility and the potential for perforation with attempted reduction. A,** Transverse view of an ileocolic intussusception demonstrated both free intraperitoneal fluid as well as fluid within the intussusception (*small white arrows*). **B,** Longitudinal view of an ileocolic intussusception demonstrated both free intraperitoneal fluid (*small white arrows*) as well as fluid within the intussusception.

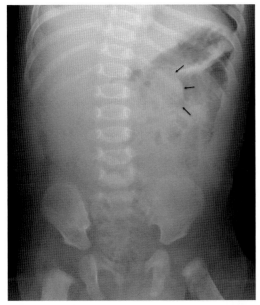

■ FIGURE 5·36 **Ileocolic intussusception on abdominal radiographs.** Supine abdominal radiograph demonstrates a soft tissue meniscus (*small black arrows*) created by the intussusception in the distal transverse colon. Note the paucity of bowel gas in the right hemiabdomen.

pain (Fig. 5-37B). Small bowel–small bowel intussusceptions are predominantly transient in nature and usually spontaneously reduce. Persistent small bowel–small bowel intussuscepts may have a lead point, similar to an ileocolic intussusception.

Imaging-Guided Reduction of Intussusception

There are several methods of increasing the pressure within the colon to reduce an intussusception while using imaging guidance. They include air insufflation with fluoroscopic guidance, contrast enema with fluoroscopic guidance, and hydrostatic reduction with ultrasound guidance. These methods are the primary therapy for intussusception, with surgery reserved for cases in which imaging-guided reduction fails or complications such as perforation occur. The method of reduction varies with each institution. I will discuss air reduction as it is my personal preference and the method used at our institution.

We use the following guidelines in preparing a patient for an attempted reduction: a working IV port, adequate hydration with IV fluids if needed, abdominal examination by an experienced physician, and consultation with the pediatric surgery service. The members of the surgical service must know that a reduction is going to be attempted, and it is preferable that they have examined the patient prior to the procedure. Contraindications for attempting pressure reduction of an intussusception include peritonitis on physical examination or pneumoperitoneum on radiographs. Findings that are not contraindications but are associated with decreased success include long duration of symptoms (>24 h) and lethargy. In a child with suspected intussusception, lethargy is a sign that the patient is potentially very ill. If a 1-year-old child does not fight you during placement of an enema tip, something is potentially wrong. Members of the surgical or emergency team should be present when performing an enema in a lethargic patient.

An air reduction requires the assistance from the X-ray technologist, as well as a Shiels intussusception air reduction system (Custom Medical Products, Maineville, OH). The key to success is generating an adequate rectal seal, so that sufficient colonic pressures can be obtained. This is

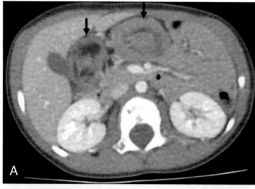

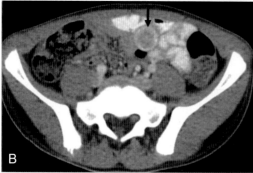

■ FIGURE 5-37 **Intussusception on abdominal CT. A,** Axial view from an abdominal CT performed for abdominal pain demonstrates a large ileocolic intussusception (*black arrows*) which can be seen in both the transverse plain (target sign) and the longitudinal plain (pseudokidney). Note the mesenteric fat within the intussusception. **B,** Axial view from an abdominal CT on a different patient than in A demonstrates an incidental small bowel–small bowel intussusception (*black arrow*). They are usually transient and spontaneously resolve.

best achieved by having the X-ray technologist hold the buttocks tightly as the radiologist takes images and insufflates the colon. Pressure generated within the colon should not exceed 120 mm Hg when the child is at rest (pressure will exceed 120 mm Hg when the patient cries or valsalvas). With air insufflation, the intussusception is encountered as a mass. The reducing intussusception moves retrograde to the level of the ileocecal valve. Criteria for successful reduction include resolution of the soft tissue mass and free reflux of gas into the small bowel (Fig. 5-38A–D).

The "mass" may get stuck at the ileocecal valve. In this case, some radiologists give the child time to rest and let the edema decrease with repeat of the air reduction in 30–60 min. This is often successful. Overall success rates for reduction enemas are greater than 85%. The risk for perforation is less than 1.0%. The risk for recurrent intussusception after a successful reduction is less than 10%, with most occurring within the first 24 hr after the reduction.

Recurrence can be treated with repeated air reduction enemas as long as the patient is clinically stable.

With air reduction, perforation has been reported to be higher in patients with clinical symptoms greater than 72 hr. Perforation has also been reported to be higher in those with a redundant colon, particularly the sigmoid colon and when air is seen dissecting within the layers of the intussusception during the reduction. A perforation during an air reduction can lead to tension pneumoperitoneum. This must be reduced immediately as it may result in circulatory collapse of the patient. This is best achieved with needle decompression. An 18-gauge needle inserted midline below the umbilicus should quickly release the tension pneumoperitoneum. The surgical service (and potentially the code team) should be immediately notified.

Meckel Diverticulum

The omphalomesenteric duct is a fetal structure that connects the umbilical cord to the portion of the gut that becomes the ileum. Any or all of the structure can abnormally persist into postnatal life, resulting in cysts, sinuses, or fistulae from the umbilicus to the ileum. Most commonly, the portion adjacent to the ileum persists and results in a Meckel diverticulum. Meckel diverticula can cause painless rectal bleeding, focal inflammation, perforation, distal small bowel obstruction, or intussusception. Bleeding occurs secondary to the presence of ectopic gastric mucosa within the diverticulum. Although most Meckel diverticula do not contain gastric mucosa, almost all of those associated with bleeding do. Therefore, the imaging modality of choice to detect bleeding Meckel diverticula is nuclear scintigraphy with technetium (Tc) 99m pertechnetate, which accumulates in gastric mucosa. Such studies demonstrate foci of increased activity within the right lower quadrant of the abdomen, similar to that within the stomach (Fig. 5-39A and B).

Meckel diverticulum can be encountered on abdominal ultrasound or CT for the evaluation of pediatric abdominal pain, more commonly than those who present with GI bleeding. On CT, there are three general patterns, including an inflamed tubular structure (that is not the appendix) with surrounding inflammatory changes. This may be present with or without perforation (Fig. 5-40A and B). The second pattern includes a distal small bowel obstruction. The actual Meckel diverticulum may not always be visualized (Fig. 5-41A and B). Third is a small bowel–small bowel intussusception often with associated small bowel obstruction.

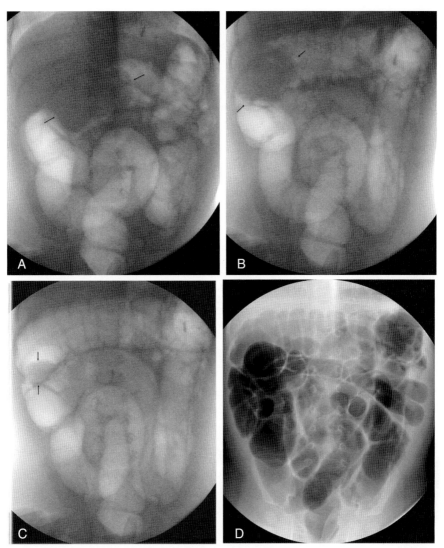

■ **FIGURE 5-38 Air reduction of an ileocolic intussusception. A,** Fluoroscopic image from air reduction shows the intussusception as a large fusiform soft tissue mass (*small black arrows*). **B,** Subsequent fluoroscopic image shows progressive retrograde motion of the soft tissue mass (*small black arrows*) toward the ileocecal valve. **C,** Further imaging shows near total resolution of the soft tissue mass (*small black arrows*). **D,** Final image from an air enema shows two criteria for a successful reduction: resolution of the soft tissue mass and reflux of air into distal small bowel.

Gastrointestinal Duplication Cysts

A duplication cyst is a congenital lesion that is intimately associated with the GI tract. They can occur anywhere along the GI tract, but most commonly occur near the terminal ileum. The majority of duplication cysts do not communicate with the lumen of the GI tract. They are usually round or oval-shaped cystic lesions with a classic bowel wall signature on ultrasound. This consists of alternating hypoechoic and hyperechoic layers that correlate with the mucosa (hyperechoic) and muscular layers (hypoechoic) (Fig. 5-42A). These cysts may present as a palpable mass on clinical exam, they may cause compression of adjacent

anatomic structures, and they may also be a lead point for bowel obstruction, intussusception, or volvulus. Duplication cysts that contain gastric mucosa can become inflamed, ulcerate, and bleed (Fig. 5-42B).

■ SWALLOWED FOREIGN BODIES

The majority of foreign bodies swallowed by children pass through the GI tract without complication. The proximal esophagus, particularly at the level of the thoracic inlet, is the most common site for a lodged foreign body (Fig. 5-43A and B). Suspected foreign body

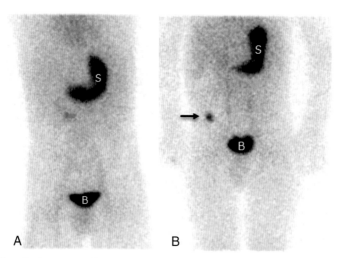

■ FIGURE 5-39 **Meckel diverticulum on nuclear scintigraphy. A,** Negative Study (Normal): Coronal view from a nuclear scintigraphy study using technetium (Tc) 99m pertechnetate. There is increased activity in the stomach (S) and bladder (B). No activity noted in the right lower abdomen. **B,** Positive Study (Abnormal): Coronal view from a nuclear scintigraphy study using technetium (Tc) 99m pertechnetate. There is increased activity in the right lower abdomen (*small black arrow*), similar to the activity in the stomach (S). This indicates the presence of ectopic gastric mucosa within a Meckel diverticulum.

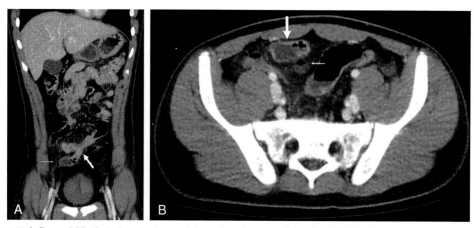

■ FIGURE 5-40 **Inflamed Meckel diverticulum with perforation on abdominal CT. A,** Coronal view demonstrates a tubular structure originating from the antimesenteric side of the distal ileum (*large white arrow*). There is a fluid-filled, dilated tip with mural enhancement (*small white arrow*). Notice the induration of the surrounding mesenteric fat. **B,** Axial view demonstrates the tip of a fluid-filled, dilated tubular structure with mural enhancement (*large white arrow*). There is induration of the surrounding mesenteric fat as well as extraluminal air (*small white arrow*) suggesting perforation.

ingestion should be evaluated with a lateral view of the airway as well as a frontal view of the chest and abdomen. This will assess the entire GI tract from the mouth to the anus. Foreign bodies, even when initially lodged, may be asymptomatic; thus, imaging is necessary to confirm their presence. Follow-up radiographs to ensure passage are sometimes obtained.

The most common foreign body encountered in pediatric patients is an ingested coin (personal experience ranks the top three as coins, button batteries, and Lego pieces). A foreign body that becomes lodged in the proximal esophagus may result in complications, such as edema, ulceration, perforation, and even a TEF. The edema and inflammatory changes surrounding a lodged esophageal foreign body may create an inflammatory mass that compresses the adjacent trachea. Such foreign bodies may present with respiratory rather than GI symptoms. These localized inflammatory changes can be seen on the lateral radiograph as increased distance caused by soft tissue density between the coin and the anterior airway (Fig. 5-44).

Lodged esophageal foreign bodies may also be a sign of underlying pathology, such as an

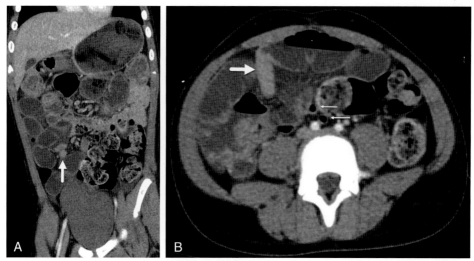

■ FIGURE 5-41 **Meckel diverticulum with small bowel obstruction on abdominal CT. A,** Coronal view demonstrates multiple fluid-filled dilated small bowel loops, consistent with a distal small bowel obstruction. The large white arrow indicates the Meckel diverticulum acting as a lead point for the obstruction. **B,** Axial view demonstrates the Meckel diverticulum (*large white arrow*) acting as a lead point for the distal small bowel obstruction. Note the separate normal air-filled appendix (*small white arrows*).

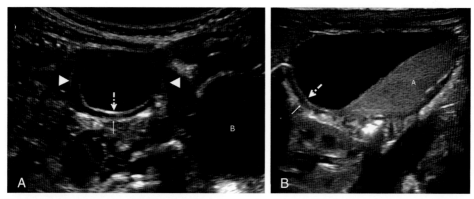

■ FIGURE 5-42 **Duplication cyst on ultrasound. A,** Transverse view from abdominal ultrasound demonstrates an oval-shaped cystic lesion (*white arrowheads*). Note "gut signature" with the inner echogenic ring resents the mucosal layer (*discontinuous white arrow*). The outer muscular layer is hypoechoic (*small white arrow*). B, bladder. **B,** Transverse view from abdominal ultrasound in a different patient than in A demonstrates an oval-shaped cystic lesion anterior to the right kidney. It has a layering echogenic fluid level (A), secondary to hemorrhage. Note "gut signature" with the inner echogenic ring resents the mucosal layer (*discontinuous white arrow*). The outer muscular layer is hypoechoic (*small white arrow*).

esophageal stricture or vascular ring that did not allow the foreign body to pass. Esophageal strictures can occur secondary to a number of causes in children, including corrosive ingestion, previous EA repair, epidermolysis bullosa, and chronic gastroesophageal reflux. Such strictures are often treated with balloon dilatation under fluoroscopic guidance.

There are several types of foreign bodies that deserve special mention: zinc pennies, multiple magnets, and button batteries.

- *Zinc pennies:* Post-1982 U.S. pennies have been constructed with a zinc-based core and copper coating (rather than the pre-1982 solid copper pennies). If retained in the stomach, the coins can corrode, allowing the zinc core to escape and react with the hydrochloric acid in the stomach to create a reaction that can lead to gastric ulceration. Radiography of such coins retained in the stomach can show irregular margins and developing radiolucent holes in the coins (Fig. 5-45). If a penny is retained in the stomach and the patient is symptomatic, the coin should be removed endoscopically.

- *Multiple magnets:* Small magnets associated with colorful children's toys are an enticing

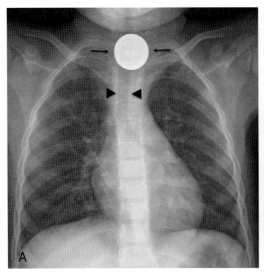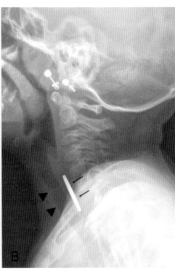

■ FIGURE 5-43 **Ingested radiopaque foreign body (coin) on radiographs. A,** Frontal view chest radiograph demonstrates a round radiopaque foreign body (*small black arrows*) lodged at the level of the thoracic inlet. The foreign body is seen in face and extends past the confines of the tracheal air column (*black arrows*), documenting that it is in the proximal esophagus. **B,** Lateral airway in same patient demonstrates a round radiopaque foreign body lodged at the thoracic inlet (*small black arrow*). The addition of a lateral airway helps to confirm that the foreign body is posterior to the tracheal air column (*black arrow heads*) and in the proximal esophagus. Note the lack of soft tissue thickening between the coin and the trachea.

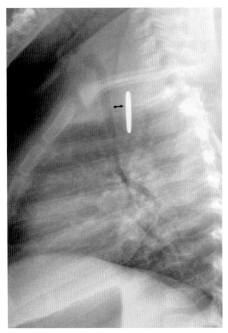

■ FIGURE 5-44 **Lodged foreign body (coin) as seen on lateral chest radiograph.** Single lateral chest radiograph demonstrates a radiopaque foreign body in the proximal esophagus. Note the soft tissue thickening between the coin and trachea (*double arrow*) indicating chronicity resulting in inflammatory tissue.

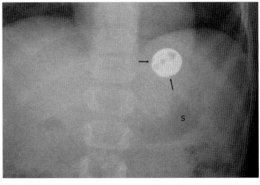

■ FIGURE 5-45 **Erosive changes of an ingested foreign body (coin).** A single frontal radiograph of the proximal abdomen demonstrates a round radiopaque foreign body in the proximal stomach (S). There are three round central erosions as well as erosions of the peripheral margins (*small black arrows*). These findings suggest a post-1982 penny.

target for ingestion. When several are ingested, they can attract each other across bowel wall, creating an obstruction. Adherent magnets are less likely to pass through the GI tract. With time, this may lead to ischemia, necrosis, obstruction, and perforation. It should be considered a surgical emergency when identified. When multiple radiopaque densities are seen lining up in tandem (stacked configuration), multiple magnets should be suspected (Fig. 5-46). These foreign bodies should absolutely be followed until complete passage, if the patient is asymptomatic and not treated surgically. Close attention to bowel gas pattern is necessary to assess for any evolving obstruction.

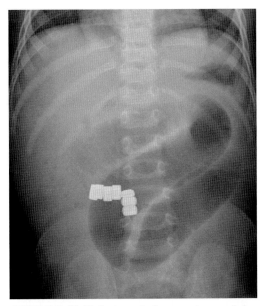

■ FIGURE 5-46 **Multiple ingested magnets on abdominal radiograph.** The frontal radiograph of the abdomen demonstrates multiple stacked radiopaque foreign bodies, suspicious for ingested magnets. The radiograph also demonstrates several dilated small bowel loops, conserving for a bowel obstruction. Ingested magnets with an obstruction is a surgical emergency.

- *Button batteries:* Button batteries are disk-shaped batteries, such as those used in cameras, watches, and hearing aids. When swallowed by children, these batteries can cause caustic injury to the mucosa, particularly when lodged in the esophagus. The shape of these batteries is slightly different from that of a coin. On a lateral view, the front edge of the battery is beveled with a central protrusion. In other words, the central portion is thicker than the peripheral portion (Fig. 5-47A). On a frontal view, the periphery may appear to have two circular edges (Fig. 5-47B). These batteries may develop corrosive holes if they are present internally for some time. The potential presence of a button battery should be communicated to the caregivers immediately to allow for expedited removal.

■ ABNORMALITIES OF THE PEDIATRIC MESENTERY

The mesentery does not have easily defined boundaries on imaging. Therefore, localization of abnormalities involving the mesentery can be difficult. The relative paucity of mesenteric fat in pediatric patients can make the detection and localization of pathology in the mesentery even more difficult than in adults, in whom fat is typically more abundant. The following criteria is helpful in localizing a process to the mesentery in children: (1) partial or complete envelopment of the SMA or SMV, (2) peripheral displacement of jejunal or ileal bowel loops, or (3) extension of the process from superocentral to inferoperipheral in a cone-like manner. Mesenteric disorders are divided into the specific patterns of involvement that can readily be identified by imaging: developmental abnormalities of

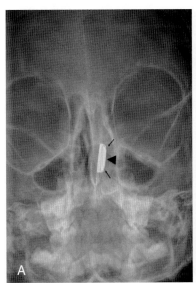
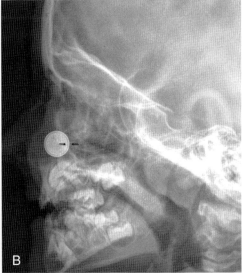

■ FIGURE 5-47 **Button battery lodged in nares on airway radiographs. A,** When viewed on end, the central portion of a button battery (black arrowhead) is thicker than the periphery, which is beveled (*small black arrows*). **B,** When viewed in the lateral position, the periphery of the button battery appears as two concentric rings (*small black arrows*).

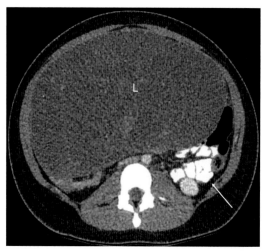

■ FIGURE 5-48 Mesenteric lymphatic malformation. Axial view from an abdominal CT demonstrates a large cystic lesion (L) with some subtle internal septations. Note the displacement of both small and large bowel to the periphery (*small white arrow*).

mesenteric rotation, diffuse mesenteric processes, focal mesenteric masses, and multifocal mesenteric masses. Abnormalities of mesenteric rotation have already been discussed.

Processes that can involve the mesentery diffusely include edema, hemorrhage, and inflammation. Diffuse mesenteric processes characteristically demonstrate replacement of mesenteric fat by soft tissue attenuation with resultant loss of vascular definition. Focal masses within the mesentery in the pediatric population can be secondary to lymphoma, mesenteric cysts, desmoids, teratomas, and lipomas. Mesenteric cysts, also known as lymphatic malformations, are developmental anomalies in which focal lymphatic channels fail to establish connections with the central lymphatic system. Lymphatic malformations are often multiseptated and quite large (Fig. 5-48).

Multifocal mesenteric masses most commonly represent lymphadenopathy. On imaging studies such as CT, mesenteric lymph nodes are considered abnormal if they are greater than 6 mm in the shortest transverse diameter. Mesenteric lymphadenopathy can be a manifestation of either a malignant neoplastic or an inflammatory process. Malignant entities include lymphoma, lymphoproliferative disorder, and metastatic disease. Lymphomatous involvement of the mesentery most often occurs in association with non-Hodgkin disease and usually involves both the mesentery and retroperitoneum. Most cases of non-Hodgkin lymphoma that involve the abdomen demonstrate lymphadenopathy rather than parenchymal masses. Mesenteric lymphadenopathy can also be caused by infectious disorders, such as tuberculosis, cat-scratch disease, or fungal infection. Central low attenuation with peripheral enhancement favors an inflammatory over a neoplastic cause. Central low attenuation of lymph nodes has been described as characteristic of tuberculosis and is present in as many as 60% of cases. With tuberculosis, it has been suggested that the mesenteric adenopathy is often more pronounced relative to the degree of retroperitoneal adenopathy.

Note that visualization of nodes smaller than 6 mm in the inferior mesentery and right lower quadrant is common in children and has no clinical significance.

Mesenteric Lymphadenitis

Enlarged mesenteric lymph nodes are frequently noted in children who present for the evaluation of abdominal pain. Enlarged mesenteric lymph nodes with no other identifiable source for the abdominal pain are attributed to mesenteric lymphadenitis. The inflammation of the lymph nodes is usually benign in etiology and self-limiting.

Patients may present with right lower quadrant pain and tenderness, nausea, vomiting, fever, and leukocytosis. Due to the overlap in clinical presentation between appendicitis and mesenteric lymphadenitis, these patients are often initially evaluated for acute appendicitis with ultrasound or abdominal CT. Common findings on imaging include a cluster of >3 enlarged mesenteric lymph nodes measuring >6 mm in the shortest transverse dimension. The cluster of nodes is most likely localized to the right lower quadrant of the abdomen, anterior to the right psoas muscle (Fig. 5-49A and B). There may be some induration of the adjacent mesentery as well as thickening of the terminal ileum. The most important finding is to document a normal appendix.

■ NEONATAL JAUNDICE

Hyperbilirubinemia or physiologic jaundice can be present in more than half of normal full-term neonates. Its presence is related to physiologic destruction of red blood cells in the polycythemic newborn. Jaundice that persists beyond 2 weeks of age will result in laboratory and imaging workup. 90% of cases are due to biliary atresia or neonatal hepatitis, with choledochal cyst as the third etiology.

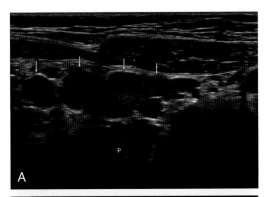

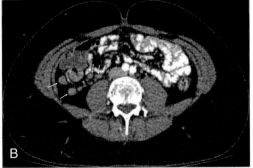

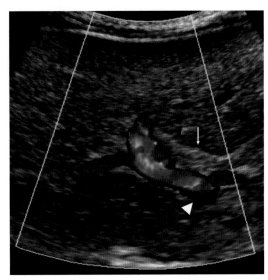

■ FIGURE 5-50 **Biliary atresia on ultrasound.** Single transverse view from a Doppler ultrasound study demonstrated a triangular echogenic structure (*small white arrow*) adjacent to the portal vein (*white arrowhead*). This is consistent with the *triangular cord sign* of biliary atresia.

■ FIGURE 5-49 **Mesenteric lymphadenitis in a patient with abdominal pain. A,** Transverse view from an abdominal ultrasound demonstrates a cluster of enlarged mesenteric lymph nodes (*small white arrows*) in the right lower quadrant of the abdomen. Note that they are anterior to the right psoas muscle (P). The appendix was normal on this exam. **B,** Axial view from an abdominal CT in a different patient as in A demonstrates enlarged mesenteric nodes in the RLQ, anterior to the right psoas muscle. The appendix was air filled and normal on this exam. Note the excessive subcutaneous fat consistent with obesity.

Biliary Atresia versus Neonatal Hepatitis

It is important to identify children with biliary atresia early, usually before 2 months of age, as they may have a higher rate of success from surgical intervention (Kasai procedure). A detailed workup is also essential to avoid unnecessary laparotomies in patients with neonatal hepatitis. These two entities have overlapping clinical, laboratory, and pathologic findings. As a result, diagnostic imaging plays an important role in differentiating between the two etiologies. In biliary atresia, there is congenital obstruction of the biliary system. Specifically, there is bile duct proliferation intrahepatically and focal or total absence of the extrahepatic bile ducts. Cirrhosis ultimately develops unless there is corrective surgery. There is an association with the abdominal heterotaxy syndromes and with Trisomy 18.

Ultrasound is the initial imaging modality in neonates with jaundice. It can exclude the presence of choledochal cysts and dilatation of the biliary system due to other causes of obstruction. Absence of a gallbladder is suggestive of biliary atresia. A small gallbladder can be seen with both biliary atresia and neonatal hepatitis and is an indeterminate finding. A normal or enlarged gallbladder helps to exclude the diagnosis of biliary atresia and therefore is supportive of the diagnosis of neonatal hepatitis. Visualization of a triangular echogenic structure in the porta hepatis, adjacent to the main portal vein, is called the *triangular cord sign* (Fig. 5-50). It is thought to be the remnant of the common bile duct in biliary atresia. Like the absence of the gallbladder, the triangular cord sign is specific for biliary atresia. Hepatic echotexture is another indeterminate factor as it can be normal or coarsened in both biliary atresia and neonatal hepatitis.

Hepatobiliary scintigraphy with Tc 99m-iminodiacetic acid derivatives remains one of the most reliable ways to differentiate between neonatal hepatitis and biliary atresia. The radiopharmaceutical is usually administered after pretreatment with oral phenobarbital, which enhances hepatocellular function. Normally, radiopharmaceutical uptake and clearance by hepatocytes exceeds cardiac blood pool tracer activity. Radiotracer can normally be visualized within the biliary tree and intestines 15 min after administration. Classically described scintigraphic appearance of neonatal hepatitis includes delayed uptake of radiotracer by hepatocytes,

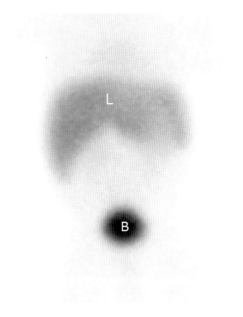

■ **FIGURE 5-51 Biliary atresia in a newborn with persistent jaundice.** Radionuclide hepatobiliary image obtained at 2 h shows prompt uptake in the liver (L). No activity is present in the gastrointestinal tract centrally. Radioactivity is also seen in the urinary bladder (B).

slow clearance of blood pool radiotracer, but eventual radiotracer excretion into bowel. In biliary atresia, radiotracer uptake and clearance by hepatocytes are adequate, with prominent hepatic activity identified, but the tracer never reaches the GI tract, even on 24-hr delayed imaging (Fig. 5-51).

An abnormal nuclear medicine scan will result in a liver biopsy. If biliary atresia is suspected on pathology, the patient will then move on to an intraoperative cholangiogram, which is the gold standard in confirming biliary atresia. Those with an abnormal cholangiogram will then have a Kasai procedure.

Choledochal Cyst

Choledochal cyst is defined as local dilatation of the biliary ductal system and is categorized into five types based on the anatomic distribution of dilatation. These types include localized dilatation of the common bile duct below the cystic duct (Fig. 5-52A and B), dilatation of the common bile and hepatic ducts, localized cystic diverticulum of the common bile duct, dilatation of the intraduodenal portion of the common bile duct (choledochocele), and multiple cystic dilatations involving both the intrahepatic and extrahepatic bile ducts (Caroli disease).

Choledochal cysts are uncommon, and the cause is unknown. They most commonly present early in life with jaundice (80%), abdominal mass (50%), or abdominal pain (50%). Ultrasound demonstrates a cystic mass in the region of the porta hepatis that is separate from an identifiable gallbladder. The presence of a dilated common bile duct or cystic duct or visualization of the hepatic duct directly emptying into the cystic mass confirms the diagnosis. In cases of a nonspecific cyst in the region of the porta hepatis, hepatobiliary scintigraphy can be used to demonstrate radiotracer accumulation within the cyst, confirming the diagnosis.

■ LIVER MASSES

Hepatic masses constitute roughly 6% of all intraabdominal masses in children, and primary hepatic neoplasms constitute about 2% of all pediatric malignancies. Primary hepatic neoplasms are the third most common abdominal malignancy in childhood, after Wilms tumor and neuroblastoma. Hepatic masses can be present at birth (congenital), neoplastic (primary or metastatic), or infectious in etiology.

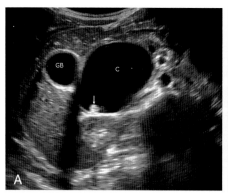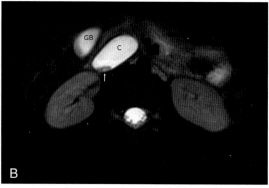

■ **FIGURE 5-52 Choledochal cyst in neonate with persistent jaundice. A,** Transverse image from an abdominal ultrasound demonstrated a large cyst (C) in the porta hepatis, medial to the gallbladder (GB). Note that there is a dependent echogenicity in the cyst (*small white arrow*) consistent with a stone. This represents a type one choledochal cyst, dilatation of the common bile duct, the most common type. **B,** Axial T2 image from an abdominal MRI in same patient shows the large cyst (C) medial to the gallbladder (GB). There are dependent stones (*small white arrow*).

Children most often present with a palpable mass on clinical exam. They may also present with abdominal pain, distension, anorexia, jaundice, paraneoplastic syndromes, hemorrhage, and congestive heart failure. Ultrasound is usually the first radiological exam performed to evaluate the clinical finding. Ultrasound will confirm the organ of origin, characterize the consistency of the lesion, and demonstrate its extent. Radiographs are limited in their evaluation of a palpable abdominal mass, but may demonstrate hepatic calcifications, bowel displacement from the right upper quadrant, or an enlarged hepatic silhouette. Ultrasound is often performed as a screening examination. Whether CT or MRI is the modality of choice for the definitive imaging of liver masses is a controversial topic. The major role of cross-sectional imaging is to define the extent of the lesion in relation to hepatic lobar anatomy, vascular and biliary structures for preoperative planning. Cross-sectional imaging is also used to monitor tumor response to chemotherapy or radiation. For most hepatic malignancies, complete tumor resection or liver transplantation is essential for cure. The types of liver resection performed include left lobectomy, left lateral segmentectomy, right lobectomy, or trisegmentectomy (right lobe and medial segment of the left lobe). Therefore, a mass must be confined to the left or right lobe or the right lobe plus the medial segment of the left lobe to be considered resectable. If a lesion does not meet anatomic requirements for resectability at initial imaging, the child is often treated with chemotherapy, with or without radiation, and then reimaged to see if resection is a viable option.

The differential diagnosis for liver masses in children is extensive and only a few of the most common etiologies will be covered in this section. Congenital masses include hepatic or choledochal cysts as well as congenital hemangiomas. Primary hepatic neoplasms include hepatoblastoma, infantile hemangioma, mesenchymal hamartoma, hepatic adenoma, hepatocellular carcinoma, lymphoma, undifferentiated embryonal sarcoma, and angiosarcoma, Metastatic lesions may be seen with Wilms or neuroblastoma. Infectious etiologies include bscesses of fungal, bacterial, or parasitic origin.

Several factors help to focus the differential diagnosis, including the age of the child, the alpha fetoprotein level, associated clinical findings, and whether the lesion is solitary or multiple on imaging. The most common hepatic tumors in children younger than 5 years of age include hepatoblastoma, hepatic hemangioma, mesenchymal hamartoma, and metastatic disease resulting from neuroblastoma or Wilms tumor.

TABLE 5-4 Causes of Pediatric Hepatic Masses
Age Less Than 5 Years
• Hepatoblastoma (+AFP)
• Congenital or infantile hepatic hemangioma
• Mesenchymal hamartoma
• Metastatic disease (Wilms, neuroblastoma)
Age Greater Than 5 Years
• Hepatocellular carcinoma (+alpha fetoprotein level)
• Undifferentiated embryonal sarcoma
• Hepatic adenoma
• Hemangioma
• Metastatic disease
Immunocompromised State
• Lymphoproliferative disorder
• Fungal infection

In children older than 5 years of age, the most common tumors include hepatocellular carcinoma, undifferentiated sarcoma, hepatic adenoma, hemangioma, and metastatic disease (Table 5-4). Liver tumors that are associated with elevated serum alpha fetoprotein levels include hepatoblastoma and hepatocellular carcinoma. Most of the remaining liver masses are not associated with an elevated serum alpha fetoprotein. The presence of multiple liver lesions favors metastatic disease, abscesses, infantile hemangiomas, lymphoproliferative disorder, or hepatic adenomas associated with a predisposing syndrome (Fanconi anemia and Gaucher disease).

Hepatoblastoma

Hepatoblastoma is the most common primary malignant liver tumor of childhood. More than half of cases occur in patients less than 1 year of age with the majority of cases occurring before the age of five. The most common presentation is a large palpable mass, usually painless, in the right upper quadrant of the abdomen. Predisposing conditions include Beckwith–Wiedemann syndrome, hemihypertrophy, familial polyposis coli, Gardner syndrome, Wilms tumor, and biliary atresia. However, most hepatoblastomas are seen in patients without associated conditions or underlying liver disease. Serum alpha fetoprotein levels are elevated in more than 90% of patients and necessary in making the appropriate diagnosis. Metastasis may occur, with the lungs as the most common site.

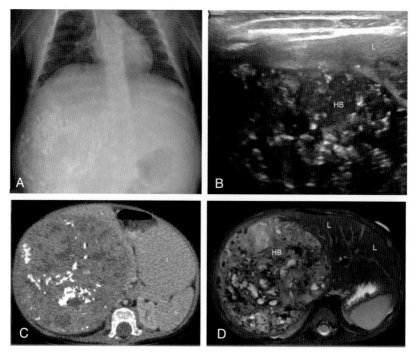

■ **FIGURE 5-53 Hepatoblastoma. A,** Supine radiograph demonstrates numerous coarse calcifications in the right upper quadrant of the abdomen. There is a paucity of bowel visualized in the right upper abdomen. **B,** Transverse image from an abdominal ultrasound demonstrates a large well-defined solid mass (HB) in the right lobe of the liver (L). Note the heterogeneity of the lesion. Numerous echogenic calcifications are present, several with posterior acoustic shadowing. **C,** Axial image from a precontrast abdominal CT demonstrates a large well-defined solid mass occupying the right lobe of the liver. The mass (HB) is heterogeneously lower in attenuation than the adjacent liver parenchyma (L). The necrotic areas are the lowest in attenuation. Note numerous high-attenuation calcifications. **D,** Axial T2 with fat saturation demonstrates the heterogeneous nature of the mass (HB) with numerous areas of necrosis (low signal) and cystic change (high signal).

Abdominal radiographs may show an enlarged hepatic silhouette, displaced bowel, or focal hepatic calcifications (Fig. 5-53A). Calcifications will be present in half of the imaged hepatoblastomas. Ultrasound will demonstrate a large, well-circumscribed, heterogeneous mass (5−53B). Hepatoblastoma can displace or invade the adjacent vascular structures, making a Doppler study an important preoperative exam. Doppler will help to identify flow within the mass as well. Hepatoblastoma may have areas of hemorrhage or necrosis which accounts for the heterogeneous appearance on imaging. The tumor is usually hypoattenuating on precontrast CT (5−53C) and will heterogeneously enhance following the administration of IV contrast. Similarly on MRI, the tumor will be hypointense on T1 with heterogeneous increased intensity on T2 varying with the degree of hemorrhage and necrosis present (Fig. 5-53D).

Childhood Liver Hemangiomas

Childhood liver hemangiomas are categorized into congenital or infantile type. Congenital hemangiomas are present at birth and tend to be solitary lesions. They usually do not grow any further after birth and will involute by 12−14 months (Fig. 5-54A and B). Conversely, infantile hemangiomas will grow during the first years of life and will spontaneously involute over the course of 1−7 years. Symptomatic cases usually present by 6 months of age. Infantile hemangiomas may be multifocal or diffuse. While they can be asymptomatic, they may also present as an abdominal mass with high-output congestive heart failure, consumptive coagulopathy (thrombocytopenia), or hemorrhage.

Infantile hemangiomas are well defined and hypoechoic on ultrasound. All modalities, including ultrasound, may demonstrate varying degrees of heterogeneity with the presence of hemorrhage and necrosis. Internal flow on Doppler will vary with the presence of shunting. On CT, they are usually low in attenuation and may contain calcification. After the administration of IV contrast, the lesion will demonstrate a peripheral somewhat nodular enhancement pattern, with delayed central enhancement. On MRI, the lesion is hypointense on T1 and hyperintense on T2 sequences (5-55A). IV contrast administration will demonstrate a

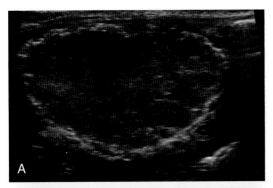

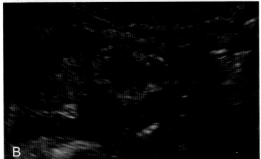

■ **FIGURE 5-54 Congenital hemangioma on ultrasound. A,** Longitudinal image of the left lobe of the liver, obtained within the first month of life, demonstrates a large oval-shaped solid mass that is heterogeneous in echogenicity. **B,** The second longitudinal image, obtained 1 year after birth, shows significant involution of the hemangioma.

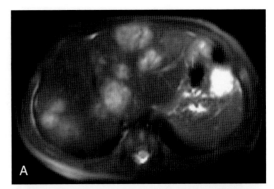

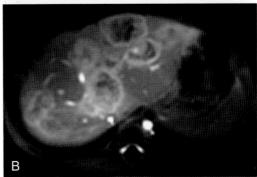

■ **FIGURE 5-55 Infantile hemangioma on MRI. A,** Axial T2 sequence with fat saturation demonstrates multiple liver lesions with increased signal. **B,** Axial postcontrast image demonstrates peripheral, nodular enhancement.

similar peripheral enhancement pattern as CT (Fig. 5-55B). The lesions may contain internal flow voids with the presence of shunting.

On all imaging modalities, the descending aorta superior to the level of the hepatic branches of the celiac artery may appear abnormally enlarged as compared to the infrahepatic aorta, due to the degree of shunting occurring within the liver.

Mesenchymal Hamartoma of the Liver

Mesenchymal hamartoma of the liver is a rare, benign, cystic liver mass that most commonly presents before 2 years of age. The lesion is considered a developmental anomaly rather than a true neoplasm. Patients usually present with a large painless abdominal mass and a normal serum alpha fetoprotein level. On ultrasound, it presents as a multiseptated cystic mass (5-56A). There is no significant internal flow on Doppler. With CT, the septations and any residual solid component will enhance with IV contrast. With MRI, the cystic components are hypointense on T1 with hyperintensity on T2 sequences (Fig. 5-56B). Treatment involves surgical resection.

■ BLUNT ABDOMINAL TRAUMA

The abdomen is the second most common site of trauma in children, cranial trauma occurring more frequently. Blunt force trauma accounts for the majority of the trauma to the abdomen. The most common etiology is motor vehicle accidents. Other causes include blunt force trauma from abuse, fall from height, full contact sports as well as a direct abdominal injury from handlebars when falling off a bike. Abdominal trauma may result in a CT of the abdomen and pelvis, FAST scan in the emergency department, or a targeted ultrasound to assess for specific solid organ injury. Ultimately, CT is the preferred imaging modality as it has the ability to get delayed images to look for active extravasation, lung windows to look for free air, and bone windows to look for acute fractures. Added benefits of CT include thin-cut axial images, sagittal and coronal reformatted images, and the ability to perform a CT cystogram to assess for bladder rupture.

There is overlap in imaging pediatric patients and adults for trauma. Similarities such as the appearance and grading of solid organ injury are not discussed in detail here. However, there are several significant differences that are emphasized in this section.

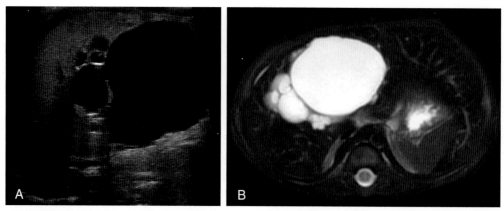

■ **FIGURE 5-56 Mesenchymal Hamartoma. A,** Transverse ultrasound demonstrates a multilobulated cystic lesion in the liver. Note the through transmission associated with the cystic lesions. **B,** Axial T2 MRI sequence with fat saturation shows cystic components with increased signal.

Solid Organ Injuries

The frequency in which solid organ injuries occur in children is as follows: liver, spleen, kidney, adrenal gland, and pancreas. Injury to multiple solid organs can occur in up to 20% of trauma cases. The majority of solid organ injuries in children are treated conservatively. Surgery is only required for a small percentage of those who are hemodynamically unstable. The size and appearance of a solid organ injury has been shown to be an inaccurate predictor of which patients will need surgery. Active extravasation of contrast from a solid organ laceration (attenuation as high as the enhancing aorta seen within the peritoneum) in concert with a poor or declining clinical state strongly predicts the need for surgery (Fig. 5-57A and B). This is the reason why trauma studies should be checked real time and the decision for delayed images made immediately to look for active extravasation. If there is any question of active extravasation, delayed images through the solid organ or whole abdomen should be obtained. The trauma service should also be notified immediately.

Heterogeneous splenic enhancement, consisting of alternating bands of high and low attenuation, can be seen when imaging early in the arterial phase of enhancement. This *zebra stripe* appearance should not be mistaken for splenic injury as it involves the spleen in a diffuse manner instead of a focal injury. If there is any question as to its etiology, delayed images through the spleen are helpful. On delayed imaging, this pattern will diminish and the spleen will have a more homogeneous attenuation.

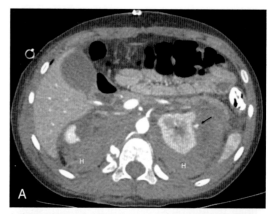

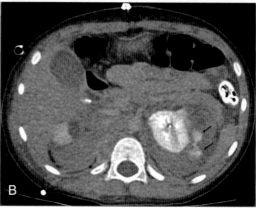

■ **FIGURE 5-57 Active extravasation on trauma abdominal CT. A,** Axial image from a contrast-enhanced trauma CT demonstrates bilateral perinephric hematomas (H) secondary to renal lacerations. There is a small focus of high attenuation (*small black arrow*) lateral to the left kidney suspicious for active extravasation. Note the attenuation is similar to that within the aorta. **B,** 10 min delayed images were obtained which demonstrated increased areas of high attenuation (*small black arrows*) lateral to the left kidney confirming active extravasation.

Bowel Injury

Bowel injury is uncommon in children with abdominal trauma. It occurs in less than 10% of cases. Bowel injury is associated with a motor vehicle accident with seat belt trauma to the abdomen. The most common CT finding includes focal bowel wall thickening secondary to mural hematoma. Findings are most often seen in the jejunum and duodenum. Rarely is there full bowel wall perforation or associated mesenteric injury.

The bowel wall thickening may be concentric (Fig. 5-58A and B) or eccentric (Fig. 5-59A and B). Other associated findings include focal bowel dilatation, prominent bowel wall enhancement, mesenteric soft tissue induration, and free peritoneal fluid in the absence of solid organ injury,

particularly fluid tracking along the root of the mesentery. More specific findings of bowel injury are less common and include free intraperitoneal air, extraluminal bubbles of gas in the vicinity of a subtle injury, and, even less common, active extravasation of enteric contrast. Most bowel injury is managed nonoperatively with bowel rest, unless the patient becomes unstable. Those that decompensate or those with frank evidence of bowel perforation or mesenteric injury will have an emergent laparotomy.

A patient who receives a direct blow to the upper abdomen, commonly by bicycle handlebars or by abuse, is at increased risk for having a duodenal hematoma with/without an associated pancreatic laceration. On CT, duodenal hematomas can be eccentric or circumferential. The attenuation can be high, low, or mixed. Duodenal hematoma most often occurs in the second or third portion of the duodenum. There may also be hemorrhage within the lumen of the duodenum (Fig. 5-59A and B).

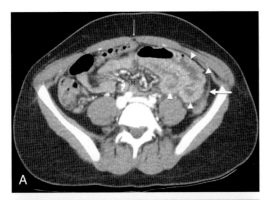
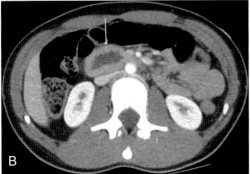

■ FIGURE 5-58 **Bowel injury on trauma abdominal CT. A,** Axial image demonstrates several loops of jejunum with concentric mural thickening (*white arrowheads*) representing bowel injury. Note the adjacent induration of the fat along the left paracolic gutter (*large white arrow*). Secondary signs of bowel injury are present including a focus of free intraperitoneal air along the nondependent anterior abdomen (*small white arrow*). There is also fluid and induration tracking along the root of the mesentery (M). The mesenteric fat should always be low attenuation in contrast to the hazy appearance on this scan. **B,** Axial image in a different patient than in A demonstrates concentric thickening (*small white arrow*) of the third portion of the duodenum secondary to handlebar injury to the proximal abdomen.

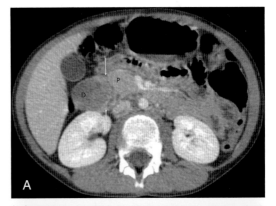
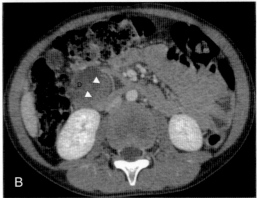

■ FIGURE 5-59 **Duodenal hematoma secondary to handlebar injury. A,** Axial trauma CT demonstrates eccentric thickening (*small white arrows*) of the medial wall of the second portion of the duodenum (D). Note the adjacent pancreatic head (P). **B,** Adjacent image demonstrates lobulated ill-defined material within the lumen of the duodenum representing hemorrhage (*white arrowheads*).

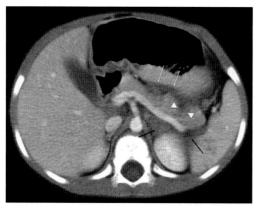

■ **FIGURE 5-60** **Pancreatic laceration on trauma CT.** Axial image demonstrates low-attenuation cleft in the tail of the pancreas (*white arrowheads*) consistent with laceration. Note that there is fluid in the lesser sac (*small white arrows*) and the left anterior pararenal space (*small black arrows*). Incidental finding is partial visualization of linear low attenuation in splenic (S) consistent with laceration.

Pancreatic Trauma

In pediatric patients, a solitary pancreatic injury is rare and is usually seen in concert with an acute injury to the liver, spleen, or duodenum. Pancreatic lacerations appear as linear low-attenuated parenchymal defects. A complete transection would be a low-attenuated linear defect extending from the anterior to the posterior margin of the organ with fluid or hematoma intervening between the two components. An actual laceration may be difficult to visualize in a young patient and peripancreatic fluid is a more sensitive finding for acute pancreatic injury. Look for fluid in the lesser sac, anterior pararenal space, or insinuating between the pancreas and the splenic vein (Fig. 5-60).

Hypoperfusion Complex

Clinical findings associated with hypovolemic shock can be masked for a longer period of time in children due to more pronounced peripheral vasospasm and tachycardia. The constellation of findings on CT in patients with hypovolemic shock has been referred to as **hypoperfusion complex** or as **shock bowel**. CT findings include intense enhancement of the bowel wall, mesentery, adrenal glands, liver, kidneys, and pancreas. Patients can also have intense enhancement and decreased caliber of the inferior vena cava and aorta. Bowel is often fluid filled and diffusely dilated (Fig. 5-61A–D). The bowel findings (bowel wall enhancement and dilatation over a diffuse distribution) should not be confused with the focal dilatation and bowel wall thickening more typical of bowel injury. In cases in which the cause of the bowel findings is unclear, identifying other findings of the hypoperfusion complex is helpful.

The CT findings of hypoperfusion complex may be identified prior to the clinical findings of shock. Radiologists should view trauma studies real time and immediately notify the trauma team of any findings associated with hypoperfusion complex. This may help the covering service prepare for or even prevent the evolution of a hemodynamically unstable patient.

■ THE IMMUNOCOMPROMISED CHILD

Children can be born with a compromised immune system (i.e., primary immunodeficiency disorder) or may develop a weakened or compromised state due to treatment for an underlying illness (i.e., therapy for malignancy, bone marrow transplantation, solid organ transplantation, or acquired immunodeficiency syndrome).

Immunocompromised children may develop several issues related to immunodeficiency (infection), thrombocytopenia (bleeding), and other therapy-related complications, including mucositis, radiation injury, and the development of a secondary neoplasm. They may also experience a higher rate of common childhood illnesses that are unrelated to the patients' primary disorder.

The GI tract is commonly involved with such processes. These patients usually present with nonspecific symptoms, which may result in an abdominal ultrasound or CT. Imaging may be requested to rule out an abscess; however, loculated fluid collections are not common in immunocompromised children. More often, the abdominal source of sepsis is related to bowel wall compromise secondary to a variety of types of enterocolitis. Common bowel diseases in immunocompromised children are listed in Table 5-5. Most of these enterocolitis are managed medically unless there is evidence of perforation (extraluminal gas, free fluid, or fluid collection). When intraabdominal abscesses are present, they are often related to systemic fungal infection with organisms such as *Candida albicans* or *Aspergillus* species. These abscesses appear as multiple small, low-attenuation lesions within the liver, spleen, or kidneys (Fig. 5-62).

Pseudomembranous Colitis

Immunocompromised patients routinely receive antibiotics and as a result, they are at risk for

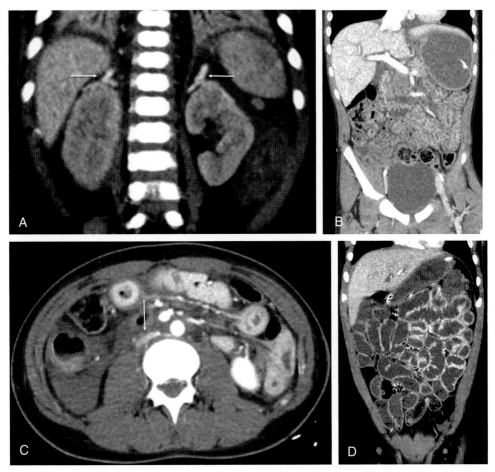

■ **FIGURE 5-61 Hypoperfusion complex on trauma CT shown in various patients. A,** Coronal image demonstrates hyperenhancing bilateral adrenal glands (*small white arrows*). **B,** Coronal image demonstrates diffuse hyperenhancement of nondilated bowel. **C,** Axial image demonstrates a flattened IVC (small white arrow). There is also hyperenhancemnt of visualized bowel. **D,** Coronal image demonstrates bowel to be diffusely fluid filled and dilated. The walls are also hyperenhancing.

developing pseudomembranous colitis. This involves the overgrowth of and toxin production by *Clostridium difficile*, after the use of antibiotics. On gross inspection of the colon, there are discrete yellow plaques (pseudomembranes) involving the mucosal surface. The plaques are usually separated by normal-appearing mucosa. In the majority of cases, there is diffuse colonic involvement (pancolitis). There is marked colonic wall thickening (average 15 mm), greater in degree than that seen in most other types of colitis. It is common for contrast material to insinuate between the pseudomembranes and swollen haustra creating an ***accordion sign***, which is highly suggestive of the diagnosis (Fig. 5-63). Because pseudomembranous colitis involves predominantly the mucosa and submucosa, the degree of inflammatory change in the pericolonic fat is often disproportionately subtle compared with the degree of colonic wall thickening.

Neutropenic Colitis

Neutropenic colitis (typhlitis, necrosing enteropathy) is a life-threatening, right-sided colitis associated with severe neutropenia. Pathologically there is necrosing inflammation of the cecum and ascending colon with associated ischemia and secondary bacterial invasion. CT shows bowel wall thickening, pericolonic fluid, and inflammation of the pericolonic fat, usually isolated to the cecum and ascending colon. In my experience, the adjacent terminal ileum is often involved as well (Fig. 5-64).

Graft-versus-Host Disease

Acute graft-versus-host disease is a process specific to bone marrow transplant recipients, in which donor T lymphocytes cause selected epithelial damage of recipient target organs.

TABLE 5-5 Computed Tomography Findings Helpful in Differentiating Bowel Diseases in Immunocompromised Children

Entity	Typical Distribution	Imaging Features
Pseudomembranous colitis	Pancolitis	Marked bowel wall thickening Nonprominent pericolonic inflammatory changes
Neutropenic colitis	Cecum, right colon, terminal ileum	Bowel wall thickening Pericolonic inflammatory changes
Cytomegalovirus colitis	Cecum, right colon, terminal ileum	Bowel wall thickening Pericolonic inflammatory changes
Mucositis	Small and large bowel	Fluid-filled, dilatated small and large bowel Thin but enhancing bowel wall Absent bowel wall thickening or adjacent inflammatory changes
Graft-versus-host disease	Diffuse small and large bowel	Mucosal enhancement Fluid-filled dilatated bowel Mild wall thickening, isolated to small bowel Prominent mesenteric inflammatory changes
Lymphoproliferative disorder	Focal involvement, typically small bowel	Marked focal bowel wall thickening Aneurysmal dilatation of bowel lumen Parenchymal (liver) masses Lymphadenopathy—mesenteric masses
Gastrointestinal bleeding	Anywhere	High-attenuation fluid or heterogeneous mass (solid thrombus) within lumen Associated underlying enterocolitis

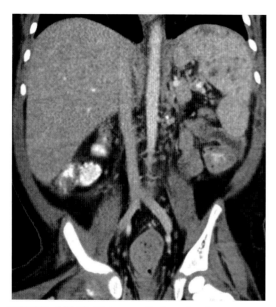

■ FIGURE 5-62 **Multiple small fungal abscesses on abdominal CT.** Coronal image from an abdominal CT in an immunocompromised child. The spleen contains numerous small low-attenuated foci consistent with fungal abscesses.

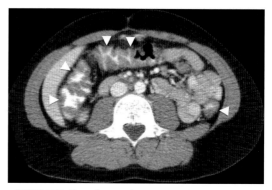

■ FIGURE 5-63 **Pseudomembranous colitis on CT.** Axial image demonstrates a pancolitis involving both the proximal and distal colon (*white arrowheads*). The oral contrast insinuates itself between the mucosal plaques and edematous haustra, creating the accordion sign. Note that the colon thickening is disproportionately greater than any inflammation of the surrounding mesenteric fat.

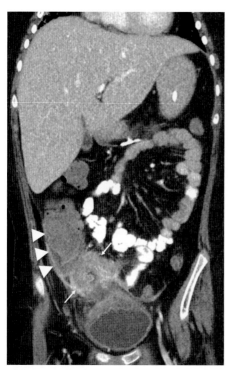

■ **FIGURE 5-64 Neutropenic colitis on CT**. Coronal image demonstrates thickening of the cecum and proximal ascending colon (*white arrowheads*). There is also associated thickening of the terminal ileum (*small white arrows*). Note the diffuse induration of the mesenteric fat and thickening of the bladder dome.

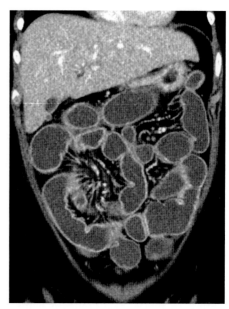

■ **FIGURE 5-65 Graft-versus-host disease on CT**. Coronal image from an abdominal CT demonstrates fluid-filled, diffusely dilated bowel throughout the abdomen. There is also thin diffuse enhancement of the mucosa.

Histopathologically, there is extensive crypt cell necrosis and, in severe cases, diffuse destruction of the mucosa throughout both the large and small bowel and replacement with a thin layer of highly vascular granulation tissue. CT findings include diffuse enterocolitis from the duodenum to the rectum. Compared with the previously discussed causes of enterocolitis, bowel wall thickening may be mild, isolated to the small bowel, or absent. More characteristically, there is abnormal bowel wall enhancement in a central, mucosal location corresponding pathologically with the thin layer of vascular granulation tissue replacing the destroyed mucosa. Both the small and large bowel are usually filled with fluid and dilated (Fig. 5-65). There is often prominent infiltration of the mesenteric fat and soft tissue attenuation.

Mucositis

Gut toxicity has been described in association with multiple chemotherapeutic agents. The damage to the mucosa, impaired ability of the bowel to regenerate its protective cell lining (mucosa), and resultant inflammation are often referred to as mucositis. Patients present with nonspecific abdominal complaints, including nausea, vomiting, and abdominal pain, and they demonstrate an ileus pattern on abdominal radiographs. The symptoms may be severe and difficult to separate clinically from the previously discussed processes. On CT, the predominant finding of mucositis is dilatated, fluid-filled loops of small and large bowel. There may be mild associated small bowel wall enhancement. Marked bowel wall thickening, predominance of colonic involvement, and marked abdominal inflammatory changes suggest other diagnoses. Treatment for mucositis is supportive.

Lymphoproliferative Disorder

Lymphoproliferative disorders are lymphoma-like diseases related to an uncontrolled proliferation of cells infected by the Ebstein–Barr virus in an immunocompromised host. Although they can occur in any immunocompromised individual, they are more commonly encountered in patients following solid organ transplantation, particularly those receiving multiorgan transplantation. The incidence is higher in pediatric versus adults transplant patients. Clinical presentation usually occurs within the first year following surgery and the etiology is thought to be due to the chronic immunosuppression related to the transplant.

Imaging findings are varied, but those involving the abdomen including focal parenchymal mass, diffuse lymphadenopathy, mesenteric mass, and

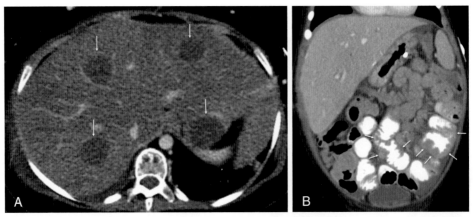

■ **FIGURE 5-66 CT findings of lymphoproliferative disorder within the abdomen. A,** Axial image, in a posttransplant patient, demonstrates four round low-attenuated lesions within the liver (*small white arrows*). **B,** Coronal image, in a different posttransplant patient, demonstrates diffuse bowel wall thickening of small bowel (small white arrows).

diffuse bowel wall thickening (Fig. 5-66A and B). In contrast to typical non-Hodgkin lymphoma, which manifests more commonly as abdominal lymphadenopathy, lymphoproliferative disorder is more often associated with parenchymal organ involvement, most commonly the liver. In solid organ transplant recipients, the distribution of disease tends to occur in the vicinity of the transplanted organ. Therefore, liver transplant recipients are more likely to have abdominal disease than are heart transplant recipients. Therapeutic options include reduction of immunosuppressive therapy, when possible, and chemotherapy.

■ COMPLICATIONS RELATED TO CYSTIC FIBROSIS

Newborn infants with CF presenting with meconium ileus have already been discussed. Older children and adults can present with a similar syndrome, distal intestinal obstruction syndrome (DIOS), also known as *meconium ileus equivalent*. These children develop obstruction secondary to inspissated, tenacious intestinal contents lodging within the bowel lumen. On radiographs, there is abundant stool within the right colon and distal small bowel and findings of obstruction (Fig. 5-67). Contrast enemas with dilute Gastrografin may be utilized to relive the obstruction. However, it should be noted that patients with CF who develop pseudomembranous colitis can develop abdominal pain and bloating, much like those with DIOS, and often do not have the diarrhea typically seen with pseudomembranous colitis. If diffuse colonic wall thickening is identified on imaging studies, the possibility of pseudomembranous colitis should be raised. In these cases, a therapeutic contrast

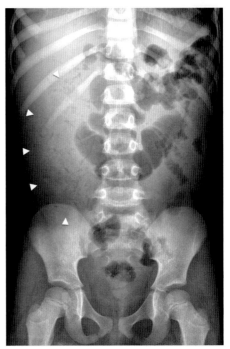

■ **FIGURE 5-67 Distal intestinal obstruction syndrome (DIOS) in patient with cystic fibrosis.** Supine radiograph of the abdomen demonstrates inspissated material in the distal ileum and proximal colon (*white arrowheads*). There are distended small bowel loops proximal to the inspissated material.

enema is contraindicated. CF patients may also develop fibrosing pathology of the colon secondary to pancreatic enzyme replacement therapy. This may result in colon thickening and strictures.

Other GI problems associated with CF include hepatic steatosis, cirrhosis, portal hypertension with varices, atrophy and fatty infiltration of the pancreas, pancreatic duct

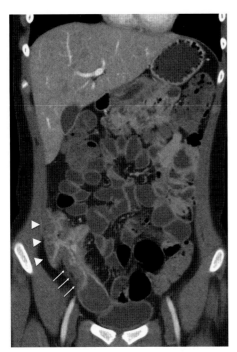

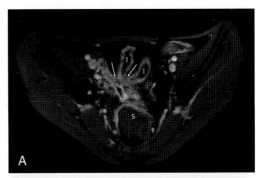

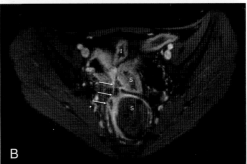

■ **FIGURE 5-68 Crohn's disease on abdominal CT.** Coronal image demonstrates thickening of a short segment of the terminal ileum (*small white arrows*). Note the fluid-filled, dilated small bowel loops proximal to the terminal ileum. There is also thickening of the cecum and proximal ascending colon (*white arrowheads*).

■ **FIGURE 5-69 Crohn's disease on abdominal MRI. A,** Axial postcontrast T1 image demonstrates enhancement of several loops of distal ileum (I) and sigmoid colon (S). There is also extensive fistulas connection between the two visualized loops of ileum and sigmoid colon (*small white arrows*). **B,** Axial image further caudal demonstrates a larger fistulas tract (*small white arrows*) between ileum and sigmoid colon.

calcifications, cholelithiasis, gallbladder wall thickening, microgallbladder, increased incidence of ileocolic intussusception, and appendicitis.

■ INFLAMMATORY BOWEL DISEASE IN CHILDREN

Inflammatory bowel disease (IBD) is far more common in the pediatric population than expected. Up to 25% of cases may occur in patients before the age of 18. Crohn's disease accounts for up to 65% of childhood IBD. In pediatric patients, Crohn's disease involves the distal small bowel and colon more than in the adult presentation (Fig. 5-68). Magnetic resonance enterography has become the study of choice for IBD due to its lack of radiation and superior ability to identify associated fistulas and strictures associated with IBD (Fig. 5-69A and B).

Imaging findings include bowel wall thickening, mucosal hyperenhancement, mural stratification (ability to see three layers), skip lesions (Crohn's disease), strictures, fistula, engorgement of the vasa recta, pericolonic inflammation, enlarged lymph nodes, abscess, and free fluid.

■ PEDIATRIC OBESITY

Pediatric obesity has reached epidemic proportions. It is estimated that up to one third of children in the United States are obese. Pediatric obesity has also become a worldwide trend. Obesity is a multiorgan system problem and has a well-documented association with several diseases of childhood, including slipped capital femoral epiphysis, glucose intolerance and type 2 diabetes mellitus, hyperlipidemia, steatohepatitis, cholelithiasis, obstructive sleep apnea, hypertension, pulmonary embolism, and psychosocial problems (poor self-esteem, depression). Many of these traditionally adult disorders are now being encountered in obese children. The challenge with obese children is to help them prevent the potential of becoming an obese adult and developing the numerous associated comorbidities.

Obesity poses multiple challenges for imaging in a pediatric setting. Image quality, imaging equipment weight limits, and diameter size limits can all be problematic with obese patients.

Some have suggested that pediatric radiologists can take an advocacy role in raising awareness of pediatric obesity by including mention of obesity, when present, in the impression of the radiology report. Written documentation of obesity in an official report can increase caregivers' and parents' awareness of a child's obesity.

SUGGESTED READING

Adeyiga AO, Lee EY, Eisenberg RL: Focal hepatic masses in pediatric patients, *AJR Am J Roentgenol* 199(4):W422–W440, 2012.

Brinkley MF, Tracy ET, Maxfield CM: Congenital duodenal obstruction: causes and imaging approach, *Pediatr Radiol* 46:1084–1095, 2016.

Callahan MJ, Talmadge JM, MacDougall RD, et al.: Selecting appropriate gastroenteric contrast media for diagnostic fluoroscopic imaging in infants and children: a practical approach, *Pediatr Radiol* 47:372–381, 2017.

Crane GL, Lee EY: Post-transplantation lymphoproliferative disorder in a child with multivisceral transplant, *Pediatr Radiol* 40, 2010.

d'Almeida M, Jose J, Oneto J, Restrepo R: Bowel wall thickening in children: CT findings, *Radiographics* 28(3):727–746, 2008.

Edwards EA, Pigg N, Courtier J, et al.: Intussusception: past, present and future, *Pediatr Radiol* 47:1101–1108, 2017.

Fields TM, Michel SJ, Butler CL, Kriss VM, Albers SL: Abdominal manifestations of cystic fibrosis in older children and adults, *AJR Am J Roentgenol* 187(5):1199–1203, 2006.

Gongidi P, Bellah RD: Ultrasound of the pediatric appendix, *Pediatr Radiol* 47:1091–1100, 2017.

Gubernick JA, Rosenberg HK, Ilaslan H, Kessler A: US approach to jaundice in infants and children, *Radiographics* 20(1):173-195, 2000.

Hameed S, Caro-Domínguez P, Daneman A, et al.: The role of sonography in differentiating congenital intrinsic duodenal anomalies from midgut malrotation: emphasizing the new signs of duodenal and gastric wall thickening and hyperechogenicity, *Pediatr Radiol* 50:673–683, 2020.

Karmazyn B, Werner EA, Rejaie B, et al.: Mesenteric lymph nodes in children: what is normal? *Pediatr Radiol* 35:774–777, 2005.

Maxfield CM, Bartz BH, Shaffer JL: A pattern-based approach to bowel obstruction in the newborn, *Pediatr Radiol* 43:318–329, 2013.

Moore MM, Kulaylat AN, Hollenbeak CS, et al.: Magnetic resonance imaging in pediatric appendicitis: a systematic review, *Pediatr Radiol* 46:928–939, 2016.

Muchantef K, Epelman M, Darge K, et al.: Sonographic and radiographic imaging features of the neonate with necrotizing enterocolitis: correlation findings with outcomes, *Pediatr Radiol* 43:1444–1452, 2013.

Olson DE, Kim YW, Donnelly LF: CT findings in children with Meckel diverticulum, *Pediatr Radiol* 39:659–663, 2009.

Orth RC, Guillerman RP, Zhang W, et al.: Prospective comparison of MR imaging and US for the diagnosis of pediatric appendicitis, *Radiology* 272:233–240, 2014.

Pakdaman R, Woodward PJ, Kennedy A: Complex abdominal wall defects: appearances at prenatal imaging, *Radiographics* 35(2):636–649, March–April, 2015.

Silva CT1, Daneman A, Navarro OM, Moore AM, Moineddin R, Gerstle JT, Mittal A, Brindle M, Epelman M: Correlation of sonographic findings and outcome in necrotizing enterocolitis, *Pediatr Radiol* 37(3):274–282, March, 2007. Epub 2007 January 16.

Sivit C: Imaging children with abdominal trauma, *Am J Roentgenol* 192:1179–1189, 2009.

Towbin AJ, Sullivan J, Denson LA, Wallihan DB, Podberesky DJ: CT and MR enterography in children and adolescents with inflammatory bowel disease, *Radiographics* 33(7):1843–1860, 2013.

Yee WH, Soraisham AS, Shah VS, Aziz K, Yoon W, Lee SK, Canadian Neonatal Network: Incidence and timing of presentation of necrotizing enterocolitis in preterm infants, *Pediatrics* 129(2):e298–304, Febuary, 2012. https://doi.org/10.1542/peds.2011-2022. Epub 2012 January 23.

CHAPTER 6

GENITOURINARY

Oscar M. Navarro

IMAGING MODALITIES

Renal Ultrasound

Ultrasound of the kidneys and bladder is the first-line imaging modality for most suspected anomalies of the urinary tract. Renal ultrasound (US) is usually performed with the patient in both the supine and prone positions. Transverse and longitudinal images are obtained of the kidney and bladder. The kidneys can be measured in both the prone and supine positions, and although measurements obtained with the patient in the prone position are more reproducible, they tend to underestimate the actual length. It is important to compare the patient's renal length with tables that plot normal renal length against age. The left and right kidneys should normally be within 1 cm of each other in length. If there is a discrepancy of more than 1 cm, an underlying abnormality should be suspected. A size discrepancy may result from a disorder that causes one of the kidneys to be too small, such as global scarring, or from a process that causes one of the kidneys to be too large, such as acute pyelonephritis or renal duplication.

The kidneys of infants have several characteristics that are different from those of older children and adults. They commonly and normally have an undulating contour secondary to persistent fetal lobulation (Fig. 6-1). The renal cortex is more echogenic than in older children and can be isoechoic or hyperechoic to adjacent liver parenchyma. Moreover, in this age range, the renal pyramids are prominent in size (Fig. 6-1), and due to their hypoechoic nature in contrast to the more echogenic renal cortex, the pyramids can be mistaken for cysts or dilation of the collecting system.

Voiding Cystourethrogram

The most common indication for a fluoroscopic voiding cystourethrogram (VCUG) is the evaluation of urinary tract infection (UTI). Other indications include voiding dysfunction, enuresis, and the work-up for hydronephrosis. VCUG can demonstrate the presence or absence of vesicoureteral reflux (VUR) and can also document anatomic abnormalities of the bladder and urethra. VCUG is performed under fluoroscopy with the patient awake. Alternatively and increasingly more commonly, ultrasound-guided VCUGs with the use of an US contrast (microbubble) agent are being performed, instead of with fluoroscopic guidance thus avoiding the radiation. Regardless of the imaging modality, the patient is catheterized under sterile conditions, typically using an 8F catheter. For fluoroscopic guidance, a precontrast scout view of the abdomen can be obtained to evaluate for calcifications, document the bowel pattern so that it is not later mistaken for VUR, and confirm the catheter position within the bladder. Contrast is then instilled into the bladder. An early filling view of the bladder should be obtained to exclude a ureterocele. Once the patient's bladder is full, bilateral oblique views are obtained to visualize the regions of the ureterovesical junctions and the expected path of the ureters to document VUR. During voiding, the male urethra is optimally imaged with the patient in the oblique projection. The female urethra is best seen on the anteroposterior view. It is critical to obtain an image of the urethra during voiding, particularly in males. Voiding images can be obtained with the catheter in the urethra as its presence does not prevent the diagnosis of posterior urethral valves. After the patient has completed voiding, images are obtained of the pelvis and over the kidneys, documenting presence or absence of VUR and evaluating the extent of postvoid residual contrast within the bladder and renal collecting systems. The use of fluoroscopy should be brief and intermittent during bladder filling. Fluoroscopic last-image hold images can often substitute for true exposures to further decrease radiation dose.

Sometimes, particularly in older children, it may be difficult to get the child to void on the table. Almost all children will eventually void, and a great deal of patience is required during such prolonged examinations. There are several maneuvers that may help the child to void. They include placing warm water on the patient's perineum or toes; placing a warm washcloth on the patient's lower abdomen; tilting the table so

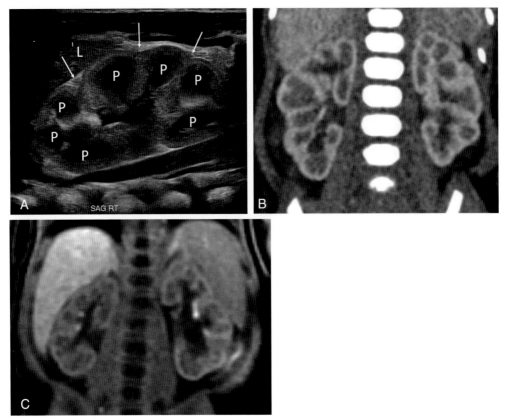

■ **FIGURE 6-1** Normal imaging appearance of neonatal kidney. **A,** Longitudinal ultrasound of a normal neonatal kidney shows fetal lobulation because of focal indentations (*arrows*) overlying the columns of Bertin. The medullary pyramids (*P*) are hypoechoic and prominent; this normal finding should not be confused with cysts or hydronephrosis. The renal cortex appears thinner when compared with older children or adults and is isoechoic to hyperechoic when compared with adjacent liver (*L*). **B,** Reformatted coronal contrast-enhanced CT image, and **C,** Coronal fat-suppressed T1-weighted MR image of normal neonatal kidneys in different patients shows similar findings.

that the head is up; letting the patient hear the sound of running water in the sink; and dimming the lights.

The expected bladder capacity of small children can be calculated by adding two to the patient's age in years and multiplying that number by 30. This yields the bladder capacity in milliliters. Obviously, this formula works only up to a certain age.

Nuclear Medicine

Technetium-99m-mercaptoacetyltriglycine (^{C}MAG3) and Technetium-99m-dimercaptosuccinic acid (^{99m}Tc-DMSA) renal scintigraphic examinations are commonly used in children. Owing to its primary active tubular excretion, ^{C}MAG3 is generally used in suspected urinary tract obstruction generally with a diuretic (furosemide) challenge. ^{99m}Tc-DMSA is most reliable to evaluate relative renal function and is used to demonstrate cortical defects in infection, infarction, and scarring.

Magnetic Resonance Urography

Magnetic resonance urography (MRU) has been increasingly used because of its superb delineation of the anatomy as a result of its intrinsic, high soft-tissue contrast resolution and multiplanar three-dimensional reconstruction capabilities. MRU is considered a "one-stop shop" examination because it can provide both anatomical and functional information in one examination without the use of ionizing radiation. MRU plays an important role in the evaluation of atypical urinary tract dilation, ureteral ectopia and genital anomalies. However, the widespread use of MRU is limited by its cost, availability, and the need for sedation.

■ URINARY TRACT INFECTION

UTI is the most common medical problem of the genitourinary system in children. The incidence of UTI is higher in girls than in boys, probably because of the short length of the female urethra. There is ongoing controversy with regard to when children with UTI should be imaged. The immediate goals of imaging children with UTI include the diagnosis of predisposing underlying congenital anomalies, identifying VUR, documenting any renal cortical damage, providing a baseline renal size for subsequent evaluation of renal growth, and establishing prognostic factors. The long-term goal is to eliminate the chance of renal damage leading to chronic renal disease and hypertension.

The *American Association of Pediatrics* recommends that the work-up of an infant with a first febrile UTI should include a renal and bladder ultrasound. Routine use of fluoroscopic or ultrasound-guided VCUG after a first febrile UTI is no longer recommended. VCUG should be obtained only if (1) US shows urinary tract dilation, scarring, obstructive uropathy, or masses; (2) any complex medical condition is associated with the UTI; (3) there are findings that suggest high-grade VUR or obstructive uropathy; or (4) there is a recurrence of febrile UTI. VCUG can be performed using fluoroscopy or ultrasound.

Acute Pyelonephritis

There is some confusion concerning the terminology used for infections of the urinary tract in children. The definition of UTI is the presence of bacteria in the urine, but the term typically refers to infections of the lower urinary tract. Acute pyelonephritis is defined as UTI that involves the kidney. Young children may present with nonspecific symptoms, such as fever, irritability, and vague abdominal pain. In older children, the findings may be more specific, such as fever associated with flank pain. In patients in whom the diagnosis is straightforward, no imaging is needed during the acute infection. US with color Doppler is probably now the most common way that pyelonephritis is imaged and shows lack of color flow in peripheral portions of the kidney. Cortical scintigraphy using ^{99m}Tc-DMSA has been advocated as being the most sensitive test for the diagnosis of pyelonephritis, showing single or multiple areas of lack of renal uptake of the radiotracer. These areas tend to be triangular and peripheral (Figs. 6-2 and 6-3). Other imaging studies that can be used to detect acute pyelonephritis include contrast-enhanced computed tomography (CT) or magnetic resonance imaging (MRI). These studies typically demonstrate lack of contrast enhancement of triangular, peripheral portions of the kidney

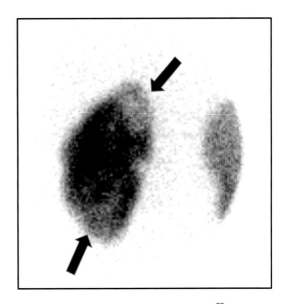

■ **FIGURE 6-2** Acute pyelonephritis. Renal ^{99m}Tc-DMSA scan shows focal, wedge-shaped areas of decreased uptake (*arrows*) in the upper and lower poles of the left kidney, consistent with pyelonephritis, in a 12-month-old girl with known bilateral vesicoureteral reflux and fever.

(Figs. 6-3 and 6-4). CT may also show a striated nephrogram. In addition, pyelonephritis can be very focal and mimic a mass on all of these studies (Fig. 6-5). US may show urothelial thickening, and both US and CT may also show asymmetric enlargement and swelling of the affected kidney as compared with the contralateral side. Sometimes these findings of pyelonephritis will be encountered during the investigation of other suspected causes of abdominal pain, such as appendicitis.

Chronic Pyelonephritis

Chronic pyelonephritis is defined as the loss of renal parenchyma resulting from previous bacterial infection. It is synonymous with renal scarring. Normally, the renal cortical thickness should be symmetric and equal within the upper, mid, and lower portions of the kidneys. The loss of renal cortical thickness as seen by ultrasound, most commonly at the renal poles, is suggestive of the diagnosis (Fig. 6-6). This should not be confused with fetal lobulation, also known as an interrenicular septum (Fig. 6-7 (old Fig. 6-7)), a normal variant. The scarring of pyelonephritis appears as indentations of the renal contour that overlie the renal pyramids, whereas in fetal lobulation the indentations overlie the columns of Bertin between renal pyramids (Fig. 6-7 (old Fig. 6-7)).

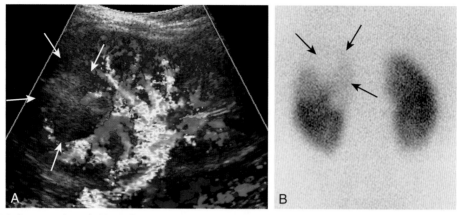

■ **FIGURE 6-3** Acute pyelonephritis on Doppler ultrasound. **A,** Longitudinal color Doppler ultrasound shows peripheral area of absent color flow in the upper pole of the left kidney (*arrows*). **B,** Corresponding nuclear scintigraphy with ^{99m}Tc-DMSA shows a wedge-shaped defect of decreased uptake (*arrows*) in the upper pole of the left kidney.

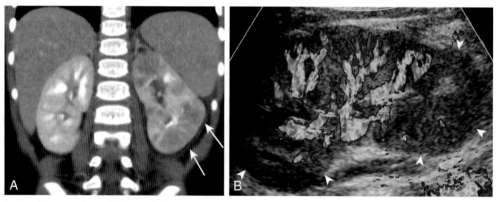

■ **FIGURE 6-4** Acute pyelonephritis on CT obtained for abdominal pain. **A,** Pyelonephritis appears as asymmetric increased volume of left kidney, with focal, wedge-like regions of hypoenhancement in the upper and lower poles of the left kidney. Note perinephric stranding with thickening of Gerota fascia (*arrows*). **B,** Corresponding color Doppler ultrasound image shows focal hyperechoic areas with loss of the corticomedullary differentiation and decreased flow in both left kidney poles (*arrowheads*).

■ POSTNATAL EVALUATION OF PRENATAL HYDRONEPHROSIS

Prenatal hydronephrosis is diagnosed in 1%−2% of all pregnancies. Many of these cases require further work-up with postnatal imaging, usually ultrasound. The first postnatal US should be done within the first month of life but not sooner than 48 h after birth because of the physiologic dehydration that occurs during this period that may result in underestimation of the degree of urinary tract dilation. Exceptions to this delay include patients with oligohydramnios, urethral obstruction, bilateral high-grade dilation, and concerns about parental noncompliance that may result in losing the patient to follow-up.

A multidisciplinary consensus group has recently proposed to standardize the terminology, grading, and follow-up protocols in these children in order to better correlate current management with decrease in the risk of postnatal uropathy and eventually improve the clinical outcomes. This consensus group proposes to use the term "urinary tract dilation" as a substitute for "hydronephrosis" as the latter can have different meanings to different practitioners. The severity of the urinary tract dilation is graded using six categories of US findings: measurement of the anteroposterior dimension of the renal pelvis (<10 mm is normal), presence and type of calyceal dilation, thickness of the renal parenchyma, appearance of the renal parenchyma, persistent dilation of ureter, and appearance of the bladder. Using these categories, patients are stratified in three risk groups and each group has follow-up recommendations regarding the timing of the second postnatal ultrasound, need for VCUG and functional

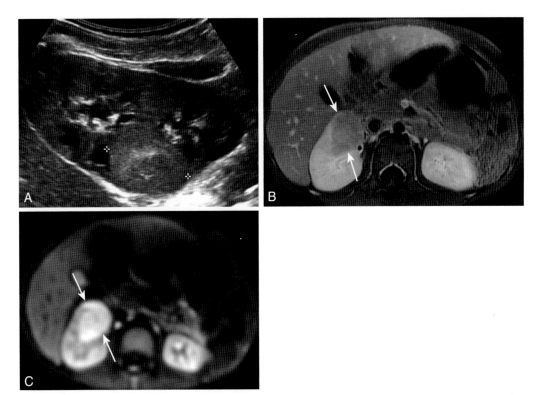

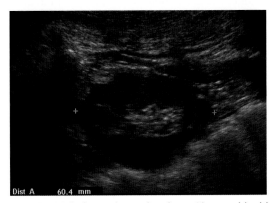

■ **FIGURE 6-5** Acute, focal pyelonephritis presenting as a mass. **A,** Longitudinal ultrasound of the right kidney shows a round heterogeneous mass (*between calipers*) with areas of increased echogenicity. **B,** Corresponding axial contrast-enhanced fat-suppressed T1-weighted MR image shows a heterogeneous mass (*arrows*) with decreased enhancement. **C,** The mass shows restricted diffusion on diffusion-weighted MR imaging.

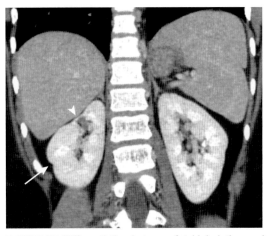

■ **FIGURE 6-6** Left renal scarring in a 10-year-old girl with high-grade vesicoureteral reflux. Longitudinal ultrasound shows the left kidney is small for age and shows diffuse irregular thinning of the renal parenchyma, most striking in the upper and lower poles, in keeping with multifocal scarring.

■ **FIGURE 6-7** Differentiation between fetal lobulation and focal scarring; both are demonstrated in the same patient. Coronal contrast-enhanced CT shows indentation and thinning of the right upper pole renal cortex directly over the medullary pyramids (*arrowhead*). This area represents focal scarring. There is also an indentation in the renal cortex between the medullary pyramids (*arrow*). This is consistent with normal fetal lobulation.

nuclear medicine scan, and indication for prophylactic antibiotics.

In about 50%−70% of prenatal urinary tract dilation cases, no specific pathology is found and the dilation is usually a transient finding without clinical repercussion. However, in approximately 30%−50% of cases, there is underlying pathology with a broad spectrum of causes that in a small group results in significant postnatal morbidity and even mortality. More common specific causes include VUR, ureteropelvic junction (UPJ) obstruction, ureterovesical junction obstruction/megaureter, and posterior urethral valves.

Vesicoureteral Reflux

VUR is defined as retrograde flow of urine from the bladder into the ureter. It can be a primary abnormality related to immaturity or maldevelopment of the ureterovesical junction. Normally, the ureter enters the ureterovesical junction in an oblique course such that the intramural ureter traverses the bladder wall for an adequate length to create a passive antireflux valve. In VUR, the angle of entrance of the ureter is abnormal and the intramural tunnel is short, allowing reflux. VUR occurs in less than 0.5% of asymptomatic children but is present in as much as 50% of children with UTI. There is an increased incidence of VUR in siblings of children with VUR and in children of parents who had VUR. VUR can also be secondary to other urinary anomalies including those that can cause bladder outlet obstruction, especially posterior urethral valves, or others such as neurogenic bladder, bladder dyssynergia and dysfunctional voiding, and prune-belly syndrome.

The importance of VUR is its association with renal parenchymal scarring. VUR is present in almost all children with severe renal scarring. In addition, a direct correlation between the grade of VUR and prevalence of scarring has been demonstrated. Other complications associated with VUR include acute pyelonephritis, interference with the normal growth of the kidney, and development of arterial hypertension.

Conventional US has a limited role in the diagnosis of VUR as it is frequently normal in cases of low-grade VUR and sometimes also in cases of high-grade VUR. On the other hand, mild degree of urinary tract dilation can be commonly found in patients without VUR. US performed after injection of microbubbles before, during, and after micturition is gaining acceptance as a modality to diagnose and grade VUR. However, VCUG remains as the most widely used modality in the assessment of VUR.

The degree of VUR is graded on the basis of several characteristics (Fig. 6-8): the level to which the reflux occurs (ureteral vs. ureteral and collecting system); the degree of dilatation; the calyceal blunting; and papillary impressions. Grade 1 reflux is confined to the ureter. Grade 2 reflux fills the ureter and collecting system, but there is no dilation of the collecting system (Fig. 6-9). Grade 3 reflux is associated with dilation of the collecting system with mild calyceal blunting. Grade 4 reflux is identified by moderate dilation of the collecting system and some tortuosity of the ureter (Fig. 6-9). Grade 5 reflux is defined by the presence of a very tortuous dilated ureter with marked dilation of the ureter and collecting system. Both grade 4 and 5 reflux can be associated with intrarenal reflux.

Most cases of low-grade VUR resolve spontaneously by the age of 5–6 years unless there is an underlying anatomic abnormality, and in these children, treatment is usually with prophylactic

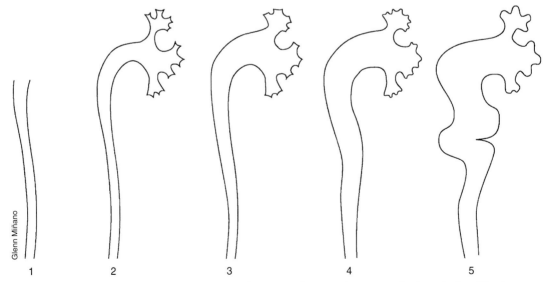

■ FIGURE 6-8 Grading system for VUR. Grade 1: Reflux is confined to the ureter. Grade 2: Reflux fills the ureter and renal collecting system without dilation. Grade 3: Reflux is associated with mild dilation of the collecting system and blunting of the calyces. Grade 4: Reflux results in moderate to marked dilation of the ureter and renal collecting system. Grade 5: Reflux results in a very tortuous, dilated ureter with marked dilation of the renal collecting system.

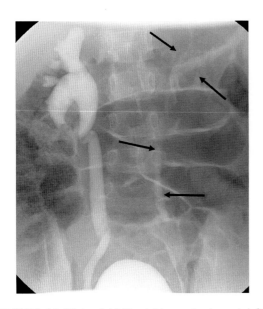

■ **FIGURE 6-9** Bilateral VUR: right, grade 4, and left, grade 2. VCUG shows reflux of contrast filling a moderately dilated right ureter and collecting system. The ureter is slightly tortuous and the calyces are blunted. On the left, the reflux of contrast results in more subtle opacification of a nondilated ureter and collecting system (*arrows*).

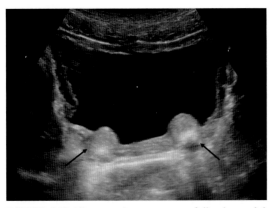

■ **FIGURE 6-10** Ultrasound appearance following minimally invasive endoscopic treatment of VUR using periureteral injection of Deflux. Transverse ultrasound image shows bilateral echogenic mounds (*arrows*) at base of bladder in region of the ureterovesical junctions.

antibiotics alone, although this is controversial. Antibiotic therapy is discontinued when the reflux has resolved. Surgical reimplantation of the ureter or submucosal injection of a bulking agent below the ureteral orifice (minimally invasive endoscopic treatment) is considered when the degree of VUR is severe, if there is evidence of renal scarring, if the VUR has not resolved over a reasonable time, or if breakthrough infections occur frequently. After periureteral injection, US will show an echogenic mound in the bladder wall in the region of the treated ureteral orifice (Fig. 6-10).

Ureteropelvic Junction Obstruction

UPJ obstruction is defined as an obstruction of the flow of urine from the renal pelvis into the proximal ureter. It is the most common congenital obstruction of the urinary tract and it is associated with an increased incidence of other congenital urinary tract anomalies including VUR and renal duplication, among others. Males are more often affected than females, and there is a predilection for the left side. In addition, UPJ obstruction may be bilateral in approximately 10% of cases, but the severity may be asymmetric. The cause of most UPJ obstructions is intrinsic narrowing at the UPJ. However, extrinsic compression secondary to anomalous vessels is also occasionally identified.

On US, there is dilation of the renal collecting system without dilation of the ureter (Fig. 6-11). The degree of dilation may be severe and associated with thinning of the renal parenchyma. Renal scintigraphy using ^{99m}Tc-MAG3 with diuretic (furosemide) challenge is often used to evaluate the severity of the UPJ obstruction. Most neonates with UPJ obstruction are characteristically asymptomatic, and the condition is usually diagnosed following postnatal US evaluation of prenatal hydronephrosis. MRU is increasingly used for better assessment of UPJ anatomy and detection of crossing vessels as well as for estimation of renal function. Children with UPJ obstruction and other congenital anomalies are predisposed to renal injury even by minor abdominal trauma (Fig. 6-12). Mild and moderate UPJ obstructions are usually managed conservatively as they tend to resolve spontaneously. However, most severe UPJ obstructions are treated surgically, with open pyeloplasty being increasingly replaced by robotic or laparoscopic pyeloplasty, with similar rates of success.

Megaureter

Megaureter is a descriptive term that indicates the presence of a dilated ureter with or without associated pelvicalyceal dilation. It is called primary if it is caused by an intrinsic ureteral anomaly and secondary if the cause is not ureteral. Four main types of primary megaureter have been described. These types include (1) obstructive megaureter, in which there is an aperistaltic segment of the distal ureter that results in a relative obstruction (Fig. 6-13). The normal more proximal ureter dilates as a consequence of the relative obstruction. It is more common on the left and in boys. Children affected with primary megaureter may present with infection or be diagnosed prenatally.

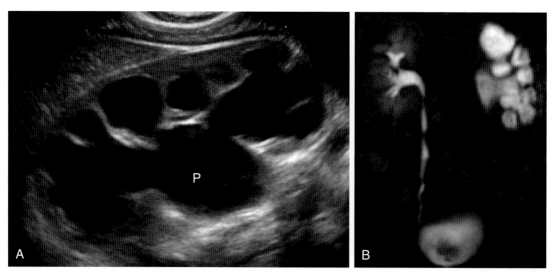

■ FIGURE 6-11 UPJ obstruction. **A,** Longitudinal ultrasound shows dilation of the calyces which connect to a central, dilated renal pelvis (*P*). There is thinning of the overlying parenchyma. The ureter was not dilated. **B,** Coronal maximum intensity projection (MIP) image from an MR urogram obtained from an acquisition performed approximately 10 min after intravenous gadolinium administration shows normal contrast excretion on the right and delayed excretion on the left with marked dilation of the collecting system and no delineation of the left ureter.

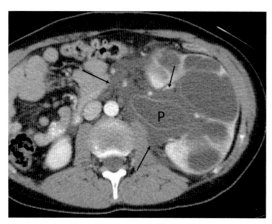

■ FIGURE 6-12 Renal injury to child with UPJ obstruction following trauma. CT shows findings of left UPJ obstruction with marked calyceal dilatation and central, dilated renal pelvis (*P*). There is a large amount of fluid (*arrows*) surrounding the renal pelvis and extending medially into the midline abdomen secondary to injury to the dilated collecting system.

US shows dilation of the ureter (>7–8 mm) above the aperistaltic segment and varying degrees of dilation of the collecting system. Other types include (2) refluxing megaureter, which is the result of VUR; (3) refluxing megaureter with obstruction, which is rare and often related to ectopic insertion of the ureter in the bladder neck; and (4) nonrefluxing, nonobstructed megaureter, which is the most common cause of a neonatal megaureter. In this latter type, no VUR or focal stenosis at the ureterovesical junction can be demonstrated. Causes of secondary megaureter include megacystis–megaureter syndrome, prune-belly syndrome, neurogenic bladder, and posterior urethral valves. Imaging algorithms are aimed to define the roles of VUR or obstruction in the presence of a megaureter.

Ureterocele

A ureterocele is defined as a cystic dilatation of the distal ureter. The dilated portion of the ureter lies between the mucosal and muscular layers of the bladder. The ureteral orifice is usually stenotic or obstructed. Ureteroceles are defined as simple or orthotopic when they are positioned at the expected orifice of the ureter at the lateral aspect of the trigone. Ureteroceles are defined as ectopic when they are associated with an ectopic insertion of the ureter. Ectopic ureteroceles can be quite large and are almost always associated with a duplicated collecting system (Figs. 6-14 and 6-15). The ureter from the upper pole moiety is the one associated with the ureterocele. On VCUG, ureteroceles appear as round, well-defined filling defect, best visualized on early filling views (Fig. 6-14). Ureteroceles may be compressed and not visualized when the bladder is distended by contrast (Fig. 6-14). Sometimes the ureteroceles can evert and appear as diverticula. On ultrasound, a ureterocele is seen as a round, anechoic intravesical cystic structure that can be connected to the distal ureter (Fig. 6-15). There can be varying degrees of dilatation of that ureter and the upper pole moiety collecting system, sometimes quite severe with associated marked parenchymal thinning (Fig. 6-15).

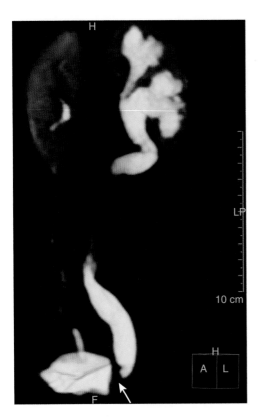

■ **FIGURE 6-13** Primary megaureter. An MIP MRU image shows narrowing of the distal ureter (*arrow*) resulting in marked dilation of the more proximal ureter and left kidney collecting system secondary to relative obstruction.

Posterior Urethral Valves

Posterior urethral valves are the most common cause of urethral obstruction in male infants. They represent abnormal mucosal folds between the urethral wall and the distal end of the verumontanum. They are identified most commonly in infancy but can be diagnosed in older children. The high back pressure can damage the kidneys and result in renal failure. Affected children can be diagnosed prenatally and present with renal failure or with UTI.

Typical US features include a thick-walled bladder with associated bilateral dilatation of the renal collecting systems and ureters (Fig. 6-16). Occasionally, a dilated posterior urethra can be identified inferior to the bladder. Perinephric fluid collections representing urinomas secondary to calyceal rupture can also be seen (Fig. 6-16). On VCUG, the posterior urethra is often very dilated (Fig. 6-16). The actual valve itself may be difficult to visualize, but it can appear as a membrane-like obstruction; however, its presence is more commonly recognized by the abrupt change of caliber at the transition from posterior to anterior urethra. The bladder is trabeculated and may have pseudodiverticula. VUR is present in approximately 50% of patients with posterior urethral valves.

Anything that relieves the increased pressure within the urinary system of patients with posterior urethral valves protects the patients

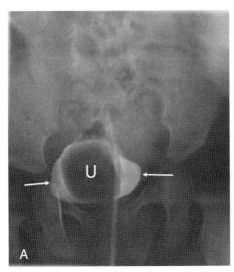
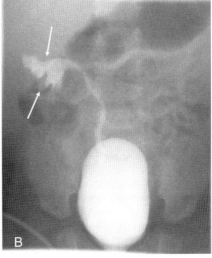

■ **FIGURE 6-14** Duplicated right renal collecting system with ureterocele and VUR into lower pole moiety. **A,** Image from VCUG obtained during early filling shows a ureterocele (*U*) as a round filling defect within the bladder (*arrows*). **B,** With further bladder filling, the ureterocele is no longer evident. There is VUR into the lower pole collecting system (*arrows*). The opacified lower pole collecting system has a "drooping lily" appearance caused by inferior displacement by a dilated, nonopacified, obstructed upper pole collecting system.

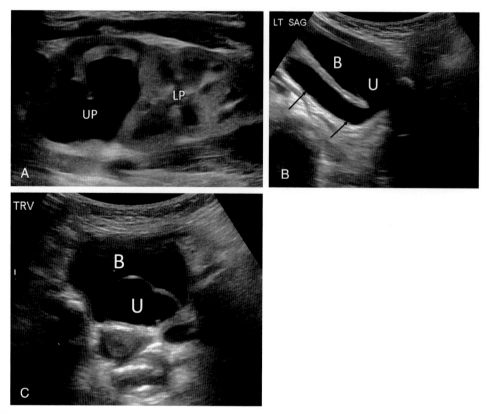

■ FIGURE 6-15 Duplicated left renal collecting system with ureterocele causing obstruction of the upper pole. **A,** Longitudinal ultrasound of the left kidney shows a markedly dilated upper pole collecting system (*UP*), secondary to an obstructing ureterocele. There is thinning of the overlying parenchyma. The lower pole moiety (*LP*) shows no dilatation of the collecting system and the parenchyma is normal. **B,** Longitudinal ultrasound, left parasagittal of pelvis shows a dilated left upper moiety distal ureter (*arrows*) leading into a ureterocele (*U*), which appears as a thin-walled cystic structure within the bladder (*B*). **C,** Transverse ultrasound better depicts the ureterocele (*U*) within the bladder (*B*) with characteristic "cyst within cyst" appearance.

from developing renal failure and is associated with a better prognosis by lowering the urinary back pressure on the renal parenchyma and decreasing the potential for renal damage. Such entities include unilateral VUR (with protection of the kidney contralateral to the reflux), large bladder diverticula, or development of intra-uterine urinary ascites. The spectrum of clinical severity is wide, and the prognosis is typically poor in cases of moderate-to-severe upper tract dilatation before 20 weeks of gestation. On the contrary, the outcome is generally favorable if the diagnosis of posterior urethral valves is made after the 24th week of gestation. It is the potential of posterior urethral valves that makes obtaining an image of the urethra during voiding a vital part of every VCUG performed on boys.

■ CONGENITAL RENAL ANOMALIES

Renal Ectopia and Fusion

Renal ectopia is defined as abnormal position of the kidney. It results from abnormal migration of the kidney from its fetal position within the pelvis to its expected position in the renal fossa. Most ectopic kidneys are found in the pelvis and are also malrotated.

Renal fusion is defined as a connection between the two kidneys. It results from failure of separation of the primitive nephrogenic cell masses into two separate left and right blastemas. With crossed fused renal ectopia, both kidneys lie on the same side of the abdomen and are fused (Fig. 6-17). In this anomaly, both ureters drain normally in their expected positions in the bladder. Single kidneys and crossed fused ectopia are commonly observed in children with VACTERL (vertebral defects, anal atresia, cardiac defects, tracheoesophageal fistula, renal and limb abnormalities) association. The most common type of renal fusion is horseshoe kidney, which occurs in approximately 1 in 400 live births. With horseshoe kidney, there is fusion of the lower pole of the two kidneys across the midline anterior to the aorta and inferior vena cava (Figs. 6-18—6-20). The connecting isthmus may consist of functional renal tissue or

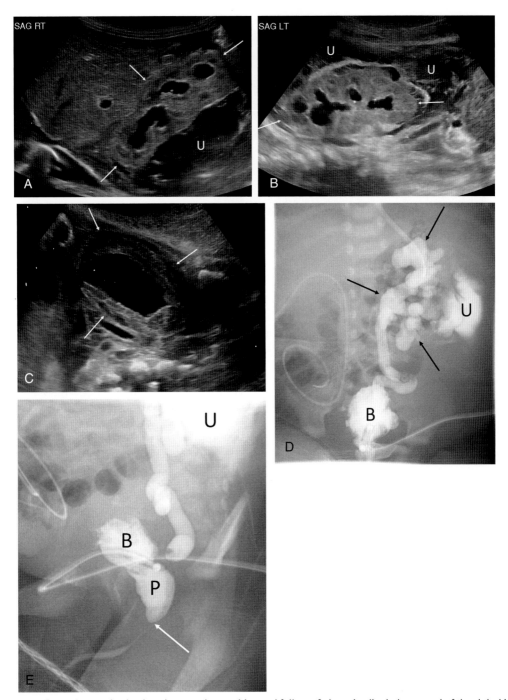

■ FIGURE 6-16 Posterior urethral valves in a newborn with renal failure. **A,** Longitudinal ultrasound of the right kidney (*arrows*) shows mild dilation of the collecting system with hyperechoic renal parenchyma. The right kidney is displaced anteriorly by a fluid collection consistent with a urinoma (*U*) secondary to calyceal rupture. **B,** Longitudinal ultrasound of the left kidney (*arrows*) shows mild dilatation of the collecting system with hyperechoic renal parenchyma. There is a large urinoma (*U*) extending into the left perinephric and pararenal spaces. **C,** Longitudinal ultrasound shows a markedly thick-walled bladder (*arrows*). **D,** VCUG performed through a vesicostomy shows trabeculated, thick-walled bladder (*B*) with pseudodiverticula. There is left VUR with dilation of the ureter and collecting system (*arrows*) with contrast extravasation into the pararenal space in keeping with urinoma (*U*) secondary to calyceal rupture. **E,** VCUG obtained during voiding shows marked dilation of the posterior urethra (*P*) with abrupt change of caliber at the site of the posterior urethral valves (*arrow*). *B,* bladder; *U,* urinoma.

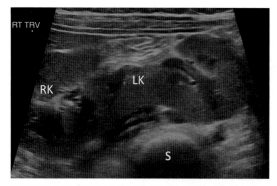

■ FIGURE 6-17 Crossed fused renal ectopia. Transverse ultrasound image shows ectopic position of the left kidney (*LK*) which lies in a somewhat transverse orientation anterior to the spine (*S*), malrotated and fused to the lower pole of the orthotopic right kidney (*RK*).

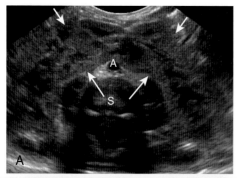

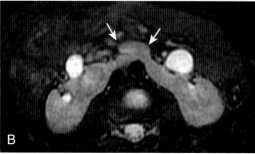

■ FIGURE 6-18 Horseshoe kidney in an infant. **A,** Transverse ultrasound shows that the right and left kidneys (*arrows*) connected by a parenchymal isthmus resulting in a horseshoe configuration. *A,* Aorta; *S,* spine. **B,** Axial contrast-enhanced MRI again shows right and left kidneys are connected by a parenchymal isthmus (*arrows*) resulting in a horseshoe configuration.

fibrous tissue. Most horseshoe kidneys are located more inferiorly than normal. Horseshoe kidneys may be seen in association with Turner syndrome (XO) and Trisomy 18. The number of ureters arising from a horseshoe kidney is variable, and they exit the kidney ventrally rather than ventromedially. Horseshoe kidneys and other types of renal fusions are at increased risk for infection, injury from mild traumatic events (Fig. 6-19), renal vascular hypertension, stone

formation, and urinary tract dilation (Fig. 6-20). There is also a slight increase in incidence of Wilms tumor. On ultrasound, the diagnosis of horseshoe kidney may be overlooked when there is obscuration of the isthmus by overlying bowel gas and when abnormalities of orientation of the kidneys are not recognized. In horseshoe kidney, the lower poles are oriented more medial than normal. It may also be difficult to measure the length of the kidneys because of the poorly defined inferior pole. Horseshoe kidneys are readily visualized on CT and MRI (Figs. 6-19 and 6-20).

Ureteropelvic Duplications

Ureteropelvic duplication refers to a broad range of anatomic variations ranging in severity from incomplete to complete. The incomplete form of duplication is more common than the complete form and is the most common anomaly affecting the renal collecting system. It occurs most often in females. With incomplete duplication, there can be a bifid renal pelvis, two ureters superiorly that join in midureter, or duplicated ureters that join just before insertion into the bladder wall. With complete duplication, there are two completely separate ureters that have separate orifices into the bladder. Ureteropelvic duplication is thought to be the result of premature division or duplication of the ureteral bud. Such duplications are five times more common unilaterally than bilaterally. On ultrasound, renal duplication may appear as a parenchymal band of similar echogenicity to the renal cortex splitting the echogenic central renal sinus into superior and inferior components (Fig. 6-21). Noncomplicated, incomplete renal duplications have little significance and should be thought of as a normal variation. Children with incomplete duplication are not at increased risk for urinary tract disease as compared with children without duplications.

In patients with complete ureteropelvic duplication, there is a higher incidence of UTI, obstruction, VUR, and parenchymal scarring. In these patients, the ureteral orifice of the upper pole moiety inserts more medially and more inferiorly than the orifice of the lower pole ureter. This is known as the Weigert–Meyer rule. The lower pole system is more prone to VUR. The upper pole system is more prone to obstruction secondary to an ectopic ureterocele (Figs. 6-14, 6-15 and 6-22).

Prune-Belly Syndrome

Prune-belly syndrome, or Eagle–Barrett syndrome, is a rare condition in which there is a triad of hypoplasia of the abdominal muscles,

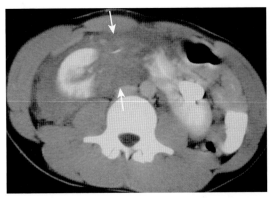

■ FIGURE 6-19 CT of horseshoe kidney with laceration due to bike handle trauma. There is an area of low attenuation (*arrows*) within the horseshoe kidney, consistent with laceration and hematoma.

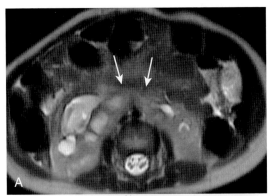

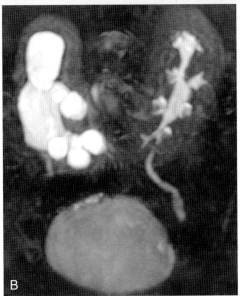

■ FIGURE 6-20 Horseshoe kidney with associated right urinary tract dilation. **A**, Axial T2-weighted and **B**, coronal MIP MR images show a horseshoe kidney with a parenchymal connection of the kidneys across the midline (*arrows*). Note dilation of the right renal moiety.

cryptorchidism, and abnormalities of the urinary tract system. The etiology of prune-belly syndrome is not fully understood. Potential urinary tract abnormalities include severe bilateral urinary tract dilation, secondary megaureter, a large capacity, trabeculated and hypertrophied bladder, and urachal diverticulum. Imaging findings include the characteristic bulging flanks secondary to abdominal wall hypoplasia and the previously described urologic manifestations (Fig. 6-23). There are multiple associated congenital anomalies. The condition affects almost exclusively boys. Even more rarely, the syndrome can be incomplete (pseudoprune-belly syndrome) in girls, who obviously cannot have cryptorchidism, and it can occur unilaterally.

■ RENAL CYSTIC DISEASE

In children, renal cysts can occur secondary to polycystic kidney disease, can be associated with a variety of syndromes, can occur secondary to cystic neoplasms, or can be related to dysplastic changes, such as multicystic dysplastic kidney (MCDK) (Table 6-1). The diagnostic criteria of and nomenclature for renal cystic disease in children have been recently standardized by an international consensus group with recommendation of using US for characterization in most cases, with MRI being reserved for selected indications. Many cystic diseases involving the kidney have a known genetic basis, and their nomenclature is clearly defined. However, these entities may be difficult to differentiate on imaging. In addition, it is important to note that although much less common than in adults, solitary simple renal cysts are not rare in children. When such unilocular, solitary cysts are encountered during the work-up for a UTI or hematuria, they are usually of no clinical significance and do not necessarily suggest an underlying developing polycystic kidney disease. As in adults, the US criteria for diagnosing a simple renal cyst include an anechoic, well-defined, round lesion; an imperceptible wall; and increased through-transmission. No central echoes or vascular flow is present within the lesion or within its walls.

Multicystic Dysplastic Kidney

MCDK is secondary to severe obstruction of the renal collecting system or ureter during fetal development. The site of the obstruction determines the imaging appearance more often resulting in the infundibular type and uncommonly in the hydronephrotic type. As implied by

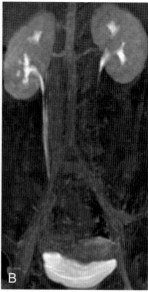

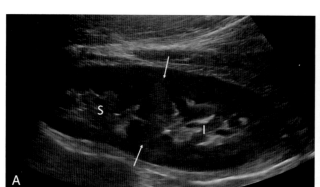

■ **FIGURE 6-21** Ureteropelvic duplication. **A,** Intrarenal duplication shown on longitudinal ultrasound as a band of parenchyma (*arrows*) of similar echogenicity to that of the renal cortex splitting the central renal sinus into separate superior (*S*) and inferior (*I*) moieties. **B,** Coronal MIP image from an MR urogram shows a duplex configuration of the right kidney with incomplete ureteral duplication as both ureters join in their mid to distal portions.

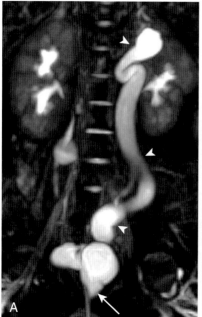

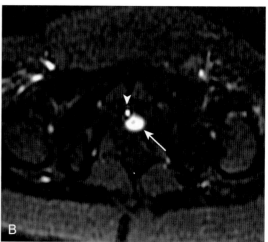

■ **FIGURE 6-22** Left ureteropelvic duplication on MR urogram. **A,** MR urogram shows marked dilatation of the upper pole collecting system and ureter (*arrowheads*), secondary to obstruction by ectopic ureter insertion (*arrow*). **B,** Axial T2-weighted MR image shows ectopic (*arrow*) low-inserting left upper pole ureter which drains into the vagina. The *arrowheads* denotes the Foley catheter coursing within the urethra.

its name, in MCDK, the renal parenchyma is dysplastic and there is formation of cysts. US is used for the diagnosis in most instances. The characteristic appearance on US is of a variable-sized kidney that is largely comprised of noncommunicating cysts of varying size without

normal renal parenchyma (Fig. 6-24). There may be hyperechoic tissue between the cysts representing dysplastic parenchyma. With MCDK, the cysts do not follow the distribution of dilated calyces, allowing differentiation from urinary tract dilation. In patients with MCDK, it is

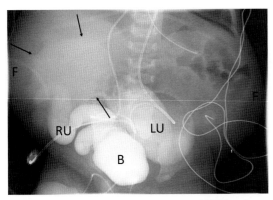

■ **FIGURE 6-23** Prune-belly syndrome. VCUG shows opacification of the bladder associated with bilateral vesicoureteral reflux. Both the right ureter (*RU*) and left ureter (*LU*) are tortuous and dilated, more severe on the left. There is marked dilation of the right kidney collecting system (*arrows*). There is also bulging of the flanks (*F*) secondary to deficient abdominal wall musculature.

✳ **TABLE 6-1** Renal Cysts in Children
Solitary simple cyst
Multicystic dysplastic kidney
Autosomal recessive polycystic renal disease
Autosomal dominant polycystic renal disease
Syndromes
Tuberous sclerosis
von Hippel–Lindau
Meckel–Gruber
Cystic neoplasms
Cystic Wilms tumor
Cystic partially differentiated nephroblastoma
Pediatric cystic nephroma

important to exclude other associated congenital anomalies of the contralateral kidney. Contra-lateral UPJ obstruction is identified in up to 12% of cases. Rarely, MCDK can be isolated to an upper or lower pole in a duplicated kidney.

Most MCDKs slowly decrease in size over time. Often the remaining residual dysplastic renal tissue will no longer be visualized by imaging techniques. Most patients are managed nonoperatively. MCDK can also predispose patients to hypertension, and if hypertension develops, nephrectomy is usually performed.

Autosomal Recessive Polycystic Kidney Disease

Autosomal recessive polycystic kidney disease (ARPKD), formerly known as infantile polycystic kidney disease, is a rare condition caused by mutations of the PKHD1 gene. It is part of the ciliopathies resulting in varying amounts of cystic disease in the kidneys and associated hepatic fibrosis. The kidneys are markedly enlarged with diffuse dilatation of the collecting ducts that result in the presence of numerous small, 1–2-mm cysts throughout the cortex and medulla. On ultrasound, the kidneys are grossly enlarged and demonstrate diffuse increased echogenicity (Fig. 6-25). Discrete cystic structures are not always identified because of the small size of the cysts. The liver usually shows increased or coarse echogenicity related to fibrosis and can be associated with cystic dilatation of the intrahepatic bile ducts (Caroli syndrome). Hepatosplenomegaly, portal hypertension, and portosystemic collaterals are not typically seen in the neonatal period and develop later in life.

Autosomal Dominant Polycystic Kidney Disease

Autosomal dominant polycystic kidney disease (ADPKD) is a dominantly inherited disease with variable penetrance. It is relatively common. ADPKD is a ciliopathy that occurs as a result of a mutation in one of two genes, polycystic kidney disease (PKD)1 and PKD2. Usually the diagnosis is made in early adulthood, when the patient presents with hypertension, hematuria, or renal failure. However, the cysts can be encountered during childhood. Some patients even present during the neonatal period, and in this scenario, the US appearance may resemble that seen in ARPKD. In the more common presentation of ADPKD during late childhood, US shows several cysts of varying sizes in both the cortex and medulla. The intervening renal parenchyma appears normal. The cysts often have a simple appearance although septated cysts or forming clusters are not rare. The cysts gradually progress in size and number with time, and the normal renal parenchyma can be compressed and destroyed. Cysts may also be found in other organs, most commonly in the liver and pancreas. There is an association between the disease and the presence of intracranial berry aneurysms (10% of cases).

■ RENAL TUMORS

Wilms Tumor

Wilms tumor, also referred to as nephroblastoma, is the most common renal malignancy in children. It accounts for approximately 8% of all childhood malignant tumors. Wilms tumor is a malignant embryonal neoplasm. Its peak incidence occurs at approximately 3 years of age, with approximately 80% of cases detected

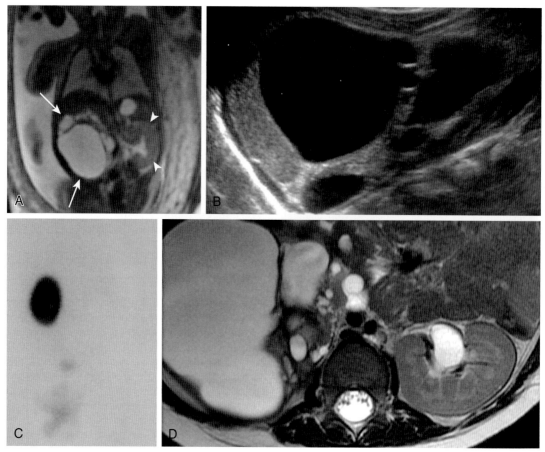

■ **FIGURE 6-24** Right MCDK. **A,** Coronal T2-weighted fetal MR image shows an enlarged right kidney (*arrows*) composed by multiple noncommunicating cysts of varying sizes. The right renal pelvis is not identified. The left kidney (*arrowheads*) is normal. **B,** MCDK shown on longitudinal ultrasound as a cluster of anechoic cysts without dominant central cyst. **C,** Scintigraphy shows normal perfusion and function of the left kidney with no renal activity on the right. **D,** Axial T2-weighted spinal MR image redemonstrates the multicystic nature of the lesion.

between 1 and 5 years of age. Wilms tumor presents most commonly as an asymptomatic abdominal mass but may present with abdominal pain, particularly when there is intratumoral hemorrhage. Although most cases of Wilms tumor occur in otherwise normal children, there is an association between the development of Wilms tumor and overgrowth disorders (congenital hemihypertrophy, Beckwith–Wiedemann syndrome), sporadic aniridia, and other malformations. Wilms tumor can be bilateral in approximately 5% of cases. Invasion of the renal vein and extension into the inferior vena cava occurs commonly in Wilms tumor. Lung metastatic disease occurs in as many as 20% of cases.

On US, Wilms tumor is typically a large, well-defined mass arising from the kidney, although smaller masses can be detected during routine surveillance of patients with predisposing conditions (Fig. 6-26). The mass is usually of increased echogenicity and may show heterogeneity related to intratumoral hemorrhage,

necrosis, or calcification. Doppler US is excellent in detecting extension of the tumor into the renal vein or inferior vena cava. It is especially important to document extension of the tumor thrombus into the right atrium because in such cases cardiothoracic surgery usually also becomes involved.

Confirmation of the lesion and evaluation of the anatomic extent of disease is usually performed using CT or MRI (Figs. 6-26–6-28). When evaluating a suspected Wilms tumor with either modality, it is important to document the following features: lymph node involvement, liver and lung metastases, involvement of the contralateral kidney by a synchronous Wilms tumor, the anatomic distribution of the intrarenal tumor, involvement of the renal vein or inferior vena cava (Fig. 6-27), and the path of the ureters in relation to the mass. Identification of the ureter as anterior or posterior to the mass is important so that the ureters are not inadvertently injured when the mass is removed.

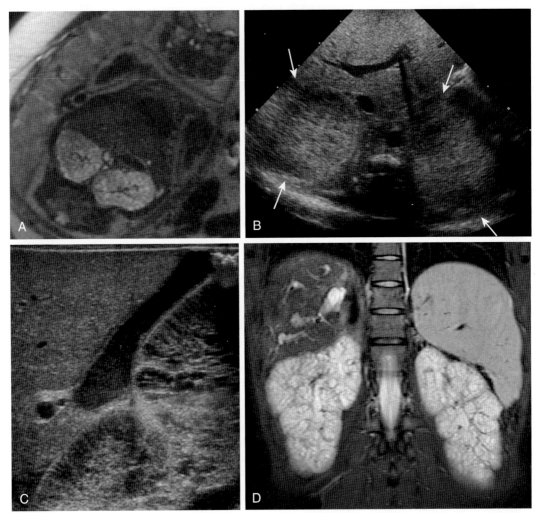

■ **FIGURE 6-25** ARPKD. **A,** Fetal MRI shows enlarged kidneys with multiple tiny cysts. There is severe oligohydramnios with a bell-shaped thoracic cage configuration related to pulmonary hypoplasia. **B,** Transverse ultrasound image shows massive enlargement of bilateral kidneys (*arrows*), which fill most of the abdominal cavity. The kidneys are of diffusely increased echogenicity, and no discrete cysts are identified. **C,** Longitudinal ultrasound scan obtained with a linear-array transducer shows to better advantage the multiple, radiating appearing, distended ducts in the pyramids and cortex. **D,** Coronal T2-weighted MR image in an older child shows enlarged kidneys with innumerable, uniform cysts. Note the inhomogeneous liver parenchyma with dilated ducts with findings consistent with congenital hepatic fibrosis.

One of the most important issues when evaluating a mass in the region of the suprarenal fossa is determining whether the mass arises from the kidney and is therefore most likely a Wilms tumor or whether it arises outside the kidney and in that case is most likely a neuroblastoma. Differential features between these two lesions are described in Table 6-2. In the case of a Wilms tumor, the mass usually appears as a well-defined, large, round mass on CT and MRI. The mass tends to grow in a ball, displacing blood vessels (Fig. 6-28) rather than engulfing

them, as does neuroblastoma. As Wilms tumor arises in the kidney, the renal parenchyma often surrounds a portion of the mass, resulting in the "claw sign" (Fig. 6-28). When the mass crosses the midline, the lesion usually passes anterior to the aorta, as compared with neuroblastoma, which can surround the aorta posteriorly and raise it anteriorly, away from the spine. Wilms tumors commonly appear to be solid, but larger lesions may have areas of heterogeneity or cystic components due to previous hemorrhage or necrosis.

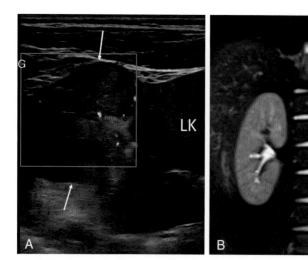

■ **FIGURE 6-26** Wilms tumor discovered during routine surveillance in a 3-year-old child with Beckwith–Wiedemann syndrome. **A,** Color Doppler longitudinal ultrasound shows a somewhat exophytic mass (*arrows*) arising from the upper pole of the left kidney (*LK*). The mass is slightly heterogeneous and mostly isoechoic to renal parenchyma with some internal vascularity. **B,** Coronal fat-suppressed T2-weighted MR image shows a lobulated, isointense to slightly hyperintense mass (*arrows*) in the upper pole of the left kidney.

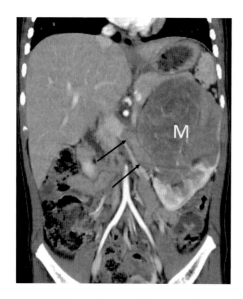

■ **FIGURE 6-27** Wilms tumor with renal vein invasion. Coronal reformatted contrast-enhanced CT image shows a large heterogeneous mass (*M*) arising from the left kidney. The left renal vein is expanded and partly occupied by tumor thrombus (*arrows*).

Nephroblastomatosis

Nephroblastomatosis is a rare entity that is related to the persistence of nephrogenic rests within the renal parenchyma after 36 weeks of gestation. These nephrogenic rests can be precursors of Wilms tumors. Most patients with nephroblastomatosis are monitored by ultrasound, MRI, or CT for the development of

Wilms tumors. On imaging, nephrogenic rests appear as plaque-like peripheral renal lesions and may be confluent (Fig. 6-29). The differentiation between nephrogenic rest and Wilms tumor is difficult. A mass that is spherical, exophytic, or larger than 1.75 cm is favored to represent Wilms tumor. On imaging follow-up of nephroblastomatosis, interval increase in size of a lesion or progressively increasing inhomogeneous enhancement as compared with the more nonenhancing nephrogenic rests also favors the diagnosis of Wilms tumor. Typically, cases of Wilms tumor associated with syndromes are the ones that develop from nephroblastomatosis.

Pediatric Cystic Nephroma

Pediatric cystic nephroma is a rare type of multicystic renal mass. This pediatric tumor is distinct from the multilocular cystic nephroma described in adult women in their fifth to sixth decades and from the cystic partially differentiated nephroblastoma, which is part of the Wilms tumor spectrum. Pediatric cystic nephroma affects primarily young boys with a median age of 19 months at time of diagnosis and it typically presents as a painless abdominal mass. This lesion is strongly associated with mutations in the *DICER1* gene, and in fact, more than half of the cases present in children with history of pleuropulmonary blastoma. Moreover, at histology, this tumor appears similar to pleuropulmonary blastoma. On ultrasound, CT, and MRI, the lesions appear as well-circumscribed, multiseptated

TABLE 6-2 Differentiating Features Between Neuroblastoma and Wilms Tumor		
Feature	**Neuroblastoma**	**Wilms Tumor**
Age	Most common before age 2 years	Peak incidence at 3 years
Calcification	Calcifications common (85% on CT) and stippled	Calcifications uncommon (15% on CT) and often curvilinear or amorphous
Growth pattern	Surrounds and engulfs vessels	Grows like ball, displacing vessels
Relation to kidney	Inferiorly displaces and rotates kidney	Arises from kidney, claw sign
Lung metastasis	Uncommon	More common (20%)
Vascular invasion	Does not occur	Invasion of renal vein and/or inferior vena cava

CT, Computed tomography.

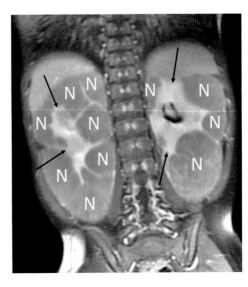

■ **FIGURE 6-29** Nephroblastomatosis. Coronal contrast-enhanced fat-suppressed T1-weighted MR image shows hypointense peripheral nephrogenic rests (*N*) in both kidneys, which are markedly enlarged. The nephrogenic rests show decreased enhancement when compared with the distorted central renal parenchyma (*arrows*).

Mesoblastic Nephroma

Mesoblastic nephroma is the most common solid renal mass in neonates. Typically, it is encountered prenatally or during the first few months of life; the mean age of diagnosis is approximately 3 months. Neonates most commonly present with a nontender, palpable abdominal mass. Histologic types include classic, cellular, and mixed types. The classic type is composed of spindle cells with benign features. The cellular and mixed types show features of infantile fibrosarcoma and exhibit a more aggressive behavior including local invasion, metastatic disease, and local recurrence after surgery. Imaging findings depend on the histologic type with a predominantly solid appearance of the classic type (Fig. 6-31) and presence of cystic changes in the cellular and mixed types.

Other Malignant Renal Tumors

Other, less common causes of malignant renal lesions include renal cell carcinoma (RCC), renal lymphoma, and rhabdoid tumor. RCC is the most common cause of renal malignancy in the second decade, although it is still much less common than in adults. There is an increased risk of developing multiple RCCs at an early age in patients with von Hippel–Lindau syndrome (VHL); therefore, all pediatric patients who develop RCC are usually screened for VHL. US, CT, and MRI typically show a

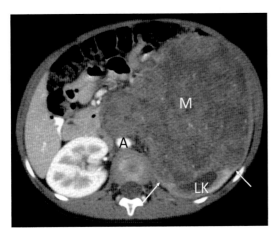

■ **FIGURE 6-28** Wilms tumor in a 5-year-old presenting with palpable abdominal mass. Axial contrast-enhanced CT image shows a large mass (*M*) arising from the left kidney (*LK*). The parenchyma of the left kidney forms a claw sign (*arrows*), which is helpful in confirming the renal origin of the mass. Note that in contrast to neuroblastoma, Wilms tumor causes displacement of the vessels rather than engulfing them, and when it crosses the midline, the mass passes anterior to the aorta (*A*) instead of posteriorly.

predominantly cystic masses (Fig. 6-30). Because the lesions cannot be differentiated from cystic partially differentiated nephroblastoma at imaging and because of the small risk of malignant transformation, surgical resection is performed.

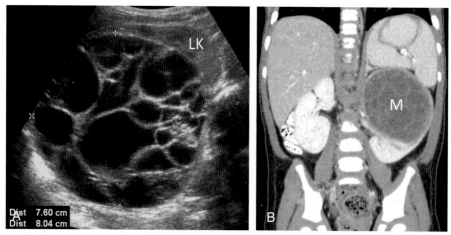

■ **FIGURE 6-30** Pediatric cystic nephroma. **A,** Longitudinal ultrasound shows a large multiseptated cystic mass (between cursors) arising from the left kidney (*LK*). **B,** Coronal reformatted contrast-enhanced CT image also shows the multiseptated cystic nature of this mass (*M*) in the upper pole of the left kidney. There is only septal enhancement of cyst walls without solid components. Further genetic testing proved *DICER1* mutation.

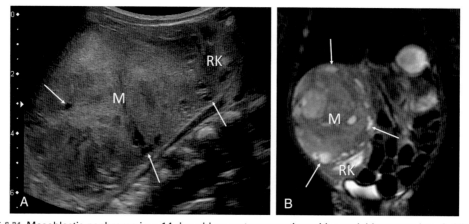

■ **FIGURE 6-31** Mesoblastic nephroma in a 14-day-old neonate presenting with arterial hypertension. **A,** Ultrasound shows a large, heterogeneous, predominantly hyperechoic mass (*M*) arising from the right kidney (*RK*). The mass contains cystic areas (*arrows*). **B,** Coronal STIR MR image also shows a large, heterogeneous right renal mass (*M*) with cystic spaces (*arrows*). Preserved right kidney (*RK*) is seen at the lower pole with some dilation of the collecting system. The most common cause of neonatal renal mass is mesoblastic nephroma. The presence of cystic spaces suggests mixed or cellular histologic types, which show a more aggressive behavior.

nonspecific solid renal mass. Calcification is more common with RCC (25%) than with Wilms tumor.

Rhabdoid tumor is a rare aggressive neoplasm more often diagnosed in children under the age of 2 years and in about 15% of cases associated with a synchronous intracranial neoplasm. They may present with palpable abdominal mass and hematuria. On imaging, it cannot be distinguished from Wilms tumor although it shows with more frequency subcapsular fluid collections (Fig. 6-32) reflecting necrosis or hemorrhage as well as intratumoral calcifications. Invasion of the renal

vein and metastasis to lymph nodes, lung, and liver can also be present.

ANGIOMYOLIPOMA

In pediatric patients, angiomyolipomas are usually associated with tuberous sclerosis. These lesions commonly demonstrate fatty components on imaging (Fig. 6-33) and may spontaneously hemorrhage. Hemorrhage from angiomyolipomas is the leading cause of death in tuberous sclerosis patients. Medical treatment with everolimus, an mTOR inhibitor, is recommended for

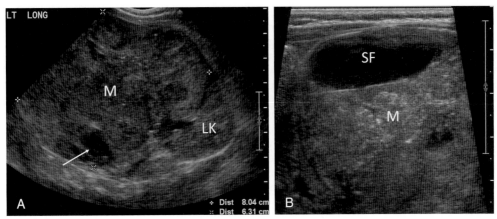

■ **FIGURE 6-32** Rhabdoid tumor in a 4-week-old child presenting with hematuria. **A,** Longitudinal ultrasound shows a large mass (*M, also denoted by the cursors*) arising from the left kidney (*LK*). The mass is heterogeneous with cystic areas (*arrow*) due to necrosis. **B,** Transverse ultrasound image obtained with high-frequency linear-array transducer from a posterior approach shows a subcapsular fluid collection (*SF*) in the posterior aspect of the mass (*M*), a common finding in rhabdoid tumor.

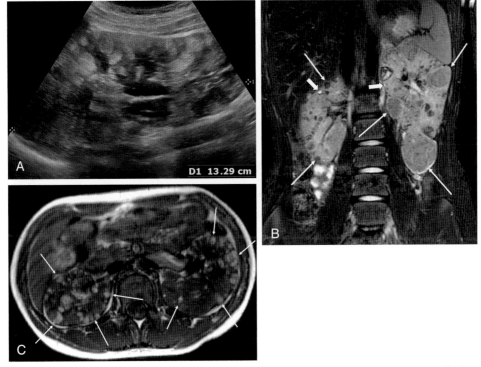

■ **FIGURE 6-33** Tuberous sclerosis. **A,** Longitudinal ultrasound of the left kidney (*between cursors*) shows neph-romegaly (length = 13.29 cm) and diffuse abnormal echogenicity due to the presence of numerous confluent hyperechoic lesions consistent with angiomyolipomas. **B,** Coronal STIR image shows a large left kidney with presence of bilateral hypointense lesions of varying size in keeping with angiomyolipomas, some of which are denoted by long arrows. There are also a few small high-signal cysts, some of which are denoted by short arrows. **C,** Axial T1-weighted image shows numerous hyperintense fat-containing lesions in both kidneys, some of which are denoted by arrows. The presence of fat is characteristic of angiomyolipomas.

enlarging angiomyolipomas larger than 3 cm in tuberous sclerosis. Angiomyolipomas larger than 4 cm in diameter often contain dysplastic arteries and aneurysms that may hemorrhage; they are commonly treated by prophylactic embolization.

On ultrasound, angiomyolipomas start as small hyperechoic foci within the kidneys during early childhood and grow into large infiltrative masses that enlarge the kidneys (Fig. 6-33). Angiomyo-lipomas can usually be diagnosed conclusively on

CT and MRI, due to the presence of intralesional fat. However, on occasions, fat-poor angiomyolipomas pose a diagnostic challenge and are difficult to differentiate from malignancy.

Tuberous sclerosis is also associated with ADPKD and renal cysts. The gene for tuberous sclerosis (TSC2 on chromosome 16) is contiguous with the PKD 1. Patients with contiguous gene syndrome have mutations that involve both genes and are at higher risk at developing hypertension and renal failure than those with tuberous sclerosis only. These patients present large cysts in large kidneys, with the cysts being more prominent than the angiomyolipomas.

Urachal Abnormalities

The urachus is an embryologic structure that extends from the apex of the bladder to the umbilicus. Normally it closes by birth. Residual urachal soft tissue is often visible postnatally at the bladder end on US and should not be misinterpreted as a pathological finding. This appears as hypoechoic nodular or fusiform solid tissue with minimal or no vascularity (Fig. 6-34).

The persistent patency of any portion of the urachus is considered an urachal abnormality. The type of the urachal anomaly present is determined by which portion of the urachus remains patent (Fig. 6-35). If the urachus remains patent in its entirety from the umbilicus to the bladder, it is a patent urachus (Fig. 6-36). A neonate with a patent urachus will have urine draining from the umbilicus. Patent urachus can be demonstrated by VCUG, fistula tract injection, or US.

If the urachus remains patent only at the bladder end of the urachus, an urachal diverticulum is present. On US or VCUG, a diverticulum

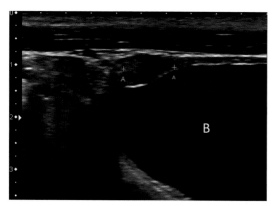

■ **FIGURE 6-34** Normal urachal remnant. Longitudinal ultrasound of the midline infraumbilical region shows a hypoechoic nodule (*between cursors*) at the anterior aspect of the dome of the bladder (*B*).

of variable size is demonstrated arising from the anterior aspect of the dome on the bladder (Fig. 6-36).

If the urachus remains patent only at the umbilical end, an urachal sinus is present. If the urachus remains patent only at its midportion and is closed at both its umbilical and its bladder ends, an urachal cyst is present. Urachal cysts may present as palpable masses but more commonly present with inflammatory changes after becoming infected. US or CT will show a cystic mass anterior and superior to the bladder dome in the midline (Fig. 6-36). Urachal carcinoma is rare in adults and extraordinarily rare in children.

Hydrometrocolpos

Genital outflow tract obstructions may lead to hydrometrocolpos or hematometrocolpos. Hydrometrocolpos is a rare condition in which there is dilation of the vaginal and uterine cavities with fluid. This occurs in response to hormonal stimulation, so it may present during infancy, secondary to maternal hormones, or during puberty. Hematometrocolpos is the accumulation of blood in a dilated vagina and uterus that occurs after menarche in patients with a genital outflow tract obstruction, often caused by imperforate hymen or transverse vaginal septum. In both hydrometrocolpos and hematometrocolpos, a fixed midline mass may be palpable; the mass can become large enough to cause ureteral obstruction and result in hydronephrosis. US demonstrates the midline abdominal mass which appears tubular or elliptical in shape. In hematometrocolpos, there is heterogeneous echogenicity secondary to the accumulation of blood products (Fig. 6-37). Because the vagina is more elastic, it becomes markedly dilated and composes the bulk of the mass. The uterus may also be dilated but cannot expand to the degree that the vagina can. Often the uterus can be identified as a small C-shaped cavity arising from the anterosuperior aspect of the distended vagina on US (Fig. 6-37). US also can reveal the degree of dilation of the urinary tract. In problematic cases, especially when there is suspicion of an associated Mullerian anomaly, MRI can be helpful in confirming the cause and the anatomy of the lesion (Fig. 6-37).

ADRENAL GLANDS

A number of pathologic processes can involve the adrenal glands in children. The most commonly encountered adrenal disorders are neuroblastoma and neonatal adrenal hemorrhage.

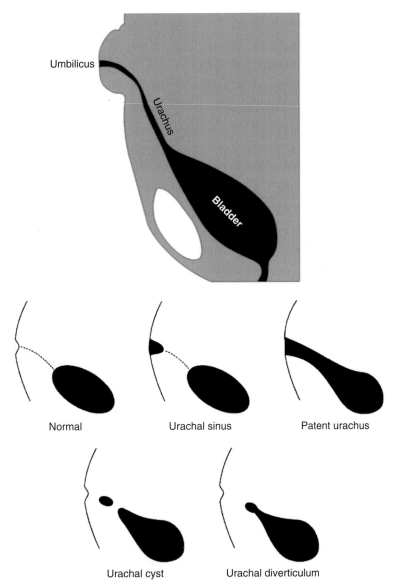

Normal   Urachal sinus   Patent urachus

Urachal cyst   Urachal diverticulum

■ **FIGURE 6-35** Urachal abnormalities. The superior image shows the urachus as a patent connection between the umbilicus and bladder during fetal life. The inferior row of images shows the potential urachal anomalies that occur when a portion or all of the urachus remains patent after birth. The type of urachal abnormality present depends upon which portion of the urachus remains patent.

Neuroblastoma

Neuroblastoma is a malignant tumor of primitive neural crest cells that most commonly arises in the adrenal gland but can occur anywhere along the sympathetic chain. It is differentiated from its more benign counterparts, ganglioneuroma and ganglioneuroblastoma, by the degree of cellular maturation. Neuroblastoma is an aggressive tumor with a tendency to invade adjacent tissues. The tumor metastasizes most frequently to liver and bone. It is the most common extracranial solid malignancy in children and the third most common malignancy of childhood, with only leukemia and primary brain tumors being more common. Approximately 90%−95% of patients with neuroblastoma have elevated levels of catecholamines (vanillylmandelic acid) in their urine, a useful diagnostic tool.

Neuroblastoma is a very unusual tumor in that the prognosis and the patterns of distribution of disease depend strongly on age. In children who are less than 18 months of age, the disease tends to spread to liver and skin. These children usually have a good prognosis. In children older than 18 months, the disease tends to spread to bone. These children have a poorer prognosis.

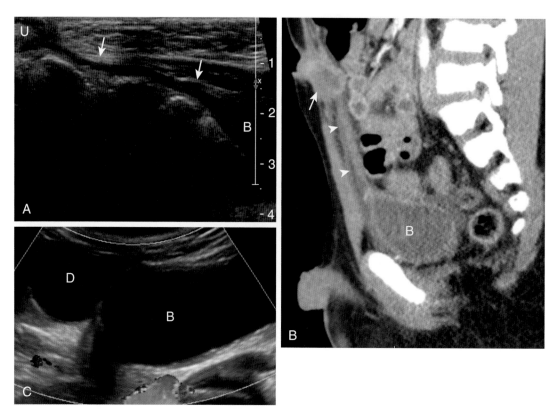

■ **FIGURE 6-36** Urachal anomalies in three different children. **A,** Patent urachus. Longitudinal ultrasound of the infraumbilical region shows patent connection between the bladder (*B*) and the umbilicus (*U*) evidenced by a hypoechoic tract (*arrows*). **B,** Infected urachal cyst. Sagittal reformatted contrast-enhanced CT image shows hypodense lesion (*arrow*) with surrounding inflammatory changes and associated tract (*arrowheads*) to the bladder (*B*). **C,** Urachal diverticulum. Longitudinal ultrasound of the infraumbilical region shows a diverticulum (*D*) extending from the superior aspect of the bladder (*B*).

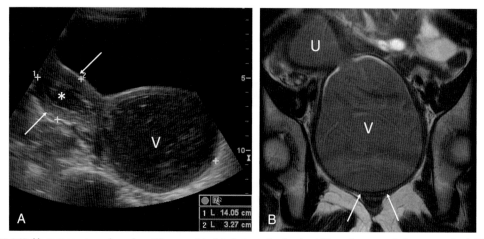

■ **FIGURE 6-37** Hematometrocolpos in a 12-year-old girl. **A,** Longitudinal midline ultrasound shows marked dilatation of the vagina (*V*), which is distended with heterogeneous hypoechoic fluid in keeping with blood products. The uterus (*arrows*) extends from the superior aspect of the dilated vagina. The uterine cavity (***) is slightly dilated with blood products as well but not nearly as much as the vaginal cavity. **B,** Coronal T2-weighted MR image shows massively dilated vaginal cavity (*V*). The uterus (*U*) extends from the superior aspect of the vagina and is deviated toward the right. The intraluminal blood products are of intermediate signal intensity. The vaginal obstruction is caused by a vaginal septum (*arrows*).

TABLE 6-3 International Neuroblastoma Risk Group Staging System

Stage	Description
L1	Localized tumor that does not involve vital structures as defined by the IRDFs and confined to one body compartment
L2	Local regional tumor with presence of one or more IDRFs
M	Distant, metastatic disease (except stage MS)
MS	Metastatic disease in children younger than 18 months with metastases confined to skin, liver, and/or bone marrow

IDRF, Image-defined risk factor. Reprinted with permission. 2009 American Society of Clinical Oncology. All rights reserved. Monclair T, Brodeur GM, Ambros PF et al.: The International Neuroblastoma Risk Group (INRG) staging system: an INRG Task Force report, *J Clin Oncol* 27:298–303, 2009.

Tumor staging is done using the International Neuroblastoma Risk Group Staging System (Table 6-3), which categorizes the tumor as stage L indicating localized disease or stage M indicating metastatic disease. Stage L is further categorized as stage L1 (Fig. 6-38) or L2 (Fig. 6-39) depending on the absence or presence of image-defined risk factors (IDRFs) (Table 6-4). IDRFs are 20 well-defined surgical risk factors, identified on imaging, that make complete tumor resection risky or complicated at the time of diagnosis. Stage MS is given to children less than 18 months of age with metastatic disease that is confined to skin, liver, and bone marrow (Fig. 6-40). Cases with cortical bone involvement demonstrated by radiography or nuclear bone scintigraphy are not considered stage MS. Patients with stage M disease have very poor prognosis and commonly require

therapy, such as bone marrow transplantation, whereas patients with stage MS disease have excellent prognosis and at many institutions are watched with imaging and receive no therapy. Other factors associated with better prognosis are listed in Table 6-5.

Although neuroblastoma may be encountered initially as a mass on abdominal radiographs or US, confirmation of the diagnosis and definition of the exact extent of disease is obtained with either CT or MRI. MRI is superior to CT on detecting bone marrow vertebral disease, chest involvement, spinal canal extension, and liver metastases. Neuroforaminal involvement is important to identify because at many institutions it will lead neurosurgery services to become involved in the surgical resection.

On CT and MRI, the tumors tend to appear lobulated with an invasive pattern of growth, surrounding and engulfing, rather than displacing, vessels such as the celiac axis, superior mesenteric artery, and aorta (Fig. 6-39). The masses are often inhomogeneous secondary to hemorrhage, necrosis, and calcifications. Calcifications are seen by CT in as much as 85% of cases (Fig. 6-39). On MRI, neuroblastoma, like most other malignancies, is hyperintense on T2-weighted images and can be heterogeneous in signal. Calcifications are less commonly seen on MRI. During the staging of neuroblastoma, most patients also undergo evaluation with metaiodobenzylguanidine (MIBG) scan as approximately 90% of neuroblastomas are MIBG avid. The role of positron emission tomography (PET) and PET-CT or PET-MR is still being defined and may be of utility in MIBG–nonavid neuroblastoma.

Other adrenal tumors that occur in childhood, but much less commonly than neuroblastoma, include pheochromocytoma and adrenocortical carcinoma.

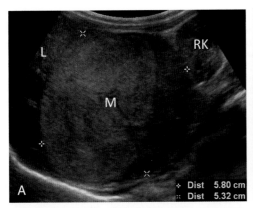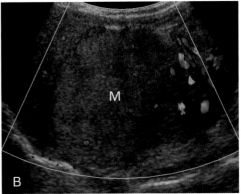

■ **FIGURE 6-38** Stage L1 neuroblastoma in a 6-month-old boy. **A,** Longitudinal ultrasound of the right suprarenal fossa shows a round, solid, echogenic mass (*M*) in between the liver (*L*) and right kidney (*RK*) indicating adrenal origin. **B,** Color Doppler ultrasound of the right adrenal mass (*M*) shows internal vascularity which is a helpful finding in the differentiation of neuroblastoma from adrenal hemorrhage in neonates. The presence of flow suggests neuroblastoma and excludes adrenal hemorrhage. However, the absence of flow does not exclude neuroblastoma.

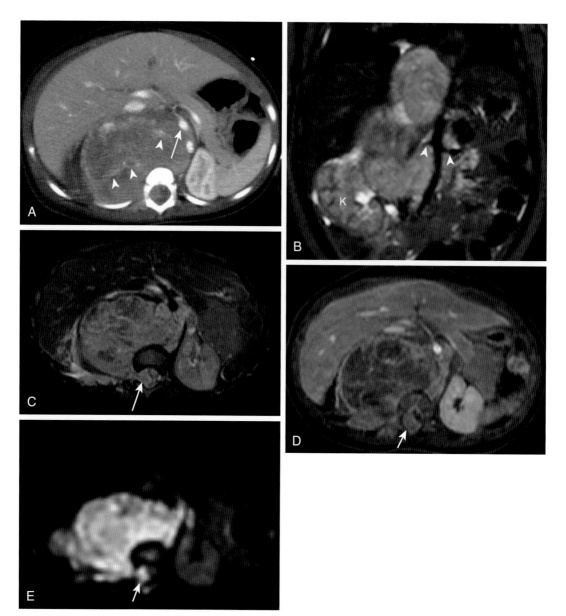

■ **FIGURE 6-39** Stage L2 neuroblastoma in a 9-month-old boy with at least three image-defined risk factors. **A,** CT shows heterogeneously enhancing retroperitoneal mass that surrounds and anteriorly displaces the abdominal aorta (*arrow*) and engulfs the origin of the celiac artery. Note the amorphous calcifications (*arrowheads*). **B,** Coronal fat-suppressed T2-weighted MR image shows the lesion crossing the midline as well as extending into the mediastinum. The lesion encircles the abdominal aorta and the origins of the bilateral renal arteries (*arrowheads*). Note inferolateral displacement of the right kidney (*K*). **C,** Axial fat-suppressed T2-weighted, and **D,** Axial contrast-enhanced fat-suppressed T1-weighted MR images show tumoral extension into the spinal canal (*arrows*), as well as encasement of the aorta and celiac axis origin. **E,** Diffusion-weighted MR image shows corresponding marked restricted diffusion and demonstrates to better advantage extension of the lesion into the spinal canal (*arrow*).

Neonatal Adrenal Hemorrhage

Adrenal hemorrhage can occur in neonates secondary to birth trauma or stress. Like neuroblastoma, adrenal hemorrhage may present as an asymptomatic flank mass and may be seen on imaging as an adrenal mass. Surgical intervention is unnecessary in adrenal hemorrhage, so differentiation from neuroblastoma is important. US may be able to differentiate the two, although often requiring serial exams. Neuroblastoma typically appears as an echogenic mass with internal vascularity on color Doppler,

TABLE 6-4 Definitions of Descriptive Terms That Determine Image-Defined Risk Factors (IDRFs)

Vital Structure	Term	Definition	IDRF
Arteries	Separation	Fat plane between artery and NBT	**No**
	Contact[a]	NBT abuts artery with no visible plane present. < **50%** of circumference of artery in contact with tumor	**No**
	Encasement	NBT abuts artery with no visible plane present. > **50%** of circumference of artery in contact with tumor	**Yes**
Veins	Flattening with visible lumen	NBT resulting in narrowing of vein with visible lumen, without complete flattening	**No**
	Flattening without visible lumen	NBT resulting in complete flattening of vein without visible lumen	**Yes**
Airway	Compression	NBT about airway and results in any deformity of airway resulting in decreased caliber of any degree	**Yes**
Spinal canal (intraspinal extension)		Either no extension into spinal canal or NBT extension that involves less than 1/3 of the volume of the canal at that level	**No**
	Invasion	NBT extension into the canal that involves > 1/3 of the volume of the canal at that level, is associated with cord compression or abnormal signal in the cord, or at the T9–T12 level (potential involvement of artery of Adamkiewicz)	**Yes**
Nonvascular vital structures	Infiltration	NBT extending into a parenchymal organ, pancreaticoduodenal block	**Yes**

NBT, neuroblastoma. [a]Note that contact of the tumor with the renal arteries or veins is automatically considered an IDRF even when encasement is not present. Adapted from Del Campos Braojos F, Donnelly LF: Practical application of the international neuroblastoma risk group staging system: a pictorial review, *Curr Probl Diagn Radiol* 48:509–518, 2019.

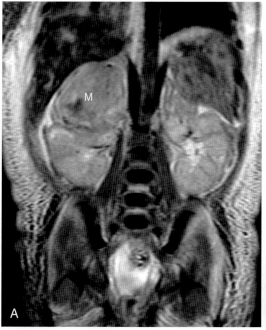

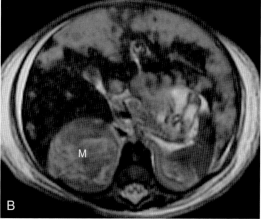

■ **FIGURE 6-40** Stage MS neuroblastoma in a neonate with palpable fullness in the abdomen. **A,** Coronal and **B,** Axial T2-weighted MR images show multiple heterogeneous masses throughout the liver parenchyma and a right suprarenal mass (*M*).

whereas adrenal hemorrhage typically appears as an avascular mass (Fig. 6-41). The internal hemorrhagic components show variable echogenicity depending on the age of the blood products, and similarly, MR signal may vary, comparable to hemorrhages elsewhere in the body. However, an avascular suprarenal mass is not diagnostic of hemorrhage as neuroblastoma

may present with similar appearance. Performing serial ultrasounds over time (follow-up in 10–14 days) is often the way of differentiating the two entities, and one can afford to wait because the prognosis for neonates with stage L1 neuroblastoma is excellent. With time, adrenal hemorrhages decrease in size and show change in the echogenicity (Fig. 6-41).

■ PELVIC MASSES

Pelvic Rhabdomyosarcoma

Rhabdomyosarcoma is the most common malignant sarcoma of childhood with a mean age at diagnosis of 5–6 years, with slight male predominance. It is a highly malignant tumor that can occur in numerous locations throughout the body but most commonly arise in the pelvis

TABLE 6-5 Features Associated With Better Prognosis in Patients With Neuroblastoma

- Age of diagnosis less than 18 months
- Histologic grade
- No extra copies of the MYCN gene
- Stage MS
- Thoracic primary

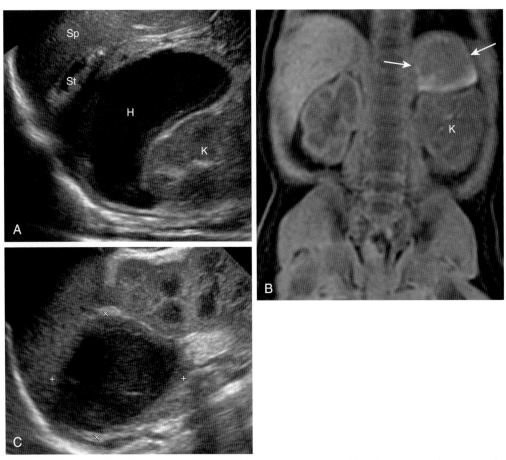

■ **FIGURE 6-41** Adrenal hemorrhage in a neonate. **A,** Initial sonogram at day 2 of life shows a complex, predominantly cystic-appearing, hypoechoic mass (*H*) in a suprarenal location. The kidney (*K*) is displaced inferiorly. *Sp,* Spleen; *St,* stomach. **B,** Coronal T1-weighted fat-suppressed MR image obtained at day 5 of life shows a complex suprarenal lesion (*arrows*) with high signal, blood degradation products consistent with an adrenal hemorrhage. The left kidney (K) is displaced inferiorly. **C,** Follow-up ultrasound from approximately 1 month later shows marked interval decrease in the size of the adrenal gland (*between calipers*), a more adreniform shape, consistent with resolving hematoma.

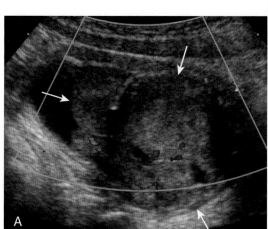
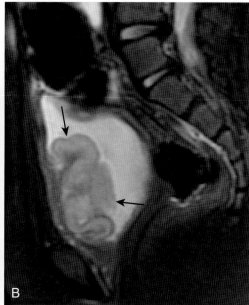

■ **FIGURE 6-42** Rhabdomyosarcoma arising from the bladder in a girl. **A,** Longitudinal ultrasound shows a large, intravesical heterogeneous mass (*arrows*) showing internal vascularity. **B,** Sagittal fat-suppressed T2-weighted MR image redemonstrates the large heterogeneous intravesical mass (*arrows*).

and genitourinary tract (23%) and head and neck (36%). Frequent locations within the genitourinary tract include the bladder (Fig. 6-42) and prostate but can also occur at the spermatic cord, paratesticular tissues, uterus, vagina, and perineum. When the lesion involves the bladder, it typically appears as a multilobulated mass, likened to a bunch of grapes, and is referred to as botryoid type. Pelvic rhabdomyosarcoma may result in hydronephrosis. Patients with cervicovaginal rhabdomyosarcoma, specifically botryoid-type embryonal, often have a cancer predisposition syndrome related to *DICER1* mutation.

Sacrococcygeal Teratoma

Sacrococcygeal teratomas typically present as large cystic or solid masses either on prenatal imaging or at birth. Less commonly they present as buttock asymmetry or a presacral mass later in childhood. They can be associated with anorectal and genital malformations. The majority are benign, but there is an increased risk for malignancy with delayed diagnosis. The mass can be primarily external, protruding from the sacral region, which is the most common type, accounting for nearly half of the cases; internal within the pelvis; or dumbbell shaped, with both internal and external components. On imaging, the lesions appear heterogeneous, with variable cystic, solid, and fatty components (Fig. 6-43).

■ ACUTE PELVIC PAIN IN OLDER GIRLS AND ADOLESCENTS

Acute pelvic pain in older girls and adolescents is a commonly encountered problem that has many possible causes. Pain can be related to menstruation, multiple ovarian pathologies, or appendicitis. Ovarian causes of pain include ovarian cysts, hemorrhagic cysts, ectopic pregnancy, ovarian torsion, endometriosis, pelvic inflammatory disease, or other masses, such as teratoma (Fig. 6-44) or other neoplasms. The high incidence and variety of pathologic processes that may involve the ovaries make US the initial imaging modality for right lower quadrant pain in girls.

Hemorrhagic cysts are a common cause of pelvic pain in adolescent girls. On US, the lesions appear as heterogeneous avascular masses that often have enhanced through-transmission. Sometimes the masses can be quite large. Ovarian cysts can also be discovered when ultrasound, CT, or MRI is performed to evaluate for appendicitis (Fig. 6-45).

Ovarian torsion, which is less common than hemorrhagic cysts, can appear on US as an enlarged and echogenic ovary secondary to

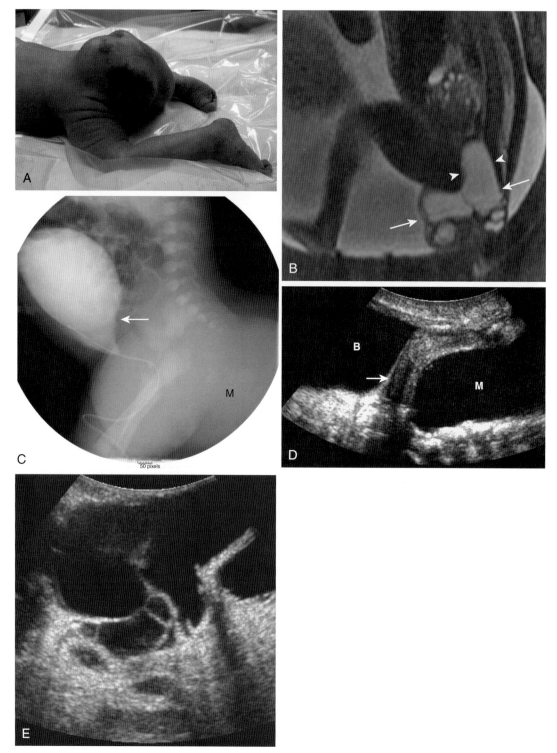

■ **FIGURE 6-43** Sacrococcygeal teratoma. **A,** Photograph of a newborn demonstrates skin-covered mass extending from buttocks region. **B,** Sagittal, T2-weighted prenatal MR image shows a multicystic mass (*arrows*) predominantly external, with component (*arrowheads*) extending within the internal pelvis. **C,** VCUG from postnatal work-up shows sacrococcygeal teratoma as a mass (*M*). Note that the bladder is displaced anteriorly (*arrow*). **D,** Longitudinal ultrasound shows that the cystic component of the mass (*M*) extends superiorly to the level of the inferior bladder (*B*). The uterus (*arrow*) is displaced posteriorly and superiorly. **E,** Ultrasound over the external portion of the mass shows its multicystic nature.

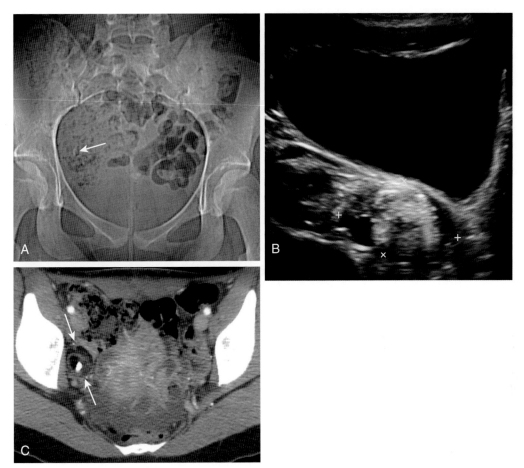

■ **FIGURE 6-44** Ovarian mature teratoma. **A,** Pelvic radiograph shows a tooth-like calcific density concerning for a teratoma in the right hemipelvis (*arrow*). **B,** Pelvic ultrasound shows an echogenic adnexal mass (between calipers) with posterior acoustic shadowing. The various interfaces in the near field, as a result of the mixture of fat and hair, obscure the remainder of the lesion, and the term *tip of the iceberg sign* is commonly used for this appearance. **C,** Corresponding CT image shows fatty tissue within the lesion (*arrows*), a typical imaging feature of mature ovarian teratomas.

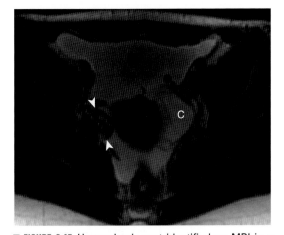

■ **FIGURE 6-45** Hemorrhagic cyst identified on MRI in a 15-year-old obese girl with right lower quadrant pain and suspected appendicitis. Axial T2-weighted MR image shows an approximately 5 × 4 cm cyst (*C*) in the left adnexal region. It is hyperintense with a crenated appearance suggestive of rupture. A moderate amount of free fluid is noted. A normal ovary is seen on the right (*arrowheads*).

edema. The follicles can have a peripheral distribution, which is highly suggestive of the diagnosis (Figs. 6-46 and 6-47). However, the most commonly encountered positive finding is asymmetric ovarian volumes, with the larger ovary located on the side of pain. Doppler US demonstration of decreased or absent blood flow is helpful in making diagnosis, but the presence of blood flow does not exclude ovarian torsion. An ovarian neoplasm, often benign, can be the present in 26% of cases of ovarian torsion (Fig. 6-47).

■ OVARIAN MASSES

Ovarian neoplasms in children are rare and are more frequently benign. The most common types are germ cell tumors, particularly mature ovarian teratoma which is often referred to as dermoid because of the predominance of ecto-dermal components (hair, skin, fat, and teeth).

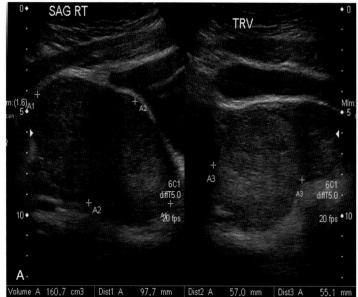

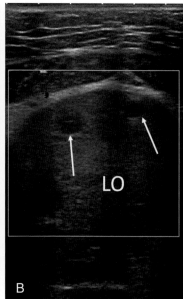

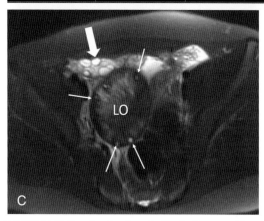

■ **FIGURE 6-46** Ovarian torsion. **A,** Dual ultrasound image, longitudinal view on the left and transverse view on the right. The ovary (*denoted by cursors*) is markedly enlarged with an estimated volume exceeding 160 cc and with diffuse increased echogenicity. **B,** Color Doppler ultrasound image shows absent flow and peripheral distribution of follicles (*arrows*) in the left ovary (*LO*). **C,** Axial fat-suppressed T2-weighted MR image of the pelvis shows an enlarged left ovary (*LO*), to the right of the midline. The ovary is of predominantly low signal intensity due to areas of hemorrhagic infarction and shows small hyperintense follicles with peripheral distribution (*thin arrows*). The normal right ovary (*thick arrow*) lies anteriorly in the right iliac fossa.

Ovarian teratoma can show varying appearances more often presenting on US as a cyst with a hyperechoic mural nodule (Rokitansky nodule) but may also contain fluid–fluid levels, fat, and calcifications, which can also be demonstrated on CT and MRI (Figs. 6-44 and 6-47). Other ovarian neoplasms are usually large at the time of presentation, can have a cystic or solid appearance, and typically do not have differentiating features at imaging. Occasionally, the clinical presentation can be helpful in suggesting a specific diagnosis. For example, ovarian granulosa cell tumor is a sex cord stromal tumor that can present with signs of precocious puberty due to production of estrogen (Fig. 6-48).

■ SCROTUM

Tumors

Most intratesticular neoplasms (>90%) are germ cell tumors with a stratification according to age. In the first decade, yolk sac tumors and teratomas are the most common types, whereas in the

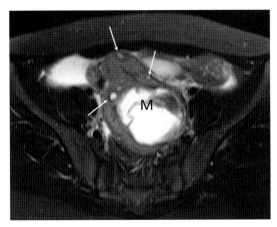

■ **FIGURE 6-47** Ovarian torsion secondary to mature ovarian teratoma in a 6-year-old girl with abdominal pain. Axial fat-suppressed T2-weighted MR image demonstrates an enlarged right ovary, which is in midline position and appears abnormally hypointense presumably due to stromal hemorrhage and necrosis. There is peripheral distribution of follicles (*arrows*). In the posterior aspect of the ovary, there is a mass (*M*) that shows hyperintense cystic areas and hypointense soft tissue representing fat, in keeping with a mature teratoma.

second decade, choriocarcinoma is the most common. Less than 10% of testicular tumors are metastatic from leukemia or lymphoma. Most primary testicular tumors present with a nontender, firm scrotal mass. US confirms an intratesticular mass (Fig. 6-49). However, there are no US findings that suggest a specific histologic diagnosis. If a scrotal mass is extratesticular in location, the most likely diagnosis is embryonal rhabdomyosarcoma arising from the spermatic cord or epididymis (Fig. 6-50).

Testicular Microlithiasis

Testicular microlithiasis appears on US as multiple punctate hyperechoic foci within the testes (Fig. 6-51), reflecting calcium deposits within seminiferous tubules. There is often no posterior acoustic shadowing because of the small size of the calcifications. The diagnosis is made when at least five microcalcifications can be seen on one US image. In children, it has a reported prevalence of 0.7%−3.8%, more often bilateral, and is typically an incidental finding. Testicular microlithiasis has a strong association with testicular neoplasms. Boys with testicular microlithiasis have approximately 22 greater odds of having a malignant germ cell tumor as compared to those without microlithiasis. However, there is controversy on the need and type of US follow-up of boys with this finding. In adults, routine surveillance with annual US is only recommended in the presence of risk factors such as previous malignancy, maldescent, small testis, and orchidopexy.

Acute Scrotum

Because of the possibility of testicular torsion, imaging of the acutely painful scrotum is an emergency. However, testicular torsion is an uncommon cause of acute scrotum. More frequent causes include torsion of the testicular (or epididymal) appendage and epididymoorchitis. Testicular hematoma is another less commonly encountered entity.

Testicular torsion occurs when the testis and cord twist within the serosal space and cause testicular ischemia. Prompt diagnosis and

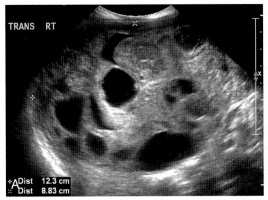
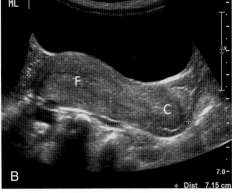

■ **FIGURE 6-48** Ovarian granulosa cell tumor presenting with abdominal mass. **A,** Transverse ultrasound shows a large right pelvic mass (*denoted by cursors*) with solid and cystic components. A normal right ovary was not seen and therefore the mass was presumed to arise from the right ovary. **B,** Longitudinal ultrasound shows an enlarged uterus (*denoted by cursors*) for the patient's age with a pubertal configuration. The fundus (*F*) has a rounded shape and is thicker than the cervix (*C*). The appearance of the uterus suggests isosexual precocity due to excessive estrogen production, a common feature of ovarian granulosa cell tumor.

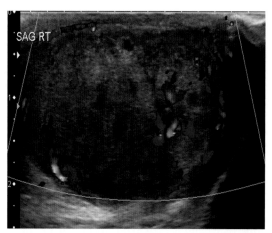

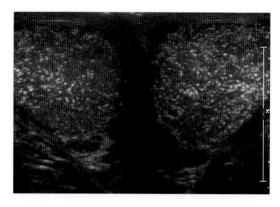

■ FIGURE 6-51 Testicular microlithiasis. Transverse ultrasound of the scrotum shows multiple punctate areas of increased echogenicity without posterior shadowing in both testicles.

■ FIGURE 6-49 Testicular yolk sac tumor in a 2-year-old boy presenting with increasing size and firm right testicle. Longitudinal color Doppler ultrasound shows diffuse involvement of the right testicle by a heterogeneous mass. There is intralesional flow, more prominent at the periphery of the mass.

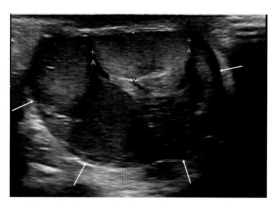

■ FIGURE 6-50 Paratesticular rhabdomyosarcoma in a 6-year-old boy presenting with scrotal enlargement. Transverse ultrasound of the right hemiscrotum shows diffuse enlargement of the epididymis (*arrows*). The right testicle (*denoted by cursors*) is displaced anteriorly.

therapy are important because preservation of the testis is possible only in patients whose torsion is relieved within 6–10 h. US with color Doppler is the modality of choice in evaluating acute scrotum and may show the whirlpool sign (Fig. 6-52) which is an abrupt spiral twist in the course of the spermatic cord at the external ring or in the scrotum and is a direct sign of testicular torsion. Other findings include absence of flow in the affected testis. Testicular flow can be present in incomplete torsion, although it is usually decreased when compared with the contralateral normal testicle. Demonstration of flow within a normal testis is more difficult in

children less than 2 years of age. Grayscale US may demonstrate a redundant spermatic cord within the scrotum as well as asymmetric enlargement and slightly decreased echogenicity of the affected testis. With progressive ischemia or infarction, hemorrhage and necrosis may cause increasing asymmetric heterogeneity (Fig. 6-53). This is a late finding.

The most common cause of acute scrotum is torsion of a testicular (or epididymal) appendage, which are normal embryonic remnants. A mass of variable echogenicity may be seen between the superior pole of the testis and the epididymis. Enlargement of an appendage to greater than 5 mm has been touted as the best indicator of torsion. Periappendiceal hyperemia and presence of testicular flow are supportive findings (Fig. 6-54). Torsion of the testicular appendage is a self-limited entity and does not require surgical management. The importance of making the diagnosis is to avoid unnecessary surgical exploration.

Epididymo-orchitis usually occurs without an identifiable cause, more commonly around puberty. In contrast to testicular torsion, in epididymo-orchitis, the affected testis and epididymis demonstrate asymmetric and sometimes strikingly increased flow on Doppler ultrasound. Grayscale US demonstrates enlargement and decreased echogenicity of the testis and epididymis. Reactive hydroceles are common.

Trauma may result in a testicular hematoma. On ultrasound, hematomas appear as avascular masses of abnormal echogenicity. Associated hematoceles are common.

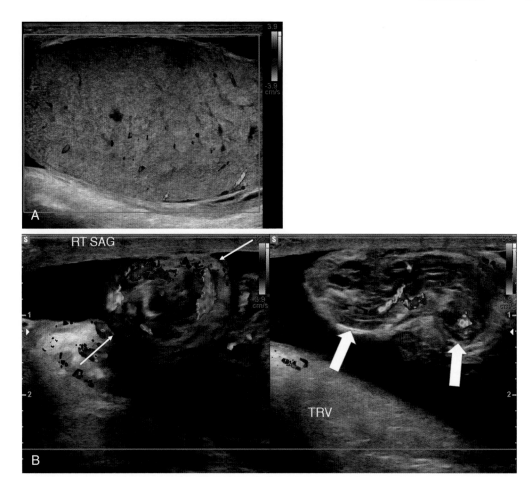

■ **FIGURE 6-52** Incomplete testicular torsion in a 13-year-old boy with intermittent episodes of right testicular pain, now with pain for 4 h. **A,** Longitudinal color Doppler ultrasound shows an enlarged right testicle and with heterogeneous echogenicity, although with flow present. **B,** Dual color Doppler ultrasound image of the right scrotum. The longitudinal view on the left shows a whirlpool sign of the spermatic cord vessels (*thin arrows*), a direct sign of testicular torsion. The transverse view on the right, just distal to the whirlpool sign, shows a redundant spermatic cord (*thick arrows*), a helpful sign in the diagnosis of testicular torsion.

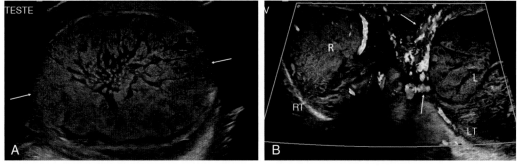

■ **FIGURE 6-53** Testicular torsion in a 13-year-old boy with a 3-day history of left testicular pain. **A,** Longitudinal ultrasound shows an abnormal left testicle (*arrows*), which is enlarged and of heterogeneous echogenicity with hypoechoic striations indicating edema and advanced ischemic changes. **B,** Transverse color Doppler ultrasound including both testicles shows enlargement, absent flow, and heterogeneous echotexture of left testicle (*L*). There is a large amount of flow (*arrows*) surrounding the left testicle, related to inflammatory reaction secondary to the necrosis. Note normal echotexture and present flow in the right testicle (*R*).

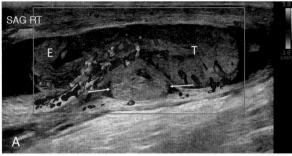
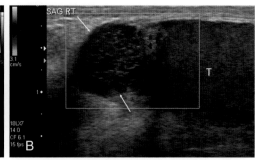

■ **FIGURE 6-54** Different appearances of torsion of the testicular appendage in two different boys. **A,** Longitudinal color Doppler ultrasound of the right scrotum shows an enlarged, predominantly hyperechoic, testicular appendage (*arrows*) adjacent to the upper pole of the testicle (*T*) and to the head of the epididymis (*E*). The enlargement and lack of flow indicate torsion of the testicular appendage. There are secondary inflammatory changes with enlargement and hyperemia of the epididymis (*E*) and hyperemia of the testicle (*T*). **B,** Longitudinal color Doppler ultrasound of the right scrotum shows enlargement and absence of flow to the testicular appendage (*arrows*). In this patient, the torsed testicular appendage shows presence of numerous tiny hypoechoic areas. *T*, testicle.

SUGGESTED READINGS

AAP subcommittee on urinary tract infection. Reaffirmation of AAP clinical practice guideline: the diagnosis and management of the initial urinary tract infection in febrile infants and young children 2–24 months of age, *Pediatrics* 138, 2016. e20163026.

Back SJ, Maya CL, Zewdneh D, Epelman M: Emergent ultrasound evaluation of the pediatric female pelvis, *Pediatr Radiol* 47:1134–1143, 2017.

Bandarkar AN, Blask AR: Testicular torsion with preserved flow: key sonographic and value-added approach to diagnosis, *Pediatr Radiol* 48:735–744, 2018.

Brisse HJ, McCarville MB, Granata C, et al.: Guidelines for imaging and staging of neuroblastic tumors: consensus report from the international neuroblastoma risk group project, *Radiology* 261:243–257, 2011.

Chung EM, Graeber AR, Conran RM: Renal tumors of childhood: radiologic-pathologic correlation part 1. The 1st decade, *Radiographics* 36:499–522, 2016.

Chung EM, Lattin GE, Fagen KE: Renal tumors of childhood: radiologic-pathologic correlation part 2. The 2nd decade, *Radiographics* 37:1538–1558, 2017.

Del Campos Braojos F, Donnelly LF: Practical application of the international neuroblastoma risk group staging system: a pictorial review, *Curr Probl Diagn Radiol* 48:509–518, 2019.

Dickerson EC, Dillman JR, Smith EA, et al.: Pediatric MR urography: indications, techniques, and approach to review, *Radiographics* 35:1208–1230, 2015.

Dillman JR, Trout AT, Smith EA, Towbin AJ: Hereditary cystic renal disorders: imaging of the kidneys and beyond, *Radiographics* 37:924–946, 2017.

Duran C, Beltrán VP, González A, et al.: Contrast-enhanced voiding urosonography for vesicoureteral reflux diagnosis in children, *Radiographics* 37:1854–1869, 2017.

Epelman M, Daneman A, Donnelly LF, et al.: Neonatal imaging evaluation of common prenatally diagnosed genitourinary abnormalities, *Semin Ultrasound CT MR* 35:528–554, 2014.

Gimpel C, Avni EF, Breysem L, et al.: Imaging of kidney cysts and cystic kidney diseases in children: an international working group consensus statement, *Radiology* 290:769–782, 2019.

Lala SV, Strubel N: Ovarian neoplasms of childhood, *Pediatr Radiol* 49:1463–1475, 2019.

Hanafy AK, Mujtaba B, Roman-Colon AM, et al.: Imaging features of adrenal masses in children, *Abdom Radiol (NY)* 45:964–981, 2020.

Lebowitz RL, Olbing H, Parkkulainen KV, et al.: International system of radiographic grading of vesicoureteral reflux: international reflux study in children, *Pediatr Radiol* 15:105–109, 1985.

McCarville MB: What MRI can tell us about neurogenic tumors and rhabdomyosarcoma, *Pediatr Radiol* 46:881–890, 2016.

Monclair T, Brodeur GM, Ambros PF, et al.: The international neuroblastoma risk group (INRG) staging system: an INRG Task Force report, *J Clin Oncol* 27:298–303, 2009.

Nguyen HT, Benson CB, Bromley B, et al.: Multidisciplinary consensus on the classification of prenatal and postnatal urinary tract dilation (UTD classification system), *J Pediatr Urol* 10:982–999, 2014.

Sung EK, Setty BN, Castro-Aragon I: Sonography of the pediatric scrotum: emphasis on the Ts—torsion, trauma, and tumors, *Am J Roentgenol* 198:996–1003, 2012.

CHAPTER 7

MUSCULOSKELETAL

Alexander J. Towbin

■ NORMAL VARIANTS AND COMMON BENIGN ENTITIES

More than in any other organ system, the normal imaging appearance of the skeletal system is strikingly different in children as compared to adults (Fig. 7-1). This is related to the changing appearance of growing and maturing bone. The most striking changes occur near the physes and apophyses. Many of the more common mistakes made in pediatric skeletal radiology are related to the misinterpretation of normal structures as being abnormal. Textbooks such as Keats's *Atlas of Normal Roentgen Variants That May Simulate Disease* are dedicated to the normal radiographic appearances and variations of bones in children. The details of all the normal changes of the maturing skeleton cannot be covered here. The following section describes several commonly misinterpreted normal variants and benign entities.

Apophyseal and Epiphyseal Irregularity

The terms *apophysis* and *epiphysis* sound similar and have similar meanings. Their differences can be confusing. The term *epiphysis* refers to the part of bone that articulates with the adjacent bone. An *apophysis* does not have an articular surface. Instead, it is a site of tendinous attachment. The growth plate, or physis, has a different appearance when associated with an epiphysis or apophysis. Epiphyseal growth plates are the primary growth centers of long bones. The physis associated with an epiphysis is oriented perpendicular to the longitudinal axis of the bone. This differs from the physis of an apophysis which is parallel to the long axis of the bone.

In the growing child, apophyses and epiphyses in various parts of the body can have variable and often somewhat irregular appearances. Separate ossicles of an apophysis can mimic fragments, irregularity can mimic periosteal reaction, and mixed sclerosis and lucency can be confused with findings of an inflammatory or neoplastic process. Common apophyses that may have this appearance include tibial tuberosity, ischial tuberosity, ischial pubic synchondrosis, posterior calcaneal apophysis (Fig. 7-2), and medial malleolus of the ankle (Fig. 7-3). Irregularity and fragmentation are commonly seen in the normal tibial tuberosity. The calcaneal apophysis can often demonstrate a strikingly sclerotic appearance (see Fig. 7-2, *C*). The ischial pubic synchondrosis can appear very prominent (see Fig. 7-1, *D*) and asymmetric.

Epiphyses can also appear irregular and even fragmented. The most common epiphyses with this irregular appearance are the distal femoral epiphysis (Fig. 7-4) and the capitellum (Fig. 7-5). It is important to recognize these irregularities as a normal stage of development and not confuse them with osteochondral lesions (in the distal femoral epiphysis or the capitellum) or with fracture (medial malleolus).

Distal Femoral Metaphyseal Irregularity

Distal femoral metaphyseal irregularity, also referred to as cortical desmoid or cortical irregularity syndrome, refers to the presence of irregular cortical margination and associated lucency involving the posteromedial aspect of the distal femoral metaphysis. It occurs in approximately 10% of boys 10–15 years of age. Although debated, its presence is thought to be related to chronic strain at the insertion of the adductor magnus muscle. While this lesion can be associated with pain, it is often discovered incidentally, and its significance lies in its striking radiographic appearance. On radiography, there is cortical irregularity along the posteromedial cortex of the distal femoral metaphysis, best seen on the lateral view (Fig. 7-6). On frontal radiographs, there may be an associated lucency (see Fig. 7-6, *B*). Familiarity with the typical location, appearance, and patient age is important so that these lesions are not confused with aggressive malignancies. Because the lesions are often bilateral, confirmation of their benign nature can be made by demonstrating a similar lesion on radiographs of the opposite knee. In problematic cases, computed tomography (CT) or magnetic resonance imaging (MRI) can be used to demonstrate the characteristic findings: a characteristic scoop-like defect with an irregular but

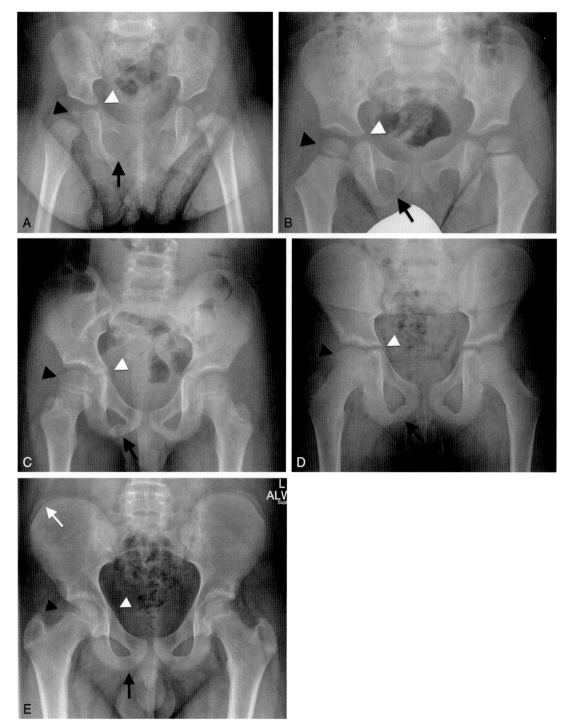

■ **FIGURE 7-1** Changes in radiographic appearance of bony structures with age. Radiographs of the pelvis are shown in different patients. **A,** At six months of age; **B,** at two years of age; **C,** at six years of age; **D,** at 10 years of age; and **E,** at 15 years of age. Note the dramatic changes in the appearance of the pelvis as structures ossify over time. At six months of age (in **A**), the femoral heads are just starting to ossify. The triradiate cartilage is open, and large portions of the ischium are not yet ossified. As children age, the femoral heads (*black arrowhead* on right femoral head) become more ossified, the ischium and pubis (*white arrow*) fuse, and the triradiate cartilage (*white arrowhead*) closes. As the ischiopubic synchondrosis (*black arrows* in **C** and **D**) closes, it can mimic a healing fracture to the untrained eye. The final portion of the pelvis to ossify is the iliac crest apophysis (in **E**, *white arrow*). This starts fusing only after the triradiate cartilage is closed.

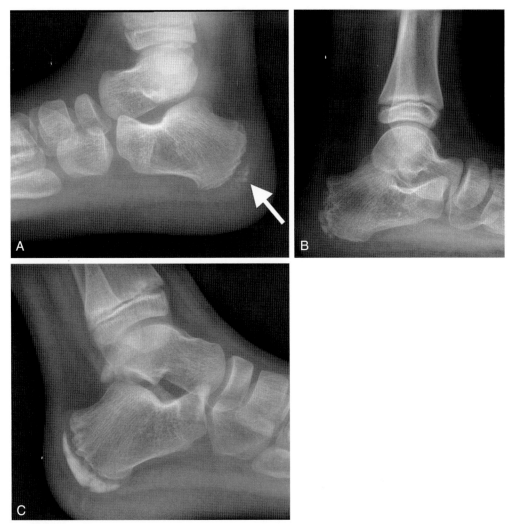

■ **FIGURE 7-2** Examples of apophyseal irregularity in the calcaneus in three separate children showing the wide variation in normal. **A,** The calcaneal apophysis (*arrow*) is just beginning to ossify in this six-year-old male. **B,** Both the metaphyseal and apophyseal edges of the calcaneus are irregular in this nine-year-old female. **C,** The calcaneal apophysis is mostly ossified in this 10-year-old male. In some children, as in this one, the normal calcaneal apophysis is sclerotic and mildly fragmented.

intact cortex; no associated soft tissue mass; and a subtle contralateral lesion.

Benign Fibrous Cortical Defects

Benign fibrous cortical defects, or nonossifying fibromas, are commonly encountered lesions of no clinical significance. They are seen in up to 40% of children at some time during development and most commonly occur between five and six years of age. The term *nonossifying fibroma* is reserved for lesions larger than 3 cm in diameter. They occur most commonly within the bones around the knee and in the distal tibia. They appear as eccentrically based, well-defined, bubbly, lucent lesions. These benign tumors have a narrow zone of transition with thin cortical rims (Figs. 7-7 through 7-9) and are typically round or oval. When the characteristic pattern is identified, no further imaging or follow-up is necessary. Occasionally a pathologic fracture can occur through the lesion (see Fig. 7-9). Over time, benign fibrous cortical defects become more sclerotic and eventually resolve (see Figs. 7-8). When imaged during this healing process, they are sometimes referred to as ossifying nonossifying fibromas.

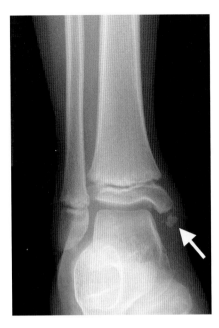

FIGURE 7-3 Apophyseal irregularity in the medial malleolus of the distal tibia. Mortise view of the ankle in a 10-year-old male shows an irregular ossification center of the medial malleolus (*arrow*). Fragmentation of the medial malleolus is almost always a part of normal development. The absence of soft tissue swelling helps to confirm that this is not related to trauma. Although there can be fragmentation of the medial malleolus, there should not be fragmentation of the distal fibula. When present, as in this case, it is related to trauma.

■ TRAUMA

Fractures in children differ from those in adults for multiple reasons. Children's bones have higher water content and are thus more pliable with a greater propensity to deform before breaking. This is akin to a new branch, or green stick, on a tree. Green sticks, with their higher water content, bend and deform before breaking.

The term *incomplete fracture* (Fig. 7-10) refers to a fracture that does not extend through the entire diameter of the cortex. Because children's bones are more elastic, incomplete fractures occur more commonly in children than adults. There are several types of incomplete fractures. *Plastic bowing deformity* (Fig. 7-11) is diagnosed when there is a greater than expected curvature of the bone after trauma without a discrete fracture line. This type of fracture occurs almost exclusively in the radius, ulna, or fibula. At times, a plastic bowing injury can be difficult to diagnose, and it is not until the follow-up image, when periosteal new bone is present, that the fracture can confidently be diagnosed. A *buckle fracture* is an incomplete fracture at the junction of the metaphysis and diaphysis along the compressive side of bone. It results in a bulge of one cortical surface. Importantly, there is no cortical disruption. Buckle fractures may be subtle and may appear only as an increase in angulation of a normally gentler curve (Fig. 7-12).

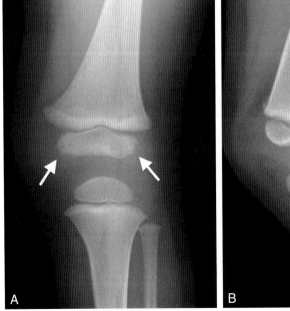

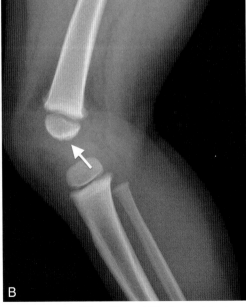

FIGURE 7-4 Epiphyseal irregularity of the distal femur. Anteroposterior (**A**) and lateral (**B**) views of the knee in a two-year-old female show developmental irregularity of the distal femoral epiphysis (*arrows*). As children age, the irregularity may become more focal and can mimic an osteochondral lesion.

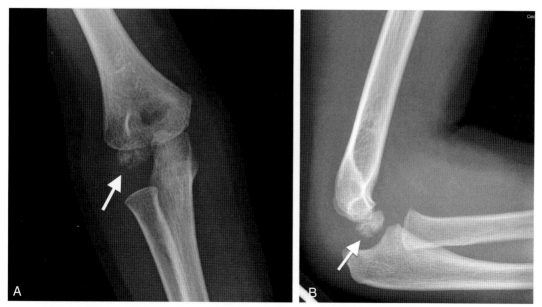

■ **FIGURE 7-5** Epiphyseal irregularity of the capitellum. Anteroposterior (**A**) and lateral (**B**) views of the elbow in a three-year-old male show developmental irregularity of the capitellum (*arrow*). The lack of soft tissue swelling and a joint effusion help to confirm that no fracture is present. Follow-up radiographs (not shown) confirmed that the findings were developmental and not related to trauma.

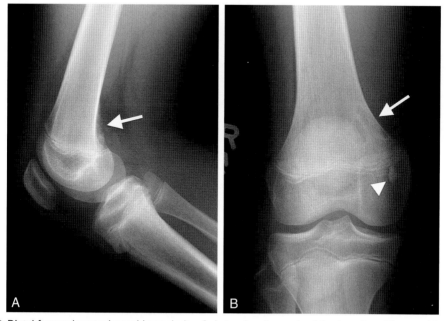

■ **FIGURE 7-6** Distal femoral metaphyseal irregularity. **A,** Lateral radiograph of the knee in a 14-year-old male shows irregularity (*arrow*) of the posterior aspect of the distal femoral metaphysis. Irregularity in this location is thought to represent chronic avulsion of the insertion of the adductor magnus muscle. **B,** On the anteroposterior view, the lesion appears as a well-marginated lucent lesion (*arrow*) along the medial aspect of the distal femoral metaphysis. In this patient, a bone island is also present in the distal femoral epiphysis (*arrowhead*).

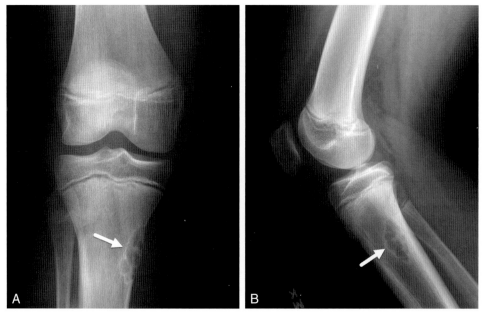

■ **FIGURE 7-7** Nonossifying fibroma. Anteroposterior (**A**) and lateral (**B**) radiograph of the knee in a 12-year-old female shows a 4.7 cm eccentrically based lucent lesion (*arrow*) with a narrow zone of transition and a sclerotic border arising from the posteromedial tibia. The eccentric location in bone and appearance is typical of a nonossifying fibroma.

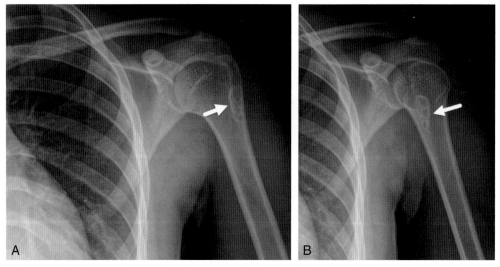

■ **FIGURE 7-8** Benign fibrous cortical defect. Anteroposterior (**A**) and lateral (**B**) radiograph of the shoulder in a 16-year-old female shows a 2.7 cm lucent lesion (*arrow*) of the proximal humerus. This lesion is eccentrically based with a narrow zone of transition and a sclerotic border. This lesion is slightly more sclerotic than the typical benign fibrous cortical defect representing early healing.

Buckle fractures are most common in the distal radius and ulna, the metacarpals and metatarsals, the phalanges, and the tibia (Fig. 7-13). Finally, a *greenstick fracture* is an incomplete fracture along the tension side of a bowing bone (Fig. 7-14). Greenstick fractures are most common in the forearm.

The potential for healing and the healing rate of fractures also differ in children and adults. Younger children heal very quickly. Periosteal reaction can be expected to be radiographically present 10–14 days after injuries in children. Children also tend to heal completely. Non-united fractures are very uncommon in children.

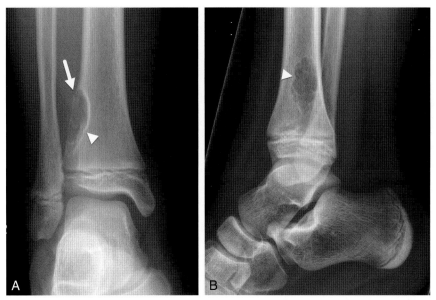

■ **FIGURE 7-9** Pathologic fracture through a nonossifying fibroma. Anteroposterior (**A**) and lateral (**B**) views of the ankle in a 12-year-old male show a pathologic fracture (*arrow*) centered in an eccentrically based lucent lesion (*arrowhead*) of the distal tibia.

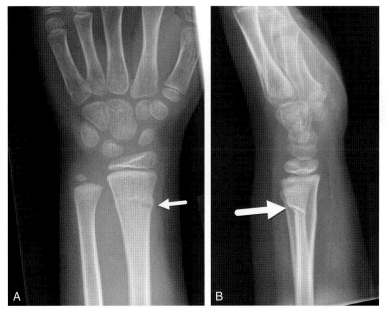

■ **FIGURE 7-10** Incomplete fracture of the radius. Anteroposterior (**A**) and lateral (**B**) radiographs of the wrist in a six-year-old female show an incomplete transverse fracture of the distal radius (*arrow*).

When describing fractures in children, the degree of displacement can help to guide the type of therapy and the need for orthopedic referral. Displacement can be described in terms of its type, direction, and magnitude. There are five main types of displacement: translation,

angulation, shortening, distraction, and rotation. The term *translation* refers to the lateral motion of the fracture fragment. *Angulation* is measured and described in relation to the apex of the curve. *Shortening* and *distraction* refer to motion along the longitudinal axis of the bone. Finally, *rotation*

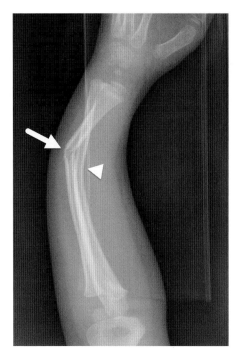

FIGURE 7-11 Plastic bowing deformity. Anteroposterior radiograph of the forearm in a three-year-old female shows a transverse fracture (*arrow*) of the distal third of the radius diaphysis and a plastic bowing deformity (*arrowhead*) of the ulna. The radius fracture is angulated with its apex directed dorsally.

is a more complex type of angulation where the motion of the fracture fragment occurs in relation to a fixed point.

Involvement of the Physis

Fractures in children may involve of the physis in up to 18% of pediatric long bone fractures. Physeal involvement requires internal fixation at a higher rate and may result in growth arrest of the affected limb. The Salter–Harris classification system is used to describe fractures that involve the physis. It divides fractures into five types according to whether there is involvement of the physis, epiphysis, or metaphysis, as determined by radiography (Fig. 7-15). Fractures classified with a greater Salter–Harris type are more likely to result in growth arrest. Type I fractures involve only the physis (Fig. 7-16). They tend to occur in children younger than five years of age. On radiography, the epiphysis may appear to be displaced in comparison with the metaphysis. However, type I fractures often reduce before the radiographs being obtained, making diagnosis extremely difficult. The potential findings of a type I fracture include soft tissue swelling adjacent to the physis, asymmetric widening of the physis, and/or displacement of the epiphysis. Salter–Harris type I injuries are

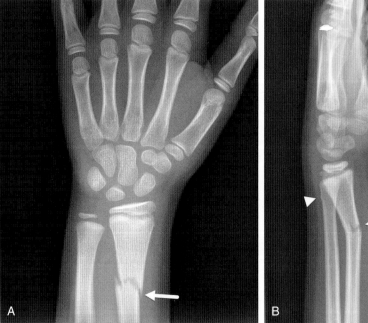
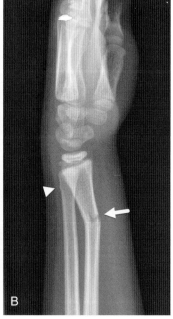

FIGURE 7-12 Buckle fracture of the distal ulna. Anteroposterior (AP) (**A**) and lateral (**B**) radiographs of the wrist in a six-year-old female show a transverse fracture of the distal radius (*arrow*) and a buckle fracture of the distal ulna (*arrowhead*). Buckle fractures can be very subtle on the AP view and occur at the junction of the metaphysis and diaphysis along the compressive side of the injury.

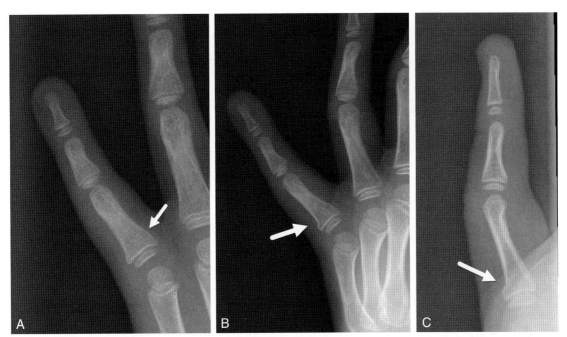

■ **FIGURE 7-13** Fracture of the proximal phalanx of the small finger. Anteroposterior (**A**), oblique (**B**), and lateral (**C**) radiographs of the small finger in a six-year-old male show a subtle contour irregularity (*arrow*) of the proximal aspect of the proximal phalanx of the ring finger. This is a common site of fracture when the finger is bent backwards.

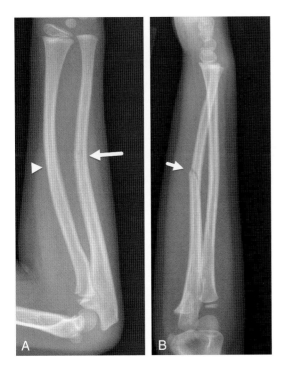

■ **FIGURE 7-14** Greenstick fracture and plastic bowing injury. Anteroposterior (**A**) and lateral (**B**) radiographs of the forearm in a four-year-old female show a greenstick fracture of the mid ulna (*arrow*) and a plastic bowing injury of the radius (*arrowhead*).

uncommon and may only occur at the distal fibula and the proximal femur (as in a slipped capital femoral epiphysis [SCFE]). Type II fractures involve the metaphysis and physis but do not involve the epiphysis (Figs. 7-17 and 7-18). They are the most common type of physeal injury, accounting for up to 75% of Salter–Harris fractures. On radiography, there is typically a triangular fragment of the metaphysis attached to the physis and epiphysis. Type III fractures involve the physis and epiphysis but not the metaphysis (Figs. 7-19 and 7-20). Type III injuries have a greater predisposition for growth arrest. Type IV injuries involve the epiphysis, physis, and metaphysis and, like type III injuries, are associated with a high rate of growth arrest (Fig. 7-21). Type V fractures consist of a crush injury to a part of or all of the physis. Like type I injuries, type V injuries are extremely difficult to diagnose. Often a diagnosis can be made only with a suspicious clinical history and comparison to the contralateral physis. With all Salter–Harris type fractures, it is important to assess the physis on follow-up images. Posttraumatic growth arrest is detected radiographically by demonstration of a bony bridge across the physis (Fig. 7-22).

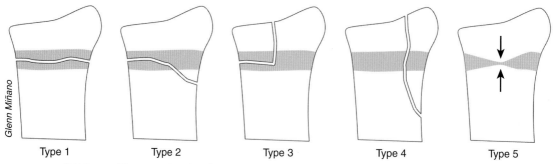

Glenn Miñano

Type 1   Type 2   Type 3   Type 4   Type 5

■ **FIGURE 7-15** Diagram showing Salter—Harris classification of fractures involving the physis.

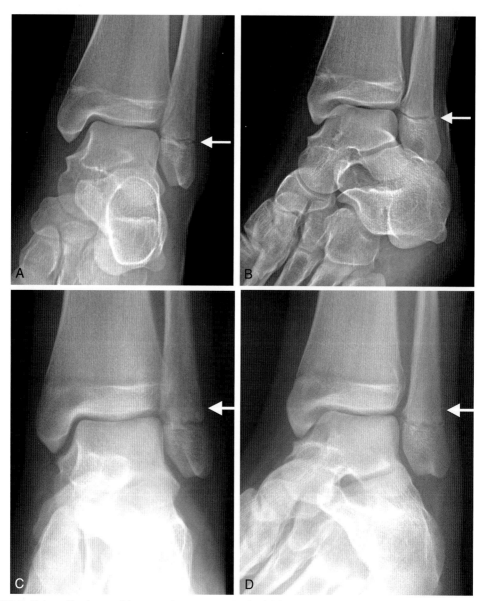

■ **FIGURE 7-16** Salter—Harris type I fracture. Anteroposterior (AP) (**A**) and oblique (**B**) radiographs of the ankle in a 13-year-old female show widening of the distal fibular physis (*arrow*) compared with the distal tibial physis. There was associated lateral soft tissue swelling. AP (**C**) and oblique (**D**) images in the same patient two weeks later show mild healing with faint periosteal new bone formation (*arrow*) adjacent to the distal fibular metaphysis.

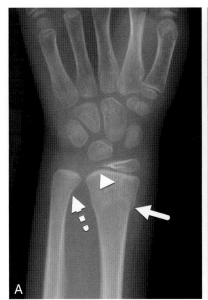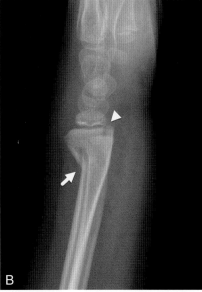

■ **FIGURE 7-17** Salter–Harris type II fracture. Anteroposterior (**A**) and lateral (**B**) radiographs of the wrist in an eight-year-old female shows an incomplete transverse fracture (*arrow*) of the distal radius. The fracture has a vertical component that extends to the physis (*arrowhead*) making it a Salter–Harris Type II fracture. A subtle incomplete transverse fracture (*dashed arrow*) of the distal ulna is also present.

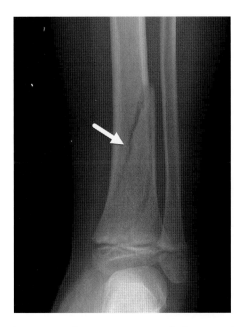

■ **FIGURE 7-18** Salter–Harris type II fracture. Anteroposterior radiograph of the lower leg in a five-year-old male shows an oblique fracture (*arrow*) of the distal tibia that extends to the physis.

Commonly Encountered Fractures by Anatomic Location

Pediatric fractures have unique features in almost all locations. The following material reviews several of the more commonly encountered areas.

WRIST

The wrist is the most common site of fracture in children. Most fractures of the distal forearm are incomplete or transverse fractures of the distal metaphysis of the radius, with or without fracture of the distal ulnar metaphysis or styloid (Figs. 7-17, 7-20, 7-21, and 7-23). It is important to assess all fractures of the distal radius for extension of the fracture line to the physis because the distal radius is also the most common area of physeal fracture (28% of physeal injuries occur in the distal radius). Vertical extension of a distal radius fracture to the physis is often subtle. However, this type of physeal extension is important for the pediatric radiologist to identify and describe as it can necessitate orthopedic referral.

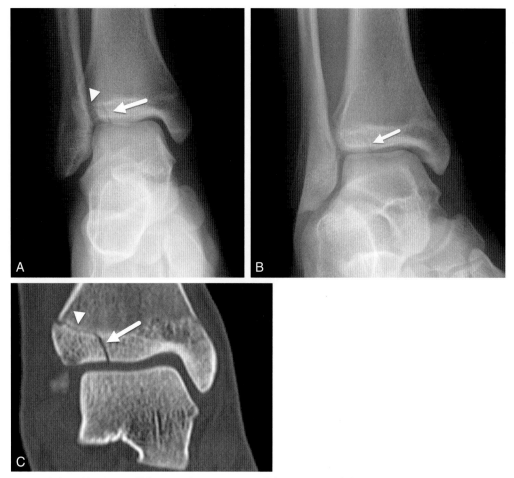

■ FIGURE 7-19 Salter–Harris type III fracture. Anteroposterior (**A**) and oblique (**B**) radiographs of the ankle in a 14-year-old male show a fracture of the epiphysis of the distal tibia (*arrow*). The fracture extends into the ankle joint. This type of fracture is termed a juvenile Tillaux fracture. Coronal computed tomography image (**C**) shows the extent of the fracture and allows for measurement of fracture displacement. A fracture gap of more than 2 mm requires internal fixation.

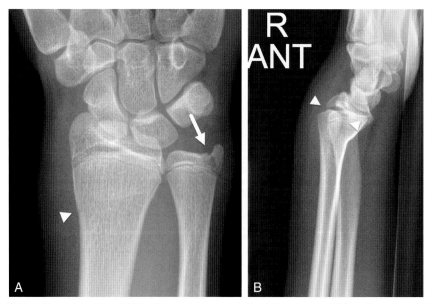

■ FIGURE 7-20 Salter–Harris type II and III fractures. Anteroposterior (**A**) and lateral (**B**) radiographs of the wrist in a 15-year-old female show a longitudinally oriented fracture (*arrow*) of the ulnar epiphysis that extends to the physis. In addition, there is an incomplete Salter Harris type II fracture (*arrowheads*) of the distal radius. The distal fracture fragment is shown to be translated palmarly on the lateral view.

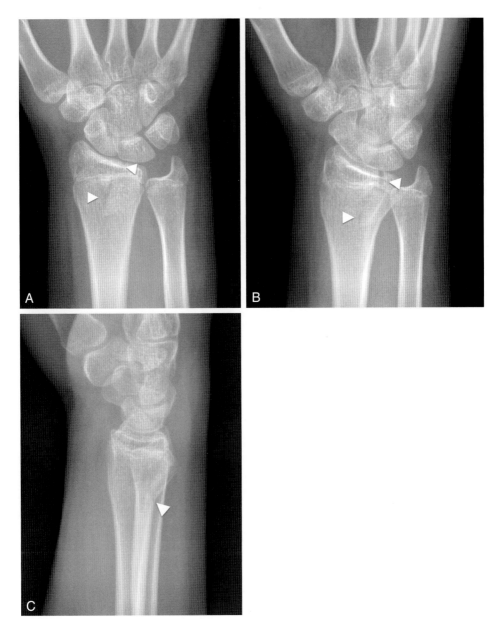

■ FIGURE 7-21 Salter–Harris type IV fracture. Anteroposterior (**A**), oblique (**B**), and lateral (**C**) radiographs of the wrist in a 12-year-old female show a complex fracture (*arrowheads*) extending from the distal radius metaphysis, through the physis and epiphysis, and into the radiocarpal joint.

Displacement or obliteration of the pronator fat pad indicates a fracture or deep soft tissue injury. The normal pronator fat pad is visualized on a lateral view of the forearm as a thin line of fat with a mildly convex border. In most distal forearm fractures, the convexity of the pronator fat pad is increased or the fat pad becomes obliterated by soft tissue attenuation.

ELBOW

There are several unusual features that make elbow injuries in children different from those in adults. In contrast to adults, in whom fracture of the radial head is the most common injury, children most commonly experience supra-condylar fractures (Figs. 7-24 and 7-25). They

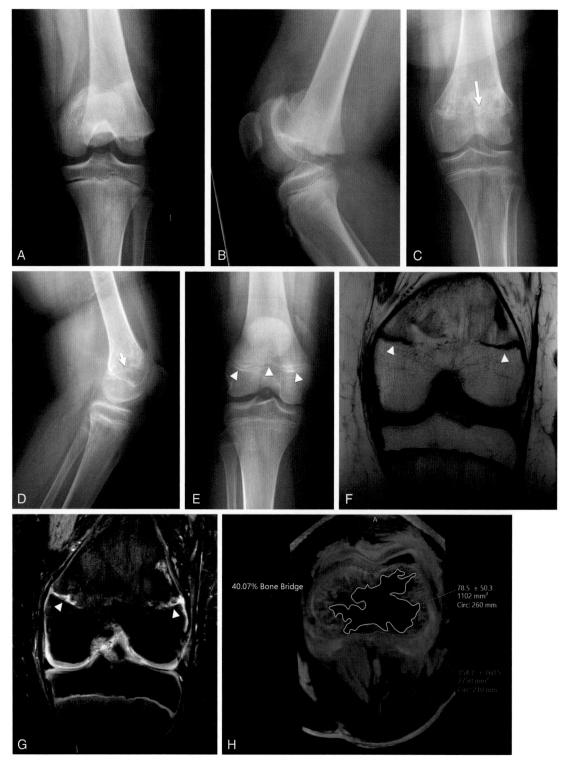

■ **FIGURE 7-22** Premature physeal fusion secondary to a Salter–Harris type II fracture. Anteroposterior (AP) (**A**) and lateral (**B**) radiographs of the knee at time of injury in a 12-year-old male show a displaced Salter–Harris type II fracture of the distal femur. The distal fracture fragment is translated ventrally by approximately 50% and rotated 90 degrees clockwise. **C,** AP and lateral (**D**) radiographs of the knee 10 months later shows premature fusion (*arrow*) of the central portion of the distal femoral physis. **E,** The normal contralateral distal femoral physis (*arrowheads*) is shown for comparison. **F,** Coronal T1-weighted magnetic resonance imaging (MRI) and intermediate-weighted cartilage sensitive sequence (**G**) confirms the premature central physeal closure. The open portion of the physis (*arrowheads*) remains visible laterally. **H,** MRI can be used to measure the percentage of the physis that has closed prematurely. This information can be used to help operative planning.

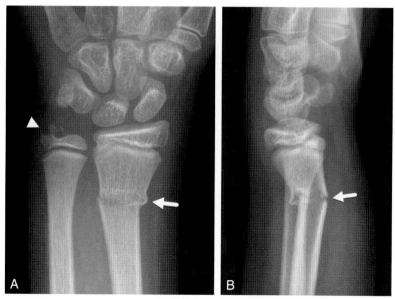

■ **FIGURE 7-23** Transverse fracture of the distal radius and ulnar styloid. Anteroposterior (**A**) and lateral (**B**) radiographs of the wrist in an 11-year-old female show transverse fractures of the distal radius (*arrow*) and ulnar styloid (*arrowhead*).

occur secondary to hyperextension that occurs when falling on an outstretched arm. As many as 25% of such fractures are incomplete and may be subtle on radiography. On radiographs, there can be posterior displacement of the distal fragment such that a line drawn down the anterior cortex of the humerus (anterior humeral line) no longer bisects the middle third of the capitellum. The fracture line is usually best seen through the anterior cortex of the distal humerus on the lateral view. A joint effusion is typically evident. Elbow effusions are identified when there is

displacement of the posterior fat pad, resulting in its visualization on a lateral view (Figs. 7-24 through 7-26). Normally the posterior fat pad rests within the olecranon fossa and is not visible on a true lateral view of the elbow. However, when an effusion is present, the posterior fat pad is elevated by the joint fluid. The anterior fat pad, which is normally visible, may become prominent and have an apex anterior convexity.

There is debate regarding the significance of a traumatic elbow effusion in the absence of a visualized fracture (see Fig. 7-26). It is often

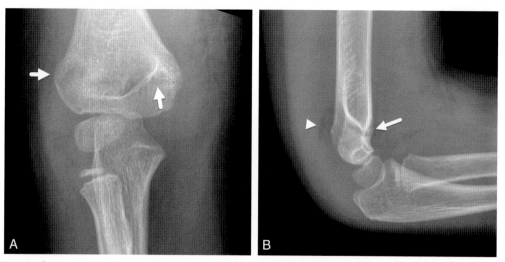

■ **FIGURE 7-24** Supracondylar fracture. Anteroposterior (AP) (**A**) and lateral (**B**) radiographs of the elbow in a six-year-old male show a supracondylar fracture (*arrows*). The fracture line is often difficult to see on the AP view. Note the large joint effusion (*arrowhead*).

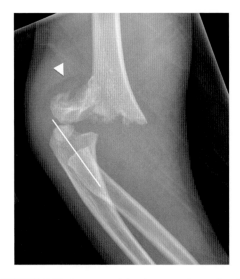

■ FIGURE 7-25 Supracondylar fracture. Lateral radiograph of the elbow in a four-year-old male shows a displaced supracondylar fracture and large joint effusion (*arrowhead*). When the fracture is this displaced, it can be difficult to determine if the elbow joint is congruent. The radiocapitellar line is used to help determine radiocapitellar alignment. This line, drawn through the longitudinal axis of the radius, should bisect the capitellum.

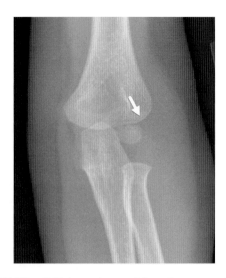

■ FIGURE 7-27 Lateral condylar fracture. Anteroposterior (AP) radiograph of the elbow in a two-year-old female shows a lateral condylar fracture (*arrow*). The fracture is usually better seen on the AP view, where there is a thin sliver of bone adjacent to the fracture line in the radial aspect of the humeral metaphysis.

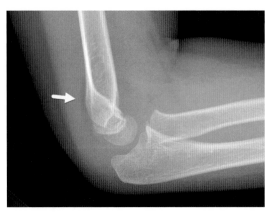

■ FIGURE 7-26 Elbow effusion. Lateral radiograph of the elbow in a five-year-old female shows a moderate joint effusion, as demonstrated by the elevation of the posterior fat pad (*arrow*). The anterior fat pad is also displaced. No fracture was present on this image or on subsequent follow-up (not shown).

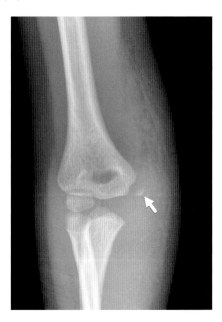

■ FIGURE 7-28 Medial epicondyle avulsion. Anteroposterior radiograph of the elbow in a five-year-old female shows avulsion of the medial epicondyle (*arrow*). There is marked medial soft tissue swelling.

taught that a joint effusion is synonymous with an occult fracture. However, studies have shown that fractures are present in 50% or fewer cases. The point is moot because traumatic injury to the elbow is treated by splinting, whether a subtle fracture is identified or not. If pain persists, a repeat radiograph is obtained at the follow-up orthopedic appointment. If a fracture is present, signs of healing are evident.

Other elbow injuries include fractures of the radial neck and lateral condyle (Fig. 7-27) and avulsion of the medial epicondyle (Figs. 7-28 and 7-29). When avulsed, the medial epicondyle may become displaced and even entrapped within the elbow joint (see Fig. 7-29). It is important to

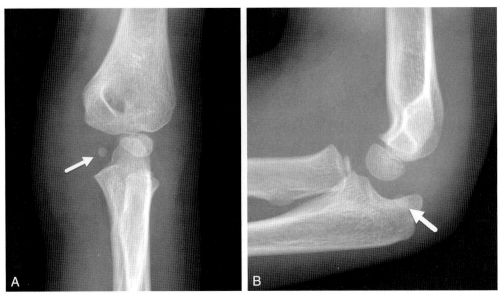

■ **FIGURE 7-29** Avulsion and entrapment of the medial epicondyle. Anteroposterior (AP) (**A**) and lateral (**B**) radiographs of the elbow in a 4-year-old female show a circular ossific density (*arrow*) overlying the elbow joint on the AP view that represents the avulsed medial epicondyle. On the lateral view, the avulsed fragment (*arrow*) is shown to be entrapped in the elbow joint. Note that the capitellum and radial head are already ossified.

know the predictable order of maturity of the elbow ossification centers so that a displaced medial epicondyle is not missed. The order can be remembered by the mnemonic CRITOE (capitellum, radial head, internal [medial] epicondyle, trochlea, olecranon, external [lateral] epicondyle).

Whenever there is a fracture of the forearm, it is important to evaluate the radial-capitellar joint for potential dislocation of the radial head. The radial head should align with the capitellum on both the anteroposterior (AP) and lateral views. If it does not, radial head dislocation should be suspected (Fig. 7-30). When a radiocapitellar

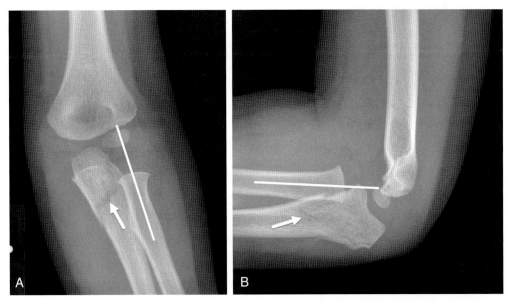

■ **FIGURE 7-30** Monteggia fracture. Anteroposterior (AP) (**A**) and lateral (**B**) radiographs of the elbow in a two-year-old male show a fracture of the proximal ulna diaphysis (*arrow*) and dislocation of the proximal radius. On the lateral view, the line drawn through the center of the radius (parallel to its long axis) does not intersect the capitellum.

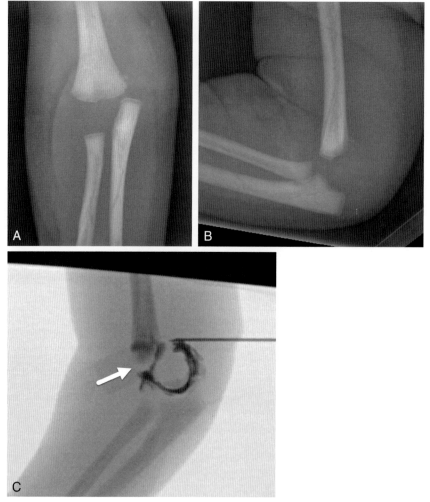

■ **FIGURE 7·31** Distal humerus physeal separation. Anteroposterior (**A**) and lateral (**B**) radiographs of the elbow in a seven-day-old male show ulnar-sided and posterior displacement of the proximal radius and ulna. This is characteristic of distal humerus physeal separation. This type of injury represents a fracture through the cartilage. **C,** Elbow arthrogram image obtained during surgical repair shows contrast outlining the cartilage of the distal humerus. The fracture (*arrow*) is visible when contrast is injected into the joint.

dislocation is present, the entire forearm should be imaged to evaluate for a Monteggia fracture. Monteggia fractures represent a fracture-dislocation injury with dislocation of the head of the radius and an associated fracture of the ulnar diaphysis (see Fig. 7-30).

Distal humerus physeal separation (Fig. 7-31) is a unique fracture seen exclusively in young children. In young infants, this represents a Salter–Harris type I fracture occurring through the distal humerus physeal cartilage. Because the fracture can occur before the capitellum begins to ossify, the fracture can be difficult to detect. On radiograph, there is usually posterior and ulnar displacement of the radius and ulna in relation to the distal humerus. This causes the forearm to not be aligned with the distal

humerus. The fracture is associated with birth trauma in neonates and child abuse in older infants.

ANKLE

The ankle is a commonly injured joint due to a combination of inversion and eversion injuries with weight bearing. There are two common fractures that are unique in adolescents, triplane fractures, and juvenile Tillaux fractures. As the name implies, a triplane fracture occurs in three planes: the coronal plane through the tibial metaphysis, the transverse plane through the physis, and the sagittal plane through the epiphysis (Fig. 7-32). Because the fracture extends through the metaphysis and epiphysis, this

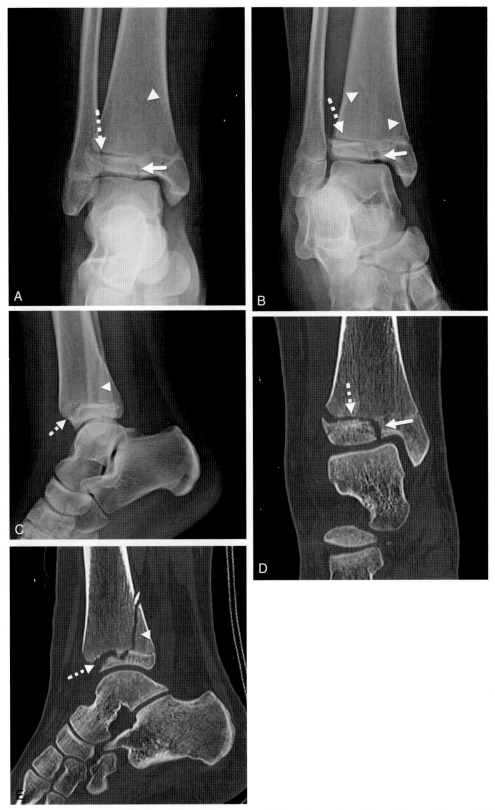

■ **FIGURE 7-32** Triplane fracture. AP (**A**), oblique (**B**), and lateral (**C**) radiographs of the ankle in a 14-year-old female show a triplane fracture of the tibia. The tibia fracture extends from the tibial metaphysis (*arrowheads*), through the physis (*dashed arrow*), and into the epiphysis (*arrow*). The metaphyseal component of the fracture is best seen on the lateral view. Coronal (**D**) and sagittal (**E**) images from a computed tomography of the ankle in the same patient shows each plane of the triplane fracture more obviously. The epiphyseal fracture component is translated laterally with a fracture gap of more than 2 mm.

is a Salter–Harris type IV fracture. Triplane fractures occur in adolescents in whom the growth plate is beginning to close. The radiologist should measure the degree of distraction of the fracture fragment as internal fixation is performed if there is more than 2-mm displacement. Often a CT is performed to evaluate the fracture and the amount of distraction more accurately. Fibular fractures are present approximately half of the time.

Juvenile Tillaux fractures are Salter–Harris type III fractures of the distal tibia. Like triplane fractures, they occur in adolescents in whom the growth plate is beginning to close. The fracture occurs because the medial tibial physis closes before the lateral physis. The differences in structural stability lead to this fracture pattern when there is abduction and external rotation of the ankle. On X-ray, there is a fracture line through the distal tibial epiphysis and widening of the medial aspect of the ankle mortise (Fig. 7-19). CT is performed to evaluate the amount of fracture distraction. Like triplane fractures, orthopedic surgeons will perform internal fixation if the fracture is distracted by more than 2 mm.

Toddler Fracture

There are several fractures referred to as toddler fractures. The most common of these is a nondisplaced oblique or spiral fracture of the tibia diaphysis (Fig. 7-33). It is often difficult to determine the vertical extent of the fracture. However, toddler fractures of the tibia can extend to the articular surface at the ankle. The radiologist should have a high index of suspicion to describe any vertically oriented lucency as extension of the fracture. Toddler fractures are relatively common and occur when a child first begins to walk. Most children present with refusal to bear weight on that extremity. Oblique views often demonstrate the fracture better than do frontal or lateral views. When diagnosing this fracture, it is important to look at the patient's age because a spiral fracture in a child who is not yet walking can be a fracture of abuse. Other types of toddler fractures include stress-type fractures involving the calcaneus or cuboid (Figs. 7-34 and 7-35).

Avulsion Fractures in Adolescents

An avulsion fracture is a structural failure of bone at a tendon or aponeurotic insertion. Adolescents are prone to avulsion fractures because of a combination of their strength, their activity or participation in sports, and their immature, growing apophyses. Avulsion fractures occur

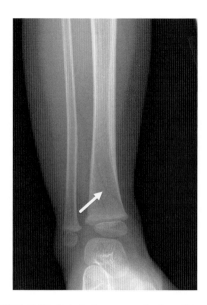

■ **FIGURE 7-33** Spiral fracture of the tibia. Anteroposterior radiograph of the ankle in an 18-month-old female shows a spiral fracture of the distal tibia (*arrow*). The fracture plane is continuous throughout its course and likely extends to the physis.

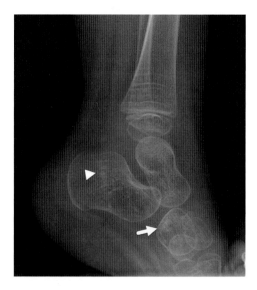

■ **FIGURE 7-34** Stress fractures of the calcaneus and cuboid. Lateral radiograph of the hind foot shows linear areas of sclerosis in the posterior calcaneus (*arrowhead*) and posterior cuboid (*arrow*). The bones are osteopenic and multiple growth recovery lines are present in the distal tibia.

because the growing apophysis and its associated physis have less structural integrity than the attaching tendon. The sites of insertion of muscles capable of generating great forces are most predisposed to avulsion injuries.

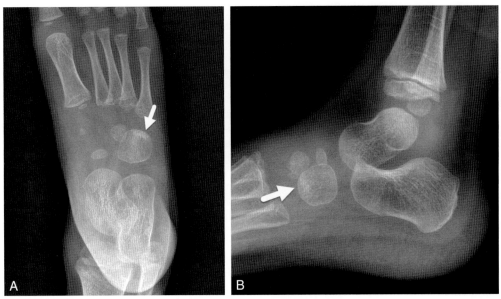

■ **FIGURE 7-35** Stress fractures of the cuboid. Anteroposterior (**A**) and lateral (**B**) radiographs focused on the hind foot and mid foot in a three-year-old male show a linear area of sclerosis in the cuboid (*arrow*) consistent with a stress fracture.

Radiologists may encounter findings of chronic avulsion when patients are imaged for pain or incidentally when imaging is performed for other reasons. The irregularity and periostitis that can be associated with chronic avulsions should not be misinterpreted as suspicious for malignancy. The most common sites of avulsion occur within the pelvis, where muscles of the abdominal wall and lower extremities attach. Common sites of pelvic apophyseal avulsions and their associated muscular attachments include the iliac crest (transversalis, internal oblique abdominalis, external oblique abdominalis; Fig. 7-36); anterior superior iliac spine (sartorius; Fig. 7-37); anterior inferior iliac spine (rectus femoris; Fig. 7-38); ischial apophysis (hamstring muscles: biceps femoris, gracilis, semi-membranosus, semitendinosus; Fig. 7-36); and lesser trochanter (iliopsoas). The radiographic findings of avulsion injuries include displacement of the ossified apophysis from its normal position and variable, often exuberant periosteal new bone formation with healing.

When involving a joint, avulsion fractures occur at the cortical insertion site of a ligament or tendon. The knee is the joint most commonly associated with an avulsion fracture. Many of these injuries occur exclusively in children and adolescents. Common sites of knee avulsion fractures and their associated tendinous or ligamentous attachments include the anterior

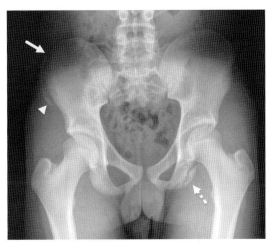

■ **FIGURE 7-36** Multiple avulsion fractures of the pelvis. Anteroposterior radiograph of the pelvis in a 16-year-old male shows asymmetric widening of the right lateral iliac crest (*arrow*). This avulsion fracture extends to include the anterior superior iliac spine (*arrowhead*). There is an additional avulsion fracture of the left ischial tuberosity (*dashed arrow*).

medial tibial spine (anterior cruciate ligament; Fig. 7-39); lateral tibial rim, also known as a Segond fracture (lateral collateral ligament; Fig. 7-40); fibular head (conjoined tendon with biceps femoris); tip of the fibular head (arcuate ligament); inferior pole of the patella, also known

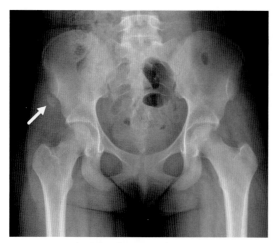

■ **FIGURE 7-37** Avulsion fracture of the anterior superior iliac spine. Anteroposterior radiograph of the pelvis in a 13-year-old female shows an avulsion fracture (*arrow*) of the right anterior superior iliac spine. The fracture fragment is translated inferiorly and laterally.

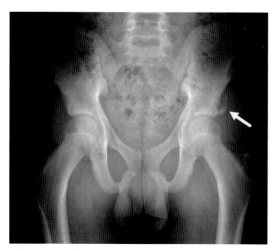

■ **FIGURE 7-38** Avulsion fracture of the anterior inferior iliac spine. Anteroposterior radiograph of the pelvis in a 14-year-old male shows a large avulsion fracture (*arrow*) of the left anterior inferior iliac spine.

as the patellar sleeve (proximal patellar tendon; Figs. 7-41 and 7-42); and tibial tubercle (distal patellar tendon Fig. 7-43). Many of these injuries present with sudden pain and a joint effusion. MRI is often indicated because these injuries are associated with other internal derangement.

Chronic fatigue or strain injuries are common in the adolescent knee and can lead to apophysitis. Apophysitis of the inferior pole of the patella at the origin of the patellar tendon is called Sinding–Larsen–Johansson syndrome (Fig. 7-44). It occurs most commonly in children between 10 and 14 years of age. Symptoms

include localized pain and swelling over the inferior aspect of the patella associated with restricted knee motion. Radiography demonstrates irregular bony fragments at the inferior margin of the patella, associated with adjacent soft tissue swelling and thickening and indistinctness of the patellar tendon. Apophysitis of the tibial tuberosity at the patellar tendon insertion is referred to as Osgood–Schlatter disease (Fig. 7-45). It is a common disorder that most often affects active adolescent boys. Symptoms include pain and swelling over the tibial tuberosity. Radiography demonstrates fragmentation of the tibial tuberosity, associated adjacent soft tissue swelling, and thickening and indistinctness of the patellar tendon.

The normal apophysis of the fifth metatarsal is frequently mistaken for an avulsion fracture. This mistake is made for two reasons. First, it is common for children with a foot injury to present with lateral foot pain. Second, avulsion fractures of the proximal fifth metatarsal, the so-called pseudo-Jones fracture, are common. The apophysis can be distinguished from a fracture based on the orientation of the lucency. The normal apophysis of the fifth metatarsal extends parallel to the long axis of the metatarsal (Figs. 7-46 and 7-47). Avulsion fractures of the fifth metatarsal occur as a result of inversion of the foot in plantar flexion such as when climbing steps. These fractures extend perpendicular to the long axis of the fifth metatarsal and may extend into the tarsal/metatarsal joint.

Child Abuse

Child abuse, also referred to as the less accusatory term, *nonaccidental trauma*, is unfortunately common. According to data from the US Department of Health and Human Services, 678,000 children were abused and 1770 killed in 2018 in the United States (https://www.acf.hhs.gov/sites/default/files/cb/cm2018.pdf). Most abused children are less than one year of age and almost all are less than six years of age. When clinical or imaging findings are suspicious for potential abuse, a radiographic skeletal survey is typically obtained. The purpose of the skeletal survey is to document the presence of findings of abuse. In young children, a head CT is often performed to identify intracranial signs of abuse. Other tests sometimes used include a repeat skeletal survey after approximately two weeks to look for healing injuries not seen on the initial skeletal survey, skeletal scintigraphy, abdominal CT, and MRI of the brain. The identification and reporting of findings of child abuse by the radiologist is an important task.

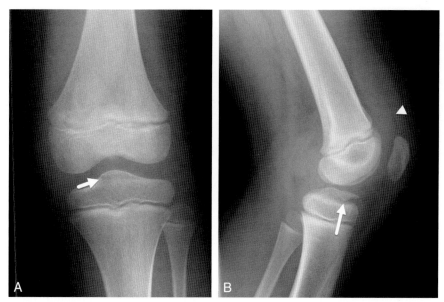

■ **FIGURE 7-39** Tibial spine avulsion fracture. Anteroposterior (**A**) and lateral (**B**) radiographs of the knee in a seven-year-old male show an avulsion fracture of the tibial spine. The avulsed fragment (*arrow*) is easier to see on the lateral view. A moderate knee joint effusion (*arrowhead*) is present.

The radiographic findings of abuse vary in their specificity. One of the highly specific findings is the presence of posterior rib fractures occurring near the costovertebral joints (Fig. 7-48). These are thought to occur when an adult squeezes an infant's thorax. Such rib fractures may be subtle before development of callus formation. The evaluation for rib fractures should be a routine part of the evaluation of the chest radiograph of any infant. Another finding

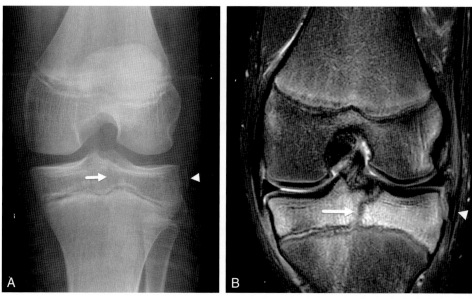

■ **FIGURE 7-40** Salter–Harris Type III fracture and Segond fracture. Anteroposterior (**A**) radiograph of the knee in a 13-year-old male shows a Salter–Harris type III fracture (*arrow*) of the proximal tibia and an avulsion fracture of the lateral aspect of the proximal tibial epiphysis (*arrowhead*). The fracture of the lateral tibial epiphysis is termed a Segond fracture. Coronal intermediate-weighted magnetic resonance imaging (**B**) highlights the Salter–Harris type III fracture (*arrow*) and Segond fracture (*arrowhead*). While a Segond fracture is usually associated with disruption of the anterior cruciate ligament, in this patient, the ligament was intact (not shown). It was thought that the Salter–Harris type III fracture protected the anterior cruciate ligament.

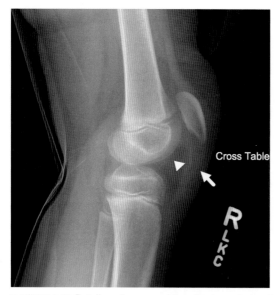

■ **FIGURE 7-41** Patellar sleeve avulsion fracture. Lateral radiograph of the knee in a nine-year-old male shows an avulsion fracture (*arrowhead*) of the inferior pole of the patella. The patellar tendon (*arrow*) is thickened and has an irregular contour suggesting that it is disrupted. In addition, the patella is higher than expected, in an alta position, and its inferior pole is tilted upward.

that is highly specific for abuse is the classic metaphyseal lesion, also known as a metaphyseal corner fracture (Fig. 7-49). This fracture occurs secondary to forceful pulling of an extremity. The broken metaphyseal rim appears as a triangular piece of bone when seen tangentially or as a crescentic rim of bone (referred to as a bucket-handle fracture) when seen obliquely. Other fractures associated with abuse include those of the scapula, spinous process, and sternum. Spiral long bone fractures in nonambulatory children are also highly suspicious. Multiple fractures in children of various ages (some with callus and some acute), as well as multiple fractures of various body parts, are highly suspicious for abuse. In fact, any fracture in an infant should be viewed with suspicion because as many as 30% of fractures in infants are secondary to abuse. Extraskeletal findings seen in abuse include acute or chronic subdural hematoma, cerebral edema (asphyxia), intraparenchymal brain hematoma, lung contusion, duodenal hematoma, solid abdominal organ laceration, and pancreatitis.

The clinical and imaging findings of abuse do not usually require a differential diagnosis. However, other entities that may cause multiple fractures or that may cause radiographic findings that could be confused with injury, such as

periosteal reaction, should always be considered. The other disorders that may present with multiple fractures in an infant are osteogenesis imperfecta (OI) and Menkes syndrome. Both entities are also associated with excessive Wormian bones and osteopenia. Rickets, caused by vitamin D deficiency, is not a cause of the fractures specific for abuse. The imaging appearance of child abuse and that of rickets do not overlap.

■ PERIOSTEAL REACTION IN THE NEWBORN

When periosteal reaction is encountered in a newborn, there are several entities that must be considered (Tables 7-1). They include physiologic new bone formation, TORCH infections (osteomyelitis), prostaglandin therapy, Caffey disease, metastatic neuroblastoma, and abuse. Physiologic periosteal new bone formation is the most common cause of diffuse periosteal new bone and can be seen in infants during the first few months of life. It typically involves rapidly growing long bones, such as the femur, tibia, and humerus. Differential features that support physiologic growth as the cause of periosteal reaction include symmetric distribution, benign appearance of the periosteal reaction, and appropriate age of the child. Radiographs may show lines of periosteal reaction paralleling the cortex of the diaphysis of the long bones. Neonates with congenital heart disease are commonly treated with prostaglandins to maintain patency of the ductus venosus. These children commonly demonstrate prominent periosteal reaction (Fig. 7-50).

TORCH Infections

The differential diagnosis for transplacentally acquired infections can be remembered by the mnemonic TORCH: toxoplasmosis, other (syphilis), rubella, cytomegalovirus, and herpes.

CONGENITAL RUBELLA SYNDROME

Rubella was once the most common transplacental viral infection. Since the introduction of the rubella vaccine, the incidence of congenital rubella has plummeted. Its features include eye abnormalities, deafness, hepatosplenomegaly, aortic and pulmonic stenosis, and intrauterine growth restriction. Bony changes are present in as many as 50% of cases.

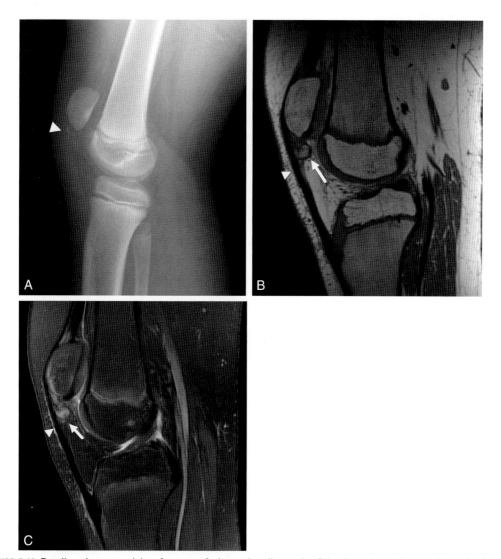

■ **FIGURE 7-42** Patellar sleeve avulsion fracture. **A,** Lateral radiograph of the knee in a 10-year-old male shows an avulsion fracture (*arrowhead*) of the inferior pole of the patella. The patella is in an alta position. The patellar tendon is taut. Sagittal T1-weighted (**B**) and fat saturated T2-weighted (**C**) magnetic resonance imaging shows the avulsed fracture fragment (*arrow*) adjacent to the inferior pole of the patella. The patellar tendon (*arrowhead*) remains partially intact. However, the fibers of the patellar tendon attached to the avulsed fragment are disrupted.

They include irregular fraying of the metaphyses of long bones and generalized lucency of the metaphyses. The findings have been likened to a celery-stalk appearance. These radiographic findings are most apparent during the first few weeks of life. The bony manifestations of rubella are currently extremely rare.

SYPHILIS

Congenital syphilis occurs secondary to transplacental infection, usually occurring during the second or third trimester. Clinical findings include hepatosplenomegaly, rash, rhinorrhea, anemia, and ascites. Bony changes are present in as many as 95% of patients but often do not appear until 6–8 weeks after the time of infection. The radiographic findings may be present before the blood serology turns positive. Findings include nonspecific metaphyseal lucent bands, serrated metaphyses, multiple fractures, lytic skull lesions, and periosteal reaction involving multiple long bones. The *Wimberger corner sign* is the most specific finding of syphilis and consists of destruction of the medial portion of the proximal metaphysis of the tibia, resulting in an area of irregular lucency. Osseous manifestations of syphilis are much more commonly encountered than those of rubella or other TORCH infections.

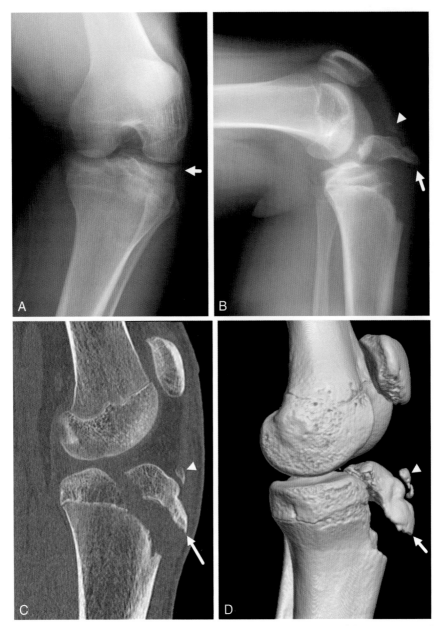

■ **FIGURE 7-43** Tibial tubercle avulsion fracture. Anteroposterior (AP) (**A**) and lateral (**B**) radiographs of the knee in a 17-year-old male show an avulsion fracture of the tibial tubercle (*arrow*). The fracture is difficult to visualize on the AP view. The best clue is that bone projects over the joint space. A second avulsion fragment is present at the patella tendon insertion (*arrowhead*). Sagittal (**C**) and three-dimensional reconstruction (**D**) from a computed tomography show how the avulsion fracture (*arrow*) of the tibial tubercle extends into the knee joint. The second avulsed fragment (*arrowhead*) has a more chronic appearance because of its rounded shape and lack of cortical irregularity at the donor site.

Caffey Disease (Infantile Cortical Hyperostosis)

Caffey disease is an idiopathic syndrome that consists of periosteal reaction shown on radiographs, irritability, fever, and soft tissue swelling over the areas of periosteal reaction. It occurs during the first few months of life. The bones most commonly involved include the mandible, clavicle, ribs, humerus, ulna, femur, scapula, and radius. Imaging shows periosteal new bone formation, sclerosis, and adjacent soft tissue swelling. The disease is self-limited and currently occurs much less commonly now than in the past for reasons that are not well-understood.

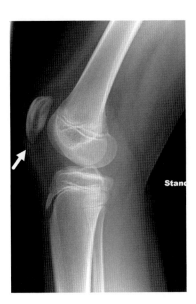

■ FIGURE 7-44 Sinding-Larsen-Johansson syndrome. Lateral radiograph of the knee in an 11-year-old female with chronic knee pain shows fragmentation of the inferior pole of the patella (*arrow*) and thickening of the origin of the patellar tendon.

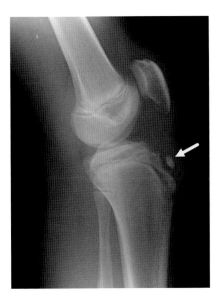

■ FIGURE 7-45 Osgood–Schlatter disease. Lateral radiograph of the knee in a 14-year-old male shows fragmentation and irregularity of the tibial tuberosity (*arrow*) at the site of the patellar tendon insertion. The patellar tendon is thickened, and there is overlying soft tissue swelling.

■ LUCENT PERMEATIVE LESIONS IN CHILDREN

A bone lesion is considered permeative when it has poorly defined borders, a wide zone of transition, and multiple small, irregular holes centrally. As in an adult, a permeative bone lesion in a child is consistent with an aggressive inflammatory or neoplastic lesion. The more common causes of a permeative lesion in a child include osteomyelitis, Langerhans cell histiocytosis (LCH), neuroblastoma metastasis, Ewing sarcoma, and lymphoma or leukemia. The differential diagnosis can be further limited by considering the patient's age (Tables 7-2). If the patient is younger than five years of age, the most likely diagnoses include osteomyelitis, LCH, and metastatic neuroblastoma. Ewing sarcoma and lymphoma are exceedingly rare in children younger than five years of age. In older children, Ewing sarcoma and lymphoma or leukemia become candidates, and metastatic neuroblastoma becomes much less likely.

Osteomyelitis

Acute osteomyelitis is a relatively common cause of clinically significant bone pathology in children. It is primarily a disease of infants and young children; one third of cases occur in children younger than two years of age, and one half of cases occur before five years of age. Because of the young age of most of the children, the presentation is often nonspecific, and diagnosis is delayed. Erythrocyte sedimentation rate is elevated in a vast majority of cases. Most cases of osteomyelitis are hematogenous in origin; many patients have a recent history of respiratory tract infection or otitis media. *Staphylococcus aureus* is the most common cause, accounting for more than 80% of cases.

Osteomyelitis tends to occur in the metaphyses or metaphyseal equivalents of children. This is related to the rich and slow-moving blood supply to these regions. Approximately 75% of cases involve the metaphyses of long bones with the most common sites being the femur, tibia, and humerus. The other 25% of cases occur within metaphyseal equivalents of flat bones such as the pelvis.

The earliest radiographic finding of osteomyelitis is deep soft tissue swelling evidenced by displacement or obliteration of the fat planes adjacent to a metaphysis. Osseous changes may not be present until 10 days after the onset of symptoms. Initial bony changes consist of poorly defined lucency involving a metaphyseal area (Fig. 7-51). Progressive bone destruction is often present. Periosteal new bone formation begins at approximately 10 days. Osteomyelitis can appear as sclerotic, rather than lucent, when it is a chronic process.

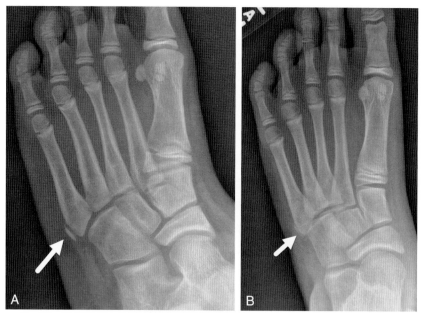

■ **FIGURE 7-46** Normal apophysis of the fifth metatarsal. Anteroposterior (**A**) and oblique (**B**) radiographs of the foot in a 12-year-old male show the normal apophysis (*arrow*) of the fifth metatarsal.

MRI has become the dominant imaging study in the work-up of osteomyelitis. Many institutions use a wide field of view T2-weighted MRI sequence to screen the affected region in symptomatic young children and then perform a more focused exam in areas of identified abnormalities. Osteomyelitis appears as an area of increased T2-weighted signal within

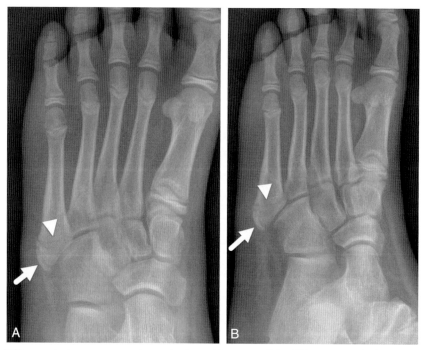

■ **FIGURE 7-47** Difference between a normal apophysis and fracture of the fifth metatarsal. Anteroposterior (**A**) and oblique (**B**) radiographs of the foot in a 12-year-old male show the normal apophysis (*arrow*) parallel to the longitudinal axis of the fifth metatarsal. A nondisplaced fracture (*arrowhead*) is also present. Fractures at this location traverse perpendicular to the longitudinal axis of the metatarsal.

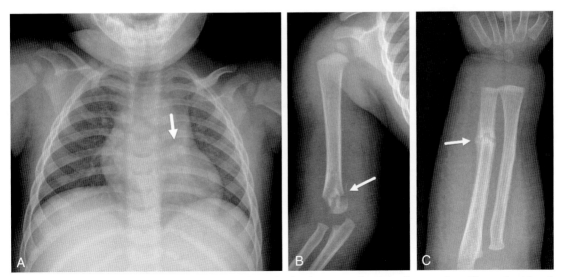

■ FIGURE 7-48 Child abuse. **A,** Frontal view of the chest obtained as part of a skeletal survey in a 13-month-old male shows a healing fracture of the left seventh posterior rib (*arrow*). **B,** Radiograph of the humerus shows an acute supracondylar fracture (*arrow*). **C,** Radiograph of the forearm shows a healing fracture (*arrow*) of the distal third of the ulna. There is considerable soft tissue swelling of the upper and lower arm.

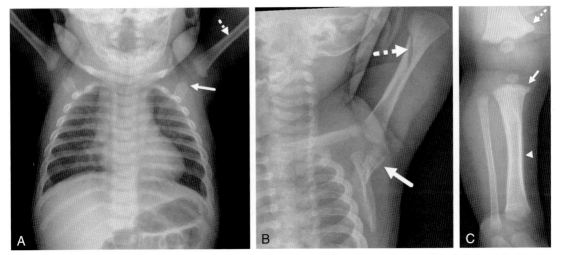

■ FIGURE 7-49 Child abuse. Anteroposterior (AP) view of the chest (**A**) and focused view of the left shoulder from an oblique view of the chest (**B**) in a four-month-old male show fractures of the left acromion (*arrow*) and left humerus (*dashed arrow*). **C,** AP radiograph of the lower leg shows classic metaphyseal lesions of the distal femur (*dashed arrow*) and proximal tibia (*arrow*). The diffuse periosteal new bone (*arrowhead*) of the tibia may be related to either a healing fracture or normal growth. The scapular fracture and classic metaphyseal lesions are both considered fractures specific for abuse.

TABLE 7-1 Differential Diagnosis for Periosteal Reaction in a Newborn
• Physiologic Growth
• TORCH infections
• Prostaglandin therapy
• Caffey disease (infantile cortical hyperostosis)
• Neuroblastoma metastasis
• Healing fractures, abuse

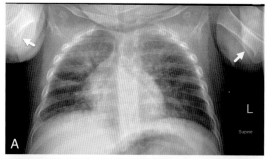

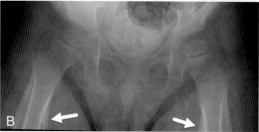

■ **FIGURE 7-50** Diffuse periosteal new bone formation. Anteroposterior radiographs of the chest (**A**) and pelvis (**B**) in a 28-month-old male with juvenile idiopathic arthritis and macrophage activation syndrome show diffuse symmetric periosteal new bone formation of the humeri and femurs (*arrows*).

✳ **TABLE 7-2** Differential Diagnosis of a Permeative Bone Lesion in a Child on the Basis of Age	
Younger than five years of Age	**Older than five years of Age**
Osteomyelitis	Ewing sarcoma
Langerhans cell histiocytosis	Lymphoma or leukemia
Neuroblastoma metastasis	Osteomyelitis Langerhans cell histiocytosis

a metaphysis. There are usually large areas of surrounding edema within the adjacent bone marrow and soft tissues. Gadolinium administration may show areas of nonenhancement suspicious for necrosis or abscess formation. Identification of subperiosteal abscesses is one of the advantages of MRI.

Skeletal scintigraphy, using technetium 99m-methyl diphosphonate, has become a much less common test to evaluate for osteomyelitis. On skeletal scintigraphy, osteomyelitis appears as a focal area of increased activity on the angiographic, soft tissue, and skeletal phase images. Skeletal scintigraphy becomes positive early after the onset of osteomyelitis and is often positive before development of changes seen on radiography. Another advantage of scintigraphy is the ability to evaluate for multiple sites of involvement.

A Brodie abscess is a unique form of osteomyelitis. It represents subacute pyogenic osteomyelitis. On X-ray or CT, a Brodie abscess appears as a focal lucent lesion surrounded by a rim of sclerosis (Fig. 7-52). Periosteal new bone formation may be present. While not always present, a tract extending from the focal lucency to the physis is considered pathognomonic. On MRI, the lesion can have variable signal appearance. The classic penumbra sign of increased T1 signal lining the rim of the abscess can help to confirm the diagnosis.

Oxacillin-resistant *S. aureus* (ORSA) deserves special mention as it accounts for over half of all cases of pediatric osteomyelitis. Patients with ORSA osteomyelitis often have a more severe infection and require more therapy than those children with oxacillin-sensitive *S. aureus*. ORSA osteomyelitis has a unique pattern on MRI, with a mottled heterogeneous appearance of the marrow (see Fig. 7-53) and extensive subperiosteal rim-enhancing collections. At times, the marrow signal abnormalities are only identified on contrast-enhanced images, where they appear as areas of absent enhancement.

Langerhans Cell Histiocytosis

LCH is an idiopathic disorder that can manifest as focal, localized, or systemic disease. It remains unclear whether the disease process is inflammatory or neoplastic. It is characterized by abnormal proliferation of Langerhans cells. The disease is twice as common in boys as in girls and occurs most commonly in Caucasians. It can occur as a single-system or multisystem disease with or without organ involvement. Organs that may be involved include the liver, spleen, lungs, and bone marrow.

Common sites of disease include bones, the skin, and pituitary. Bone is the most common site of disease, occurring in up to 80% of patients. Up to half of all lesions occur in the skull (Fig. 7-54), with the remaining sites of involvement scattered throughout the appendicular skeleton, including the proximal limbs (20%), pelvis and scapula (12%), vertebral bodies (10%), and the distal limbs (5%). On radiograph, lesions appear as a well-demarcated, lytic lesion without peripheral sclerosis. Skull lesions may have a beveled edge when viewed *en face* or a target appearance when viewed straight on because of uneven destruction of the inner and outer tables

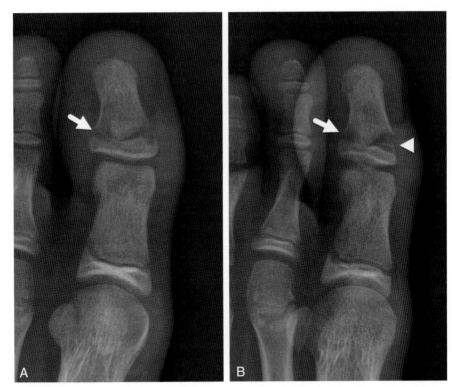

■ **FIGURE 7-51** Osteomyelitis of the great toe. Anteroposterior (**A**) and oblique (**B**) radiographs of the great toe in an 11-year-old male show a poorly defined lytic lesion (*arrow*) of the metaphysis of the distal phalanx of the great toe. The medial physis of the distal phalanx is widened to a greater degree than the lateral aspect, and there is a small Salter–Harris type II fracture (*arrowhead*). The initial injury occurred one week before these films were obtained.

of the skull. When the spine is involved, a classic finding is vertebral plana (vertebral destruction with severe collapse; Fig. 7-55).

A child who presents with a lesion suspicious for LCH should be evaluated whole body positron emission tomography (PET)-CT to identify other osseous lesions and to identify pulmonary involvement. If needed, MRI or diagnostic CT can better characterize intraabdominal organ involvement. When PET-CT is performed, affected areas show increased uptake.

Ewing Sarcoma

After osteosarcoma, Ewing sarcoma is the second most common primary bone malignancy in children. It is an aggressive, small, round, blue cell tumor similar to primitive neuroectodermal tumor. Ewing sarcoma most commonly occurs in the second decade of life. The most common sites of involvement, in decreasing order of frequency, are the femur, pelvis, tibia, humerus, and ribs. Two thirds of cases involve the pelvis or lower extremity. While Ewing sarcoma most commonly occurs in long bones, it has a greater propensity for flat bones compared with other primary bone malignancies.

The radiographic appearance of Ewing sarcoma is variable. Most lesions involve the metaphysis, but diaphyseal involvement is more common than in other bone malignancies. Most lesions have an aggressive appearance: a lucent lesion with poorly defined borders and a permeative appearance in the cortex (Figs. 7-56 and 7-57). Aggressive-appearing periosteal new bone formation (spiculated, onion skin, Codman triangle) is commonly present. However, Ewing sarcoma can appear predominantly sclerotic in as many as 15% of cases. MRI demonstrates a destructive bony mass, often with an associated soft tissue component. The five-year survival rate for those with Ewing sarcoma is 82% in those with localized disease and 39% in those in whom metastatic disease is present. Metastases primarily occur in other sites of bone and the lungs.

Metastatic Disease

In children, most cases of metastatic disease result from small, round, blue cell tumors.

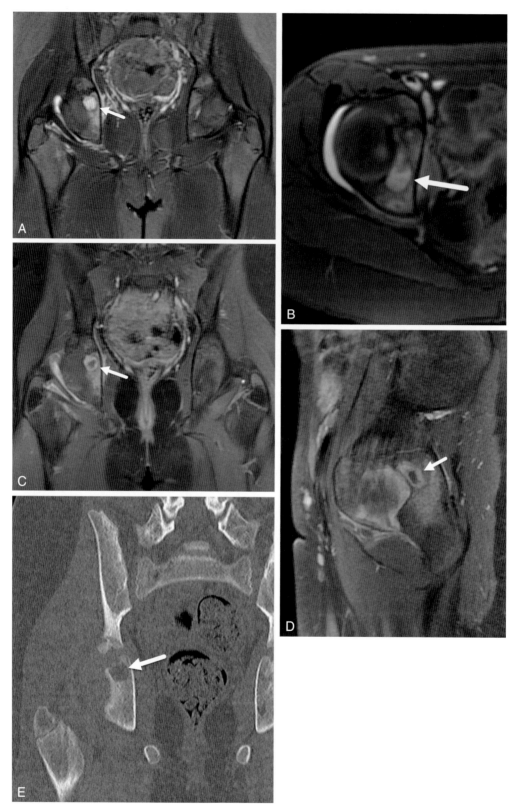

■ **FIGURE 7-52** Brodie abscess of the ischium. Coronal (**A**) and axial (**B**) fat saturated T2-weighted and coronal (**C**) and axial (**D**) fat saturated T1-weighted postcontrast magnetic resonance images in a seven-year-old female show a heterogeneous abscess (*arrow*) in the right ischium. The central portion of the abscess does not enhance after contrast administration. The increased T2 signal surrounding the abscess represents marrow edema. **E,** Coronal computed tomography image shows the abscess (*arrow*) in the superior aspect of the right ischium adjacent to the triradiate cartilage.

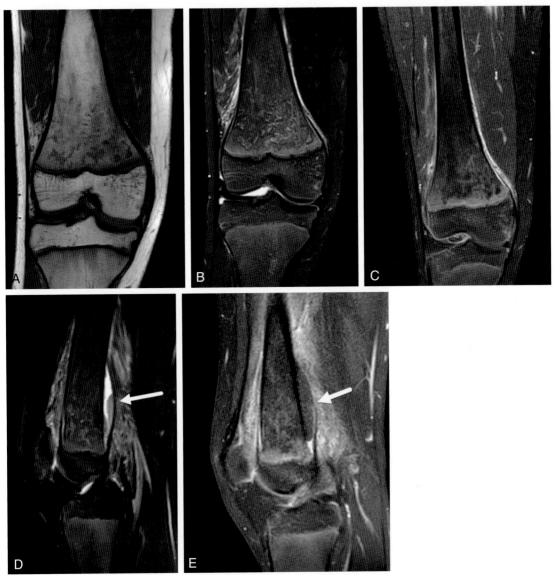

■ **FIGURE 7-53** Oxacillin-Resistant *Staphylococcus aureus*. Coronal T1-weighted (**A**), coronal fat saturated T2-weighted (**B**), and postcontrast fat saturated T1-weighted (**C**) images of the distal femur in a 12-year-old male shows the classic mottled heterogeneous signal of the marrow cavity. Sagittal fat saturated T2-weighted (**D**) and postcontrast fat saturated T1-weighted (**E**) images shows a similar mottled appearance of the marrow with a large subperiosteal abscess (*arrow*) along the posterior surface of the femur.

The most common primary neoplasms to metastasize to bone are neuroblastoma and leukemia or lymphoma. In any child younger than three years of age with a neoplastic bony lesion, metastatic neuroblastoma (Figs. 7-58 and 7-59) should be considered and is much more likely than a primary bone neoplasm. Leukemia and lymphoma may deposit in the regions of the metaphyses and cause bony destruction. The appearance is often that of lucent metaphyseal bands (Figs. 7-60 and 7-61). These nonspecific bands are often referred to as leukemic lines. Primary bone lymphoma is rare in children.

■ FOCAL SCLEROTIC LESIONS IN CHILDREN

There are multiple causes of focal sclerotic bone lesions in children. The more common causes are listed in Tables 7-3.

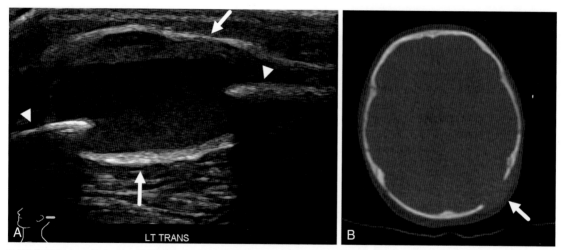

■ **FIGURE 7-54** Langerhans cell histiocytosis. **A,** Ultrasound of the scalp in a six-month-old male with a palpable mass shows a homogeneous soft tissue mass (*arrows*) that has caused destruction of the skull (*arrowhead*). **B,** Axial computed tomography (CT) image from a positron emission tomography (PET)/CT through the skull lesion shows the soft tissue lesion (*arrow*) and the skull defect.

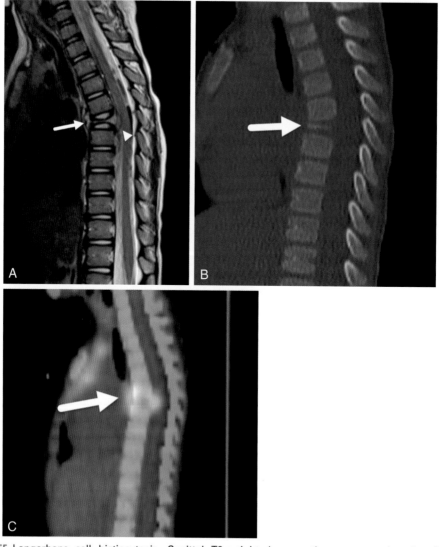

■ **FIGURE 7-55** Langerhans cell histiocytosis. Sagittal T2-weighted magnetic resonance imaging (**A**), sagittal computed tomography (CT) (**B**), and sagittal fused positron emission tomography (PET)/CT (**C**) of the thoracic spine in a three-year-old female show flattening of the T6 vertebral body (*arrow*). Although the vertebral body is barely perceptible, the posterior elements are intact.

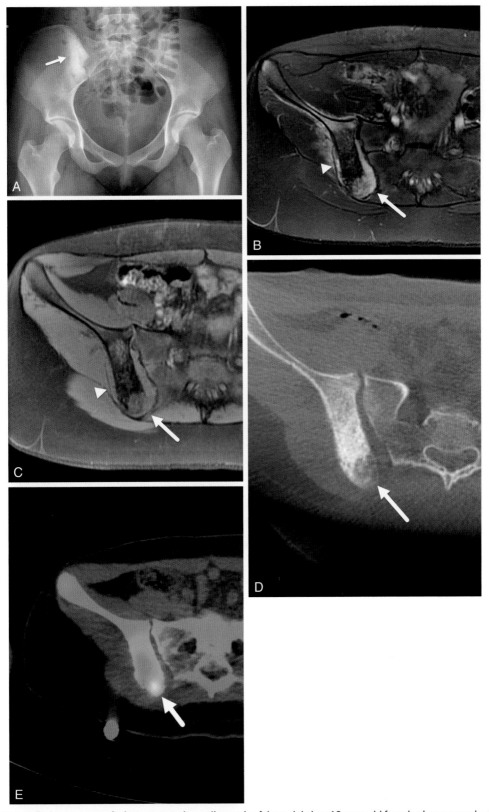

■ **FIGURE 7-56** Ewing sarcoma. **A,** Anteroposterior radiograph of the pelvis in a 16-year-old female show a poorly defined region of sclerosis (*arrow*) in the iliac bone adjacent to the sacroiliac joint. (**B**), Axial fat saturated T2-weighted and axial fat saturated T1-weighted postcontrast (**C**) magnetic resonance images shows an infiltrative mass (*arrow*) in the posterior aspect of the right iliac bone. The mass uplifts the periosteum (*arrowhead*) medially and laterally. **D,** Axial computed tomography (CT) image shows the poorly defined region of sclerosis of the iliac bone surrounding the lytic mass (*arrow*). **E,** Axial 18f Fluorodeoxyglucose positron emission tomography (PET)/CT shows uptake in the tumor (*arrow*).

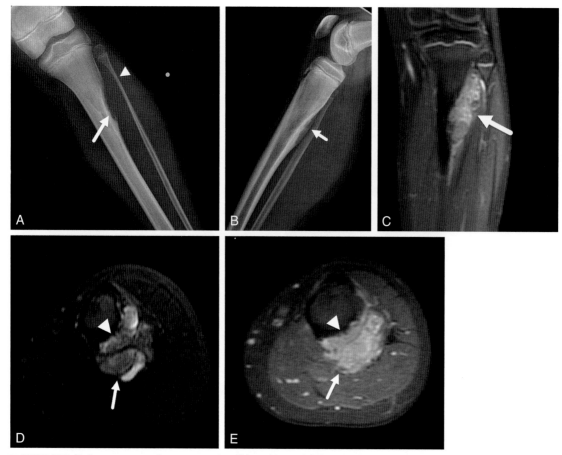

■ **FIGURE 7-57** Ewing sarcoma. Anteroposterior (**A**) and lateral (**B**) radiographs of the lower leg in a nine-year-old female show a lytic lesion (*arrow*) along the proximal and lateral aspect of the tibia. The lesion has aggressive features with fine spicules of new bone. While not visible, there is suggestion of a large soft tissue mass because of the thinning of the proximal fibula (*arrowhead*). **C,** Coronal fat saturated T1-weighted postcontrast magnetic resonance imaging shows the soft tissue component of the tumor (*arrow*) extending between the tibia and fibula highlighting the findings on the radiograph. Axial fat saturated T2-weighted (**D**) and axial fat saturated T1-weighted postcontrast (**E**) magnetic resonance images show the large soft tissue mass (*arrow*) arising from the tibia. The tibial cortex (*arrowhead*) is irregular with spicules of new bone present.

Osteoid Osteoma

Osteoid osteoma is a relatively common bone lesion. Most cases occur within the second decade of life and patients usually present with pain. Classically, the pain is worse at night and is relieved by nonsteroidal anti-inflammatory medication. The lesions are more common in boys. The cause is unknown, and it is currently unclear whether the lesion is a benign neoplasm or an inflammatory lesion. Most commonly, osteoid osteomas occur within the cortex of the metadiaphysis or diaphysis of the long bones of the lower extremities.

On radiography, an osteoid osteoma appears as a lucent cortical nidus surrounded by an area of reactive sclerosis (Fig. 7-62). By definition, the nidus is less than 2 cm in diameter. Lesions larger than 2 cm are referred to as osteoblastoma. Classically, a punctate radiodensity is identified within the central lucency (a dense dot within a lucent area, surrounded by sclerotic density). CT is used to further characterize the lesion because the punctate central radiodensity and lucency are often better demonstrated on CT than on radiography, and it defines the anatomic position of the nidus. CT can be used as guidance for percutaneous ablation or drill removal of the osteoid osteoma. MRI can also be used to diagnose and characterize the lesions. Skeletal scintigraphy demonstrates a "double-density" sign of intense increased uptake by the nidus, surrounded by less intense but abnormally

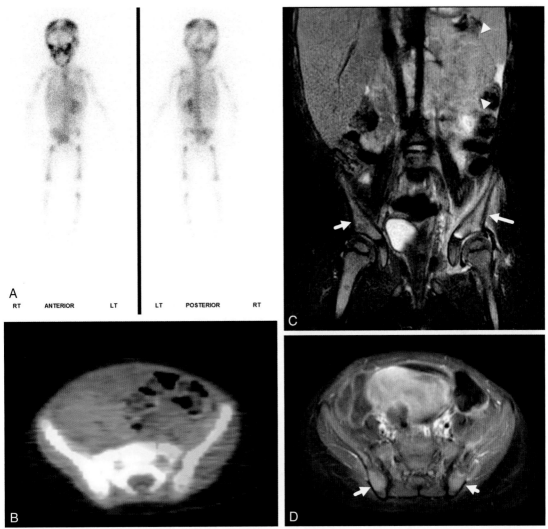

■ **FIGURE 7-58** Metastatic neuroblastoma. **A,** I 123 MIBG scan in the anterior and posterior projection in a 19-month-old female with neuroblastoma shows extensive metastatic disease throughout the skeleton. Any bone uptake is indicative of metastatic disease. The most intense area of uptake is in the skull. **B,** Axial fused I 123 MIBG SPECT/CT of the pelvis shows an abnormal radiotracer uptake in the pelvis. This is more pronounced on the right. **C,** Coronal fat-saturated T2-weighted magnetic resonance imaging (MRI) shows abnormal marrow signal (*arrows*) in the pelvis. On this image, the abnormal marrow is more pronounced on the left. The large left upper quadrant soft tissue mass (*arrowhead*) is partially imaged. **D,** Axial fat-saturated T1-weighted postcontrast MRI shows abnormal enhancement of the posterior aspect of the right and left iliac bone (*arrows*).

increased uptake by the surrounding sclerotic bone. Single-photon emission computed tomography (SPECT)-CT helps to increase the sensitivity of detecting subtle lesions.

Stress Fracture

A stress fracture is defined as an injury resulting from repetitive trauma. It occurs when a new or intense activity has recently been initiated. The most common sites of stress fractures in children, in decreasing order of frequency, are the tibia, fibula, metatarsals, and calcaneus.

A stress fracture appears on radiographs as a transverse or oblique band of sclerosis or as a lucent line surrounded by sclerosis or periosteal new bone formation. Periosteal new bone formation may be the only finding. In the tibia, the most common location is the proximal posterior cortex, although the anterior cortex can also be involved. In the calcaneus, there is typically a vertical sclerotic band paralleling the posterior cortex. Calcaneal stress fractures most commonly occur when a child has had a cast removed after a preceding lower extremity injury and returns to activity after a period of prolonged disuse (see

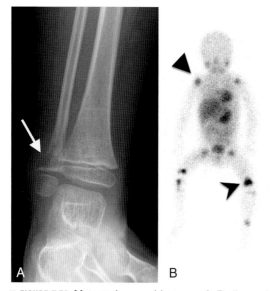

■ FIGURE 7-59 Metastatic neuroblastoma. **A,** Radiograph of the ankle in a five-year-old male with neuroblastoma shows a destructive lesion of the left fibula (*arrow*). The lesion is lucent and expansile. The nearby trabeculae are coarsened. **B,** I 123 metaiodobenzylguanidine (MIBG) scan in the anterior projection show focal areas of uptake in the shoulders (*arrowhead*), proximal and distal femurs (*chevron arrowhead*), proximal tibias, and distal left fibula.

linear structures with surrounding high T2-weighted signal edema.

Osteosarcoma

Osteosarcoma is the most common primary bone malignancy of childhood. It occurs in patients between 10 and 15 years of age and is more common in boys than in girls. Although most cases of osteosarcoma arise in otherwise healthy children, there are certain predisposing conditions, such as hereditary retinoblastoma, Li-Fraumeni syndrome, and previous radiation therapy. Osteosarcoma is a malignant lesion that uniquely gives rise to neoplastic osteoid and bone. Most osteosarcomas arise from the medullary cavity, although the lesion may arise from the surface of bone. The latter scenario gives rise to the periosteal and parosteal forms. The most common sites for development of osteosarcoma are the metaphyses of long bones. More than 60% of cases of osteosarcoma arise in the region of the knee (distal femur or proximal tibia).

The radiographic appearance of osteosarcoma is dependent on the amount of bony destruction and new bone formation. The lesions are

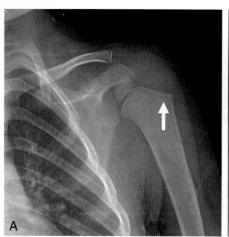

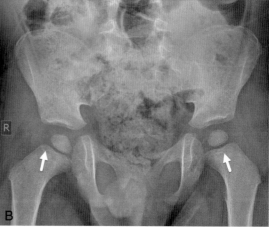

■ FIGURE 7-60 Leukemic lines. **A,** Anteroposterior (AP) radiograph of the shoulder in a two-year-old male with acute lymphoblastic leukemia shows a thin metaphyseal lucency (*arrow*) of the proximal humerus. **B,** AP radiograph of the pelvis shows thin metaphyseal lucencies (*arrows*) of the proximal femurs.

Figs. 7-34 and 7-35). Skeletal scintigraphy demonstrates a stress fracture as an area of focal increased uptake days to weeks before the development of radiographic findings. CT may be helpful in demonstrating the linear nature of the lesion when trying to evaluate whether a sclerotic lesion is a stress fracture, osteoid osteoma, or osteomyelitis. Stress fractures may be identified on MRI when it is performed to evaluate for pain. They appear as low-signal

typically large at the time of presentation. The destructive component of the tumor is demonstrated by lucent destruction of a metaphysis with aggressive features (aggressive periosteal reaction, poorly defined borders). Tumoral bone is seen in more than 90% of cases of osteosarcoma and helps to differentiate this tumor from other types of bone malignancies (Fig. 7-63). One feature that helps to differentiate tumoral bone from sclerotic reactive bone is that tumoral bone

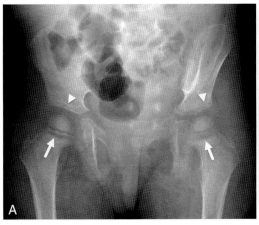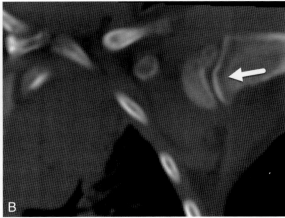

■ **FIGURE 7-61** Leukemic lines. **A,** Anteroposterior radiograph of the pelvis in a two-year-old female with acute lymphoblastic leukemia shows a metaphyseal lucencies of the proximal femoral metaphyses (*arrows*) and the superior acetabulum (*arrowhead*). **B,** Coronal computed tomography of the left shoulder shows a metaphyseal lucency (*arrow*) of the proximal humerus metaphysis.

✳ **TABLE 7-3** Common Causes of Focal Sclerotic Lesions in Children
• Osteoid osteoma
• Chronic osteomyelitis
• Stress fracture
• Osteosarcoma

extends beyond the expected confines of the normal bone. In most cases of osteosarcoma, there is a large soft tissue mass present at the time of diagnosis. In poorly differentiated, aggressive lesions, tumoral bone may not be present and the lesion may appear as a nonspecific, aggressive lucent lesion.

MRI is used to depict the relationship between the soft tissue mass and adjacent nerves and vascular structures as well as to evaluate the extent of bone and soft tissue involvement for presurgical planning. The extent of marrow abnormality, soft tissue mass, and cortical destruction is well-demonstrated as abnormal increased T2-weighted signal on MRI. However, MRI is not accurate in differentiating peritumoral marrow edema from tumor-involved marrow. Therefore, all abnormal signal in the marrow are generally considered to be involved by tumor for the sake of surgical planning. It is important to image the entire length of the bone involved by the tumor, from joint to joint, because osteosarcoma can occasionally have skip lesions. Identification of such skip lesions affects surgical planning. Surgery in conjunction with chemotherapy is standard therapy. Limb salvage

procedures are currently being performed in as much as 80% of patients.

The five-year survival of patients diagnosed with osteosarcoma has increased to 77% in recent years. However, patients with early metastases continue to have a poor prognosis. MRI has been shown to be useful in documenting chemotherapeutic response by demonstrating decrease in the size of the soft tissue mass and the amount of peritumoral edema. The best predictor of survival is the percentage of tumoral necrosis following chemotherapy. Patients with more than 90% necrosis have an 80%−90% chance of achieving a long-term cure. The most common type of metastatic disease is pulmonary (lung nodules), which is evaluated by CT. Lung metastases can appear calcified or ossified. Skeletal metastatic disease is reported to be present in as many as 15% of patients and is evaluated by skeletal scintigraphy or PET-CT.

■ MULTIFOCAL BONE LESIONS IN CHILDREN

The presence of multifocal involvement narrows the differential diagnosis for bone lesions in children (Tables 7-4). Osteomyelitis, LCH, and metastatic disease have already been discussed. In addition, there are several hereditary syndromes that cause multifocal bone lesions in children.

In multiple hereditary exostoses (osteochondromatosis), there is a propensity to develop multiple bilateral osteochondromas. Osteochondromas appear as bony growths that arise from the metaphysis and are continuous with the

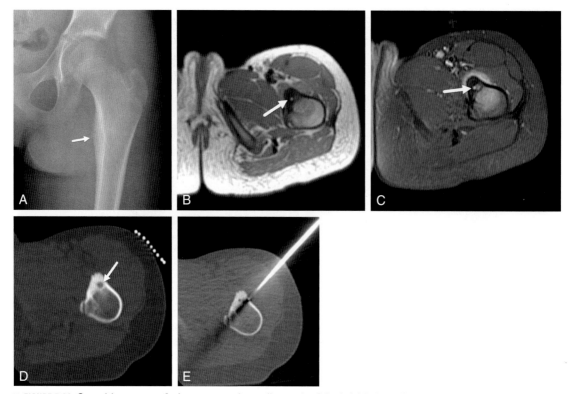

■ **FIGURE 7-62** Osteoid osteoma. **A,** Anteroposterior radiograph of the left hip in a nine-year-old female shows a faint lucent lesion in the medial cortex of the proximal femur (*arrow*). There is associated diffuse cortical thickening of the medial surface of the proximal femur. Axial T1-weighted (**B**) and axial fat-saturated T1-weighted postcontrast (**C**) magnetic resonance images show a small tumor nidus (*arrow*) along the anteromedial surface of the femur. The nidus is associated with focal cortical thickening. **D,** Axial image from a computed tomography (CT) scan shows a small lucent lesion (*arrow*) in the anterior cortex of the femur. There is a tiny central focus of sclerosis within the nidus. The anterior cortex is thickened. **E,** Axial CT image shows an ablation needle extending into the nidus.

adjacent bony cortex (Fig. 7-64). When pedunculated, they point away from joints. The most common location is the bones surrounding the knee. With osteochondromatosis the lesions can lead to multiple problems, including limb shortening, leg length discrepancy, bowing and deformity, compression of adjacent nerves and vessels, and malignant degeneration into chondrosarcoma (5%). Concerning features for the development of chondrosarcoma include new onset of pain or lesion growth. In adults, MRI is used to evaluate at-risk lesions to help to identify malignant degeneration. Although evaluation of the thickness of the cartilaginous cap is important in adults, it is not a useful marker in children because the cartilage is normally thicker around growing bone.

In Ollier disease (enchondromatosis), there are multiple enchondromas (Fig. 7-65). Although they most commonly occur bilaterally, it is possible for all the lesions to be located on one side of the body. Solitary enchondromas tend to occur in the hands and feet, whereas lesions of enchondromatosis tend to be located within the

metaphyses of long bones. With growth, the lesions may take on an oblong or flame-shaped, linear configuration perpendicular to the physis. When solitary lesions occur in long bones, they can have a more sclerotic appearance (Fig. 7-66). Malignant degeneration to chondrosarcoma occurs in approximately 30% of patients. When soft tissue venous malformations are seen in conjunction with multiple enchondromas, the syndrome is called Maffucci syndrome (Fig. 7-67). In those patients, phleboliths may be seen within the soft tissue masses on radiographs. Patients with Maffucci syndrome have an even higher risk of malignant degeneration (up to 40% of patients) than those with Ollier syndrome and are also at increased risk for malignant neoplasms of the abdomen and central nervous system.

McCune—Albright syndrome is the presence of polyostotic fibrous dysplasia, café au lait spots, and endocrine abnormalities. The most common endocrine abnormality is precocious puberty in girls. Polyostotic fibrous dysplasia most commonly involves the facial bones, pelvis, spine,

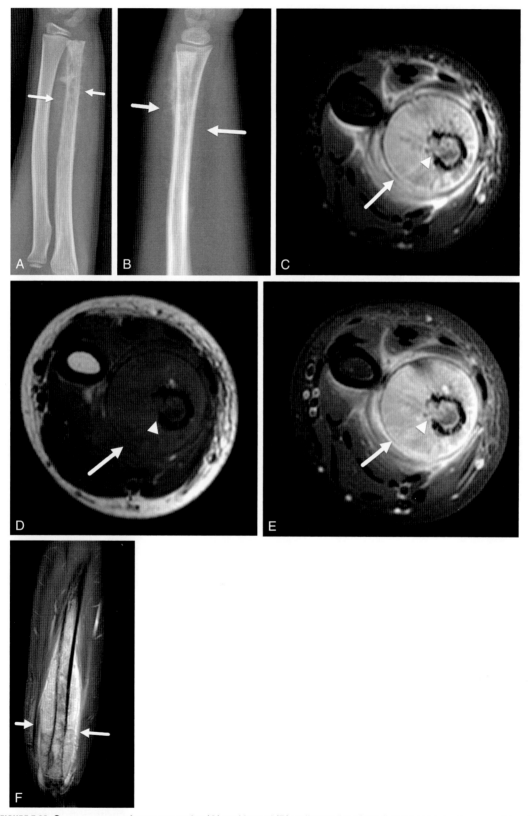

■ **FIGURE 7-63** Osteosarcoma. Anteroposterior (**A**) and lateral (**B**) radiographs of the forearm in a seven-year-old male show a large mass of the distal ulna. The ulna has a poorly defined mass with a permeative matrix and extensive speculated periosteal new bone. Axial fat-saturated T2-weighted (**C**), axial T1-weighted (**D**), and axial fat-saturated T1-weighted postcontrast (**E**) magnetic resonance images show a large soft tissue mass (*arrow*) surrounding the ulna. The ulnar cortex appears as a dark ring in the center of the mass. The mass arises from the bone and extends through a large cortical defect (*arrowhead*). **F,** Sagittal fat-saturated T1-weighted postcontrast magnetic resonance imaging shows the extent of the tumor (*arrows*).

✳ TABLE 7-4 Multifocal Bone Lesions in Children
• Multifocal osteomyelitis
• Langerhans cell histiocytosis
• Metastatic disease
• Multiple hereditary exostoses (osteochondromatosis)
• Enchondromatosis (Ollier disease, Maffucci syndrome)
• Polyostotic fibrous dysplasia (McCune–Albright syndrome)
• Neurofibromatosis

classic description is that of "ground-glass" matrix, which is a smudged and somewhat dense appearance of the central portion of the lesion. Periosteal reaction should be present only if there is a pathologic fracture.

◼ CONSTITUTIONAL DISORDERS OF BONE

The term *constitutional disorder of bone* refers to any developmental abnormality of bone resulting in diffuse skeletal abnormality. OI, skeletal

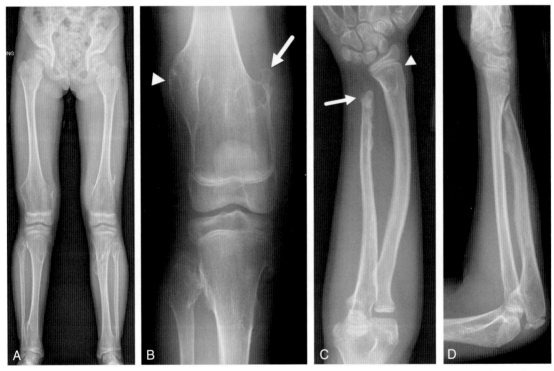

◼ **FIGURE 7-64** Multiple hereditary exostoses. **A,** Anteroposterior (AP) radiograph of the lower extremities a 13-year-old female shows multiple exostoses. **B,** AP radiograph of the right knee shows multiple lesions on each bone. The fibular lesions have a more sessile appearance, whereas the some of the femoral and tibial lesions are sessile (*arrowhead*) while others are pedunculated (*arrow*). AP (**C**) and lateral (**D**) radiograph of the forearm show multiple sessile osteochondroma of both bones. A Madelung deformity is also present with shortening of the ulna (*arrow*), ulnar deviation of the epiphysis of the radius (*arrowhead*), and bowing of the diaphysis of the radius.

and proximal humeri (Fig. 7-68). When the lesions affect the femur, patients can have an exaggerated coxa vara deformity referred to as a shepherd crook deformity. The fibrous dysplasia lesions tend to be unilateral in patients with McCune–Albright syndrome. Many patients present with pathologic fracture by 10 years of age. There is no predisposition to malignancy. Fibrous dysplasia has a variable appearance radiographically. It can be purely lytic or sclerotic and can be expansile or nonexpansile. The

dysplasias, and mucopolysaccharidoses fall into this category.

Osteogenesis Imperfecta

OI represents a group of eight different genetic disorders that result in the formation of abnormal type 1 collagen. In all types, there is osteopenia and a propensity for fracture. The different types of OI range in severity from mild to severe. The more severe types are usually

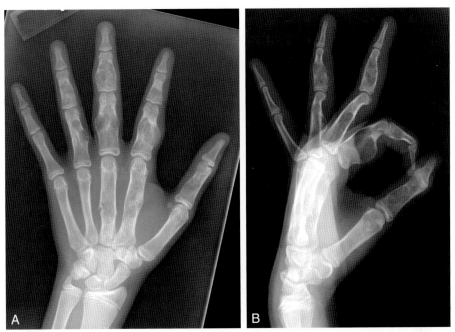

■ FIGURE 7-65 Ollier disease. Anteroposterior (**A**) and lateral (**B**) radiographs of the left hand in a 13-year-old female show multiple expansile lucent lesions affecting the first through fourth rays.

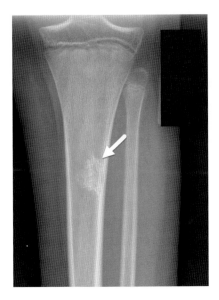

■ FIGURE 7-66 Solitary enchondroma. Anteroposterior radiograph of the lower leg in a 12-year-old male shows a sclerotic, geographic lesion (*arrow*) of the proximal tibia.

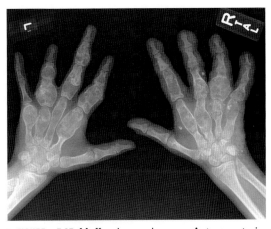

■ FIGURE 7-67 Maffucci syndrome. Anteroposterior radiograph of the hands in a 15-year-old female shows multiple enchondromas of the majority of bones of the hand. Each lesion is expansile with a heterogeneous internal matrix. Some of the lesions have a typical ground-glass matrix, whereas others have features more typical of a chondroid matrix. In addition to the bone lesions, the fingers are deformed with obvious soft tissue abnormality and calcifications.

lethal in the prenatal period. Types I—V have an autosomal dominant mode of inheritance, whereas types VI—VIII are autosomal recessive. Patients with moderate to severe disease have evidence of multiple fractures of various ages. In such cases, other findings, such as osteopenia, should be clues to a diagnosis of OI rather than child abuse. In moderate to severe cases, there are thick tubular bones (Fig. 7-69) that result from the healing of multiple fractures, resulting in short-limb dwarfism. OI patients are commonly treated with bisphosphonate therapy

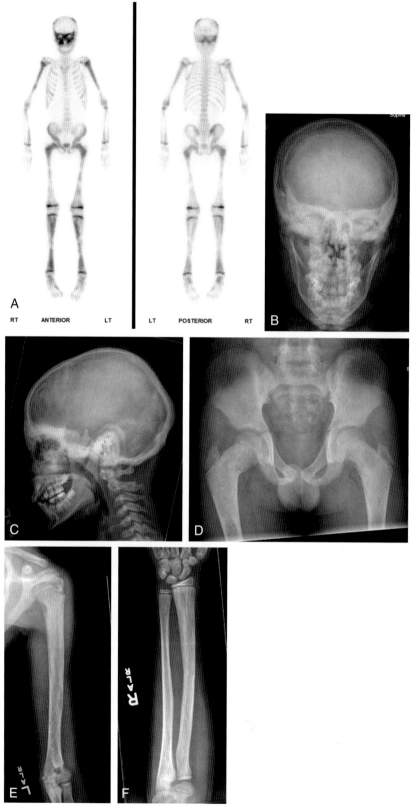

■ FIGURE 7-68 McCune–Albright syndrome. **A,** Anterior and posterior projection from a Tc 99m MDP bone scan in an 11-year-old male shows abnormal uptake in multiple bones throughout the body. The radiotracer uptake is most pronounced in the mid face. Anteroposterior (AP) (**B**) and lateral (**C**) radiographs of the skull show cortical thickening and sclerosis of the anterior skull base. **D,** AP radiograph of the pelvis shows poorly defined lesions in both proximal femurs with a smudgy internal matrix. The right hip has a varus configuration also known as a shepherd crook deformity. AP radiographs of the humerus (**E**) and forearm (**F**) diffuse lesions throughout the bones. The lesions have a mixed appearance. Portions are sclerotic while other portions have a smudgy internal matrix. There is mild expansion of the humerus and radius.

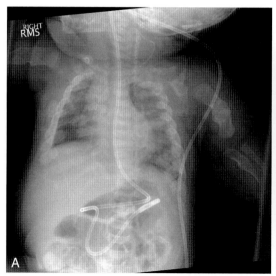
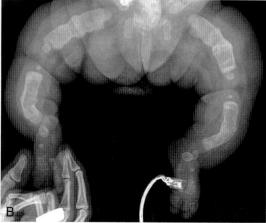

■ **FIGURE 7-69** Osteogenesis imperfecta. Anteroposterior radiograph of the chest (**A**) and lower extremities (**B**) in a newborn female show multiple fractures of virtually every bone. Many of the fractures are healing, giving the bones a thickened appearance.

to increase bone calcium deposition. Such therapy can result in a striking pattern of alternating sclerotic and lucent bands within the metaphyses of fast-growing bones. Multiple Wormian bones (small ossicles along the cranial sutures) and thin skin are also commonly noted in association with OI (Fig. 7-70). Type I and III OI are associated with blue sclera.

Osteopetrosis

Osteopetrosis is a rare bone disorder in which the osteoclasts are defective in resorbing and remodeling bone. As a result, bone is laid down and not resorbed. This results in dense bony sclerosis. There is often a bone-within-bone appearance on radiographs (Fig. 7-71). The skull

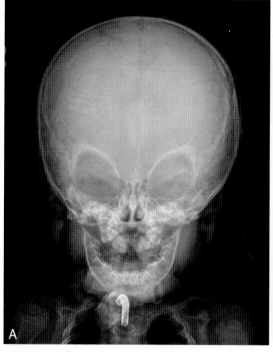
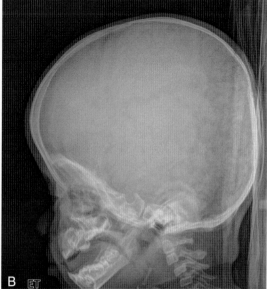

■ **FIGURE 7-70** Osteogenesis imperfecta. Anteroposterior (**A**) and lateral (**B**) radiographs of the skull show multiple Wormian bones.

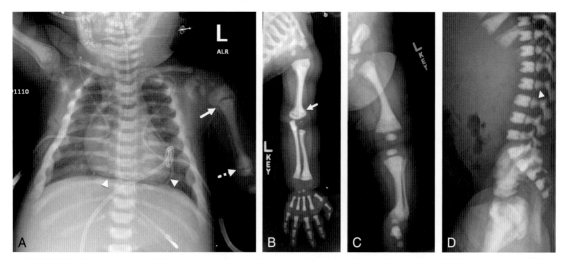

■ **FIGURE 7-71** Osteopetrosis. **A,** Anteroposterior radiograph of the chest in an 11-month old female shows diffuse periosteal reaction of the right and left humerus. Fractures are present in the proximal (*arrow*) and distal (*dashed arrow*) aspect of the left humerus. The bones are diffusely sclerotic. Pneumopericardium (*arrowhead*) is also present after pericardiocentesis. Radiographs of the upper extremity (**B**), lower extremity (**C**), and lumbosacral spine (**D**) show diffuse sclerosis of bones with extensive periosteal new bone formation giving a bone-in-bone appearance. In the spine, the bone-in-bone appearance is most visible in the pedicles (*arrowhead*). There is a fracture (*arrow*) of the distal humerus. Many of the long bones are bowed.

base is thickened and encroachment upon cranial nerves is a common complication. Although the total body calcium stores are increased, serum calcium levels are often paradoxically low, and radiographic findings of superimposed rickets are not uncommon. Lack of normal marrow space results in pancytopenia, which often leads to complications and death.

Skeletal Dysplasias

There are many different skeletal dysplasias, most of which are quite rare. In most cases, pediatric radiologists can identify that a dysplasia is present, describe the salient findings, and recommend further genetic testing be performed. In some instances, the pattern of dysplasia is pathognomonic, and the radiologist can suggest a presumptive diagnosis. The text by Taybi and Lachman is useful to help identify patterns of dysplasia and formulate a differential diagnosis. That said, it is useful to understand the more common patterns of dysplasia and a methodology for a practical work-up of affected patients.

Radiographic evaluation of dysplasia requires images of the skull, spine, thorax, pelvis, extremities, and hands. An important feature for categorization is identifying whether the extremities are shortened and, if so, which portion is short. Extremity shortening can be classified as rhizomelic, mesomelic, or acromelic. *Rhizomelic* refers to proximal shortening (humerus, femur) and is seen in achondroplasia (Figs. 7-72 and 7-73) and thanatophoric dwarfism (Fig. 7-74).

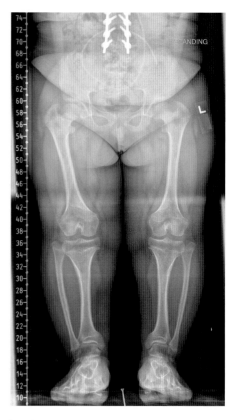

■ **FIGURE 7-72** Achondroplasia. Anteroposterior radiograph of the lower extremities in an 11-year-old female shows shortened bones of the legs, affecting the femurs to a greater degree than the lower legs. In addition, there is metaphyseal flaring of all bones, shortened femoral necks, and relative overgrowth of the trochanters. The pelvis shows shortened iliac bones and horizontal acetabular roofs.

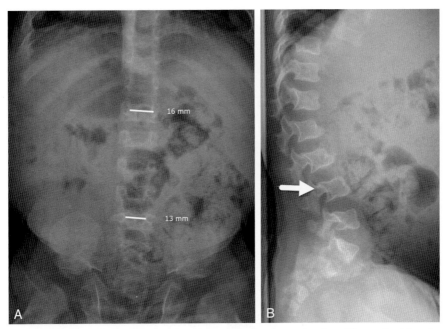

FIGURE 7-73 Achondroplasia. **A,** Anteroposterior view of the lumbar spine in a 20-month-old male shows narrowing of the interpedicular distance more inferiorly (*lines*—16 mm at L1 and 13 mm at L5). **D,** Lateral view of the lumbar spine shows shortening of the pedicles (*arrow*), making the spinal canal narrowed.

Mesomelic refers to middle narrowing (radius-ulna, tibia-fibula). Most of the mesomelic dysplasias are quite rare. *Acromelic* refers to distal shortening and is seen with asphyxiating thoracic dystrophy (Jeune syndrome); Fig. 7-75) and chondroectodermal dysplasia (Ellis—van Creveld syndrome). Other features helpful in categorizing dysplasias include determining whether there is skull enlargement, short ribs, abnormal vertebral bodies, and an abnormal pelvic configuration. The pelvis may demonstrate abnormalities in the configuration of the iliac wings or in the appearance of the acetabulum. The iliac wings may be abnormally tall or short or may have a squared appearance. The acetabular roof may appear horizontal (a decreased acetabular angle). *Trident acetabulum* refers to a pattern in which the acetabulum has three inferior pointing spikes resembling an upside-down trident. This is a buzzword for Jeune syndrome but also can be seen in Ellis—van Creveld syndrome and thanatophoric dysplasia. Some of the more common dysplasias and their radiographic manifestations are described in Tables 7-5.

ACHONDROPLASIA

Achondroplasia is discussed in greater detail because it is the most common short-limbed dwarfism. It is an autosomal dominant disease in which the heterozygous form demonstrates

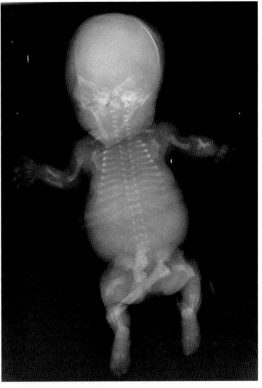

FIGURE 7-74 Thanatophoric dwarfism. Anteroposterior (radiograph of a stillborn female show severe shortening of all long bones. The femurs are bowed and have a telephone receiver configuration.

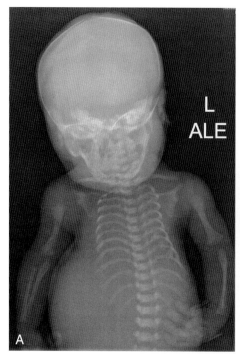

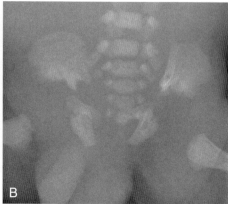

■ **FIGURE 7-75** Asphyxiating thoracic dystrophy (Jeune Syndrome). **A,** Anteroposterior (AP) radiograph of a stillborn child shows severe shortening of the ribs. The abdomen seems to protrude because of the small size of the thorax. **B,** AP radiograph of the pelvis shows a trident configuration of the iliac bone around the acetabulum.

the clinical manifestations, and the homozygous form is lethal. Patients with achondroplasia have rhizomelic limb shortening (see Figs. 7-72 and 7-73). They also have craniofacial disproportion, an enlarged skull, a small skull base, and a small jugular foramina and a foramen magnum. The latter may result in brainstem compression. In the spine, the vertebral bodies are short in their anterior-to-posterior diameter with a bullet-shaped configuration. The disk spaces appear too tall. There is a decrease in the interpedicular distance (left to right), with this distance being narrower in the more inferior lumbar spine than in the more superior lumbar spine (the opposite of normal; see Fig. 7-73, *A*). The pedicles are also short in the anterior-to-posterior diameter. Because of these findings, patients with achondroplasia are prone to spinal stenosis. The shortened long bones show metaphyseal flaring. In infancy, there is commonly space between the middle fingers, resulting in a trident appearance of the hand. The iliac bones are shortened and the acetabular roof is horizontal (a decreased acetabular angle), making the iliac bones resemble tombstones.

Mucopolysaccharidoses

Mucopolysaccharidoses are a group of hereditary disorders manifested by defects in lysosomal enzymes. They include such disorders as Hunter, Hurler, and Morquio syndromes. The skeletal findings in this group of diseases are similar and have been referred to as dysostosis multiplex (Fig. 7-76). The vertebral bodies are oval and often have a beak extending from the anterior cortex (see Fig. 7-76, *C*). The beak is in the midportion of the vertebral bodies in Morquio syndrome (M for middle and Morquio) and in the inferior portion in Hunter or Hurler syndrome. Beaking is most prominent in the lumbar vertebral bodies. There can be focal kyphosis (gibbous deformity; see Fig. 7-76, *D*) at the thoracolumbar junction because of a shortened T12 or L1 vertebral body. The shape of the vertebral bodies in achondroplasia, Hurler disease, and Morquio syndrome is often confused (Fig. 7-77). The clavicles and ribs are commonly thickened in patients with Hunter or Hurler syndrome. The ribs are narrower posteromedially, giving them a "canoe paddle" appearance.

The appearance of the pelvis is essentially the opposite of that in achondroplasia. The iliac wings are tall and flared, and the acetabuli are shallow (increased acetabular angles; see Fig. 7-76, *E*). The femoral heads are dysplastic, and femoral necks are gracile and demonstrate coxa valga (loss of angle between the neck and the shaft of the femur). The hands have a characteristic appearance that includes proximal

TABLE 7-5 Radiographic Manifestations of Several Skeletal Dysplasias

Dysplasia	Type of Extremity Shortening	Pelvis	Short Ribs	Spine	Enlarged Skull	Other
Achondroplasia	Proximal	Squared iliac wings Small sacroiliac notch Decreased acetabular angle (looks like tombstones)	Yes	Short vertebral bodies Narrow interpedicular distance	Yes	Metaphyseal flaring
Thanatophoric dysplasia	Proximal	Squared iliac wings Decreased acetabular angle Trident acetabulum	Yes	Platyspondyly	Yes	Early death Metaphyseal flaring "Telephone receiver" femurs
Chondrodysplasia punctate	Proximal	Normal	No	Stippled epiphysis	No	Stippled epiphyses
Asphyxiating thoracic dystrophy (Jeune)	Distal	Decreased acetabular angle Trident acetabulum	Yes	Normal	No	Very short ribs Respiratory distress Metaphyseal irregularity and beaking
Chondroectodermal dysplasia (Ellis–van Creveld)	Distal	Decreased acetabular angle Trident acetabulum	Yes	Normal	No	Polydactyly, abnormal nails Congenital heart disease Amish community
Cleidocranial dysplasia	All	Squared iliac wings Decreased acetabular angle Widened pubic symphysis	No	Abnormal ossification	Yes	Absent or small clavicles Widened pubic symphysis Wormian bones
Camptomelic dysplasia	All	Tall, narrow iliac wings Increased acetabular angle	No	Ossification defects	Yes	Bowing of long bones (campto = bent limb) Airway obstruction

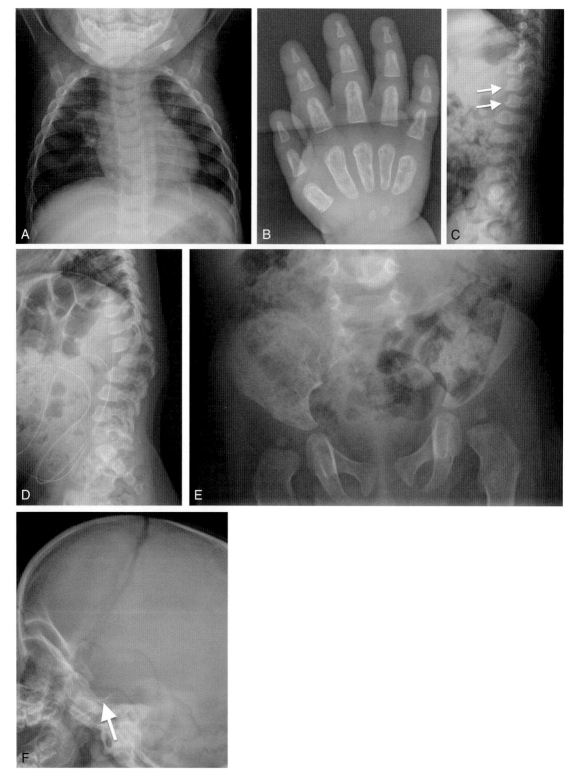

■ **FIGURE 7-76** Hurler syndrome. **A,** Anteroposterior (AP) radiograph of the chest in a one-year-old male with Hurler syndrome shows thickening of the ribs. The ribs are narrower in their posteromedial aspect. **B,** AP radiograph of the hand shows proximal tapering of the metatarsal bones. **C,** Lateral radiograph of the thoracolumbar spine shows anterior beaking along the inferior aspect of the T12 and L1 vertebral bodies (*arrows*). **D,** Lateral radiograph of the spine obtained 1.5 years later shows a focal kyphosis at this location. **E,** AP radiograph of the pelvis shows tall and flared iliac wings with shallow acetabula. **F,** Lateral view of the base of the skull shows a J-shaped pituitary fossa (*arrow*).

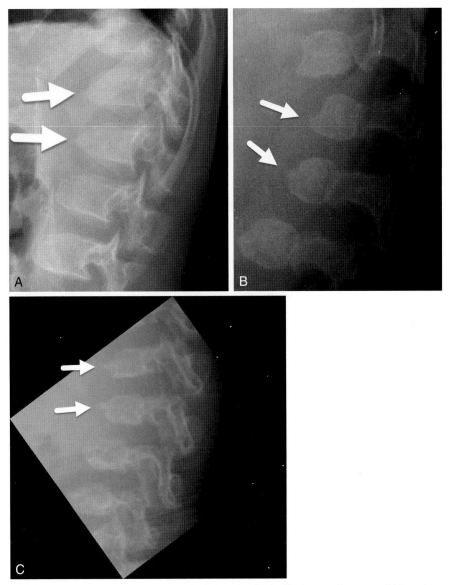

■ **FIGURE 7-77** Appearance of the vertebral bodies in Achondroplasia, Hurler syndrome, and Morquio syndrome. **A,** Lateral radiograph of the lumbar spine in a five-year-old male with achondroplasia shows bullet-shaped vertebral bodies (*arrows*). **B,** Lateral radiograph of the lumbar spine in a six-month-old male with Hurler syndrome shows beaking (*arrows*) of the inferior portion of the vertebral bodies. **C,** Lateral radiograph of the lumbar spine in a 15-year-old male with Morquio syndrome shows beaking (*arrows*) of the middle portion of the vertebral bodies.

tapering of the metacarpal bones (see Fig. 7-76, B). The pituitary fossa can have a J-shaped appearance (see Fig. 7-76, F).

■ HIP DISORDERS

There are several unique abnormalities that can involve the pediatric hip.

Developmental Dysplasia of the Hip

Development dysplasia of the hip (DDH) refers to a condition related to abnormal development and configuration of the acetabulum and to increased ligamentous laxity around the hip. The cause is debated. DDH is more common in females (in a ratio of as much as 9:1), in whites, and in children born in breech deliveries. One third

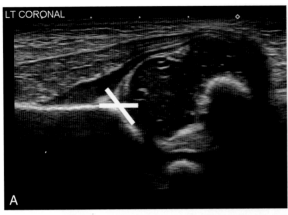
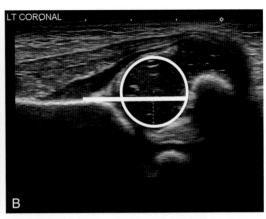

■ **FIGURE 7-78** Developmental dysplasia of the hip. **A,** Ultrasound of the left hip in a two-week-old female shows a shallow acetabulum. The alpha angle, measured as the acute angle between the horizontal line of the iliac bone and the diagonal line of the acetabular roof, is 55 degrees. **B,** Ultrasound of the left hip shows decreased coverage of the left hip. The line drawn along the iliac bone only covers 38% of the femoral head (*circle*).

of children with DDH are affected bilaterally. Clinical evaluation for DDH is part of routine neonatal screening. Neonates may demonstrate asymmetric gluteal folds, limited abduction, or a positive clunk felt on Ortolani (relocation) or Barlow (dislocation) maneuvers. If not detected and treated in infancy, DDH can lead to chronic abnormalities of the hip.

Ultrasound is used to evaluate the hips of infants who have clinical findings suggestive of DDH. Both the morphology of the acetabulum and any abnormal mobility of the hip are evaluated. Because there is physiologic ligamentous laxity during the first days of life, it is better to wait until after two weeks of life before performing hip ultrasound. The static morphologic evaluation is performed with the ultrasound probe coronal to the hip. Stress (Barlow) maneuvers are performed while evaluating the hip in the axial plane. On the static coronal view, the anatomy simulates that seen on a frontal radiograph of the pelvis (Fig. 7-78). On such a view, the iliac bone appears as a horizontal echogenic line on the left (more cranial) side of the image. This line should bisect the femoral head. A dislocated femoral head will be positioned posterior and lateral to the iliac line. The angle created between lines drawn along the straight part of the iliac bone and the acetabular roof form the alpha angle (see Fig. 7-78). Normally the alpha angle is greater than 60 degrees (55 degrees in newborns). In DDH, the acetabulum is shallow, resulting in a decreased alpha angle on ultrasound. This correlates with an increased acetabular angle on radiographs (see subsequent material). A decreased alpha angle may be followed on repeat static ultrasound during therapy to evaluate for morphologic improvement.

DDH can also be evaluated by radiography. Radiographs are particularly useful after the femoral heads begin to ossify around three months of age, rendering ultrasound of limited value. In addition, it is important to know the radiographic findings of DDH so that such abnormalities may be identified when seen incidentally on other neonatal imaging studies that include the hips, such as abdominal radiographs. Because the femoral head and portions of the acetabulum are cartilaginous and not directly visualized on radiographs of the pelvis in the newborn period, landmarks are used to determine whether the hip is dislocated. With increasing age and ossification of the femoral head, direct visualization of a dislocated femoral head can be seen. Lines used to evaluate for DDH include the Hilgenreiner line, Perkin line, Shenton arc, and acetabular angle (Fig. 7-79). The **H**ilgenreiner line is a **h**orizontal line drawn through the bilateral triradiate cartilages, touching the inferior medial aspect of each acetabulum. A second line is then drawn connecting the inferior medial and superolateral aspects of the acetabulum, outlining the acetabular roof. The angle made between these two lines is the acetabular angle. Normally the acetabular angle is just less than 30 degrees at birth and decreases to 22 degrees at one year of age. With DDH, acetabular angles are abnormally increased. Another cause of increased acetabular angles is neuromuscular disorders. Abnormally decreased acetabular angles can be seen during the first year of life in Down syndrome and in multiple dysplasias, including achondroplasia (see Fig. 7-72). The vertical line of **Per**kin is drawn such that it is **per**pendicular to the Hilgenreiner line and traverses the superolateral corner of the

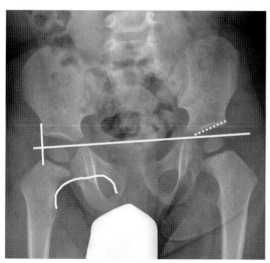

FIGURE 7-79 Normal pelvis. Anteroposterior radiograph of the pelvis in a 24-month-old male is used to highlight the normal lines of the pelvis. Hilgenreiner line is a horizontal line drawn connecting the triradiate cartilage. Perkin line is then drawn perpendicular to this line, starting from the lateral aspect of the acetabulum. The acetabular angle (*dashed line*) is calculated as the angle between Hilgenreiner line and the lateral margin of the acetabulum. Finally, Shenton arc is a continuous smooth arch connecting the medial cortex of the proximal metaphysis of the femur and the inferior edge of the superior pubic ramus.

acetabulum. When the femoral head is ossified and visible, it should lie medial to the Perkin line in the lower inner quadrant. When dislocated, the femoral head is usually in the upper, outer quadrant. When the head is not ossified, the Perkin line should bisect the middle third of the metaphysis. If the metaphysis is lateral to this position, the hip is subluxed or dislocated (Fig. 7-80). The Shenton arc is a continuous smooth arch connecting the medial cortex of the proximal metaphysis of the femur and the inferior edge of the superior pubic ramus. In DDH and dislocation, the arc is discontinuous (see Fig. 7-80).

Chronic Hip Subluxation

In patients with neuromuscular disorders, such as cerebral palsy, development of progressive hip subluxation or dislocation may occur. Radiographs (Fig. 7-81) are used to evaluate how much the bony acetabulum covers the femoral head (percentage of coverage), degree of coxa valga (loss of angle between the neck and shaft of the femur), and presence of complete dislocation. The proximal femoral migration percentage can be used to assess the degree of subluxation and to monitor it with time.

Proximal Focal Femoral Deficiency

Proximal focal femoral deficiency (PFFD) is a congenital disorder consisting of a range of hypoplasias to variable absence of the proximal portions of the femur (Fig. 7-82). In its most severe form, the acetabulum, femoral head, and proximal femur may be absent. A varus deformity is commonly associated with the deficiency. It is important not to confuse the milder forms of PFFD with developmental dysplasia of the hip. In the latter, the femur is of normal length. PFFD can be associated with ipsilateral fibular hemimelia and deformity of the foot.

Septic Arthritis

There are many potential causes of painful hips in children (Tables 7-6). Many of these diagnoses present at specific ages, so the differential diagnosis can often be limited based on age (see Tables 7-6).

Septic arthritis is the most urgent diagnosis to exclude in a patient with a painful joint because delay in diagnosis can lead to destruction of the joint. In children, septic arthritis is thought to occur most commonly as a result of extension of infection from the adjacent metaphysis. In younger children, it usually occurs secondary to bacterial sepsis, and the most common organisms are *S. aureus* (more than 50% of cases) and group A streptococci. Most cases of septic arthritis are monoarticular and involve large joints. The hip is the most common joint involved, followed by the knee.

In septic arthritis of the hip, children usually present with pain, limp, or failure to bear weight. Radiographs of the pelvis and hips are obtained to exclude other diagnoses. The primary radiographic finding of septic arthritis is asymmetric widening of the hip joint space by more than 2 mm on a nonrotated film (Fig. 7-83). The joint spaces are evaluated by measuring the distance between the teardrop of the acetabulum and the medial cortex of the metaphysis of the femur. Unfortunately, this finding, although important when positive, is neither sensitive for a joint effusion nor specific for septic arthritis. Fluid tends to accumulate in the anterior recess of the hip joint before displacing the femur laterally. When septic arthritis is associated with osteomyelitis or another cause of soft tissue swelling, displacement or obliteration of the fat pads surrounding the hip may be noted. These include the obturator internus, gluteus muscle, and iliopsoas fat pads. Abnormalities of the fat pads are also neither sensitive nor specific. Therefore, a normal pelvic radiograph in no way excludes a

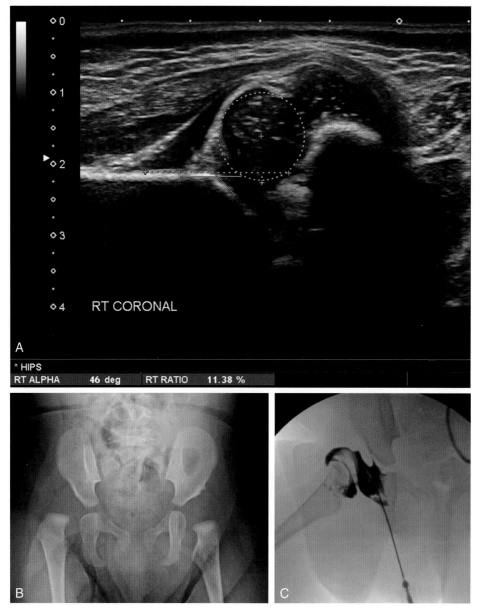

■ **FIGURE 7-80** Developmental dysplasia of the hip. **A,** Ultrasound of the right hip in a 17-day-old female shows flattening of the acetabulum with an alpha angle of 46 degrees. The hip is subluxed with only 11% coverage of the femoral head. **B,** Anteroposterior radiograph of the pelvis at six months of age shows continued findings of right hip dysplasia. While neither femoral head is ossified, the right femoral head is subluxed superiorly and laterally, and the right acetabulum is shallow. **C,** Right hip arthrogram performed at eight months of age during cast fixation shows the cartilaginous femoral head subluxed superiorly and laterally.

diagnosis of septic arthritis, and an abnormal radiograph does not cinch the diagnosis.

The presence of hip joint effusion can be evaluated by ultrasound. The probe is placed longitudinally, anterior to the hip joint. Asymmetric widening of a hypoechoic space between the shaft of the proximal femur and the joint capsule is diagnostic of a joint effusion (Fig. 7-84). The absence of fluid does exclude a diagnosis of septic arthritis. When fluid is present, ultrasound guidance can be used to tap the effusion. There are causes of joint effusion other than septic arthritis. They include toxic synovitis, noninfectious arthritis, and Legg-Calvé-Perthes (LCP) disease.

In the setting of suspected septic arthritis or osteomyelitis, many institutions have instituted a screening MRI examination with a wide field of

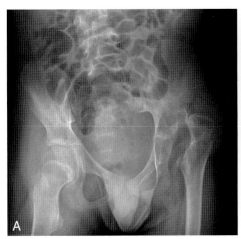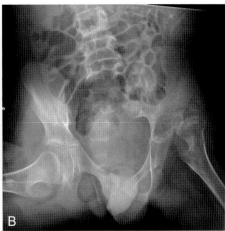

■ FIGURE 7-81 Chronic hip dislocation. Anteroposterior radiograph of the pelvis in a 13-year-old male shows chronic dislocation the left hip. The femoral head is displaced superiorly and laterally and articulates with the iliac bone. The left acetabulum is flattened. Both hips have a valgus configuration. This is more severe on the left.

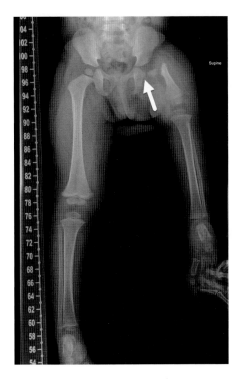

■ FIGURE 7-82 Proximal focal femoral deficiency. Anteroposterior radiograph of the lower extremities in a two-year-old male shows a shortened and irregular left femur (*arrow*). The left femoral head (*arrow*) articulates with the acetabulum. There is fragmentation of the proximal femur with a pseudoarticulation.

✳ TABLE 7-6 Potential Causes of Hip Pain in Children	
Diagnosis	**Typical Age at Presentation**
Septic arthritis	Any age; most common in infants and teenagers
Toxic synovitis	<10 years of age
Osteomyelitis	<5 years of age
Langerhans cell histiocytosis	Any age, but pelvic bone involvement typically seen in those <5 years of age
Slipped capital femoral epiphysis	12–15 years of age
Legg-Calvé-Perthes disease	5–8 years of age
Juvenile rheumatoid arthritis	1–3 years of age
Ewing sarcoma	Second decade
Osteoid osteoma	Second decade

view to identify the area of abnormality. A more focused examination is then performed in the abnormal area.

Toxic Synovitis

Toxic synovitis is the most common cause of acute hip pain in children younger than 10 years of age. It occurs most commonly in children between four and seven years of age and typically follows an upper respiratory infection. Affected children present with pain or limping, have a joint effusion, have no findings of organisms in joint aspiration, and have symptoms that subside with rest (Fig. 7-85). It is a diagnosis of exclusion

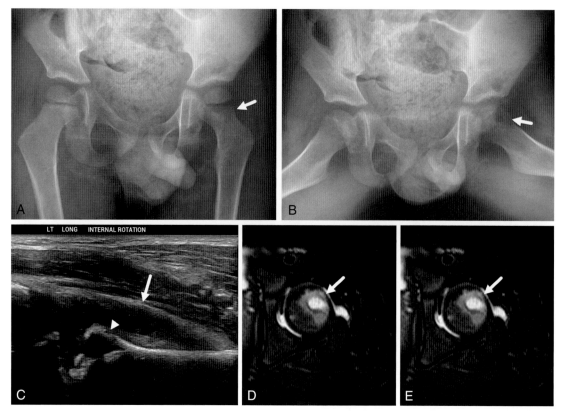

■ **FIGURE 7-83** Septic hip. Anteroposterior **(A)** and frog leg lateral **(B)** radiographs of the hip in a six-year-old male show a lucency (*arrow*) in the proximal left femoral metaphysis. The proximal femoral physis is mildly widened. **C,** Ultrasound of left hip shows an effusion (*arrow*) extending. The synovium is thickened, and there is complexity of the effusion. A cortical defect (*ar*) is also present in the proximal femoral metaphysis with an abnormal region of hypoechoic bone deep to the defect. Axial fat-saturated T2-weighted **(D)** and axial fat-saturated T1-weighted **(E)** magnetic resonance images show an intraosseous abscess (*arrow*) in the proximal femur. The T2-weighted image highlights the joint effusion.

and is always in the differential diagnosis of septic arthritis.

Legg-Calvé-Perthes Disease

LCP disease is idiopathic avascular necrosis of the proximal femoral epiphysis. It occurs more commonly in boys than in girls (4:1), most commonly in whites, and typically between five and eight years of age. Affected children present with pain in the groin, hip, or ipsilateral knee. The disease can be bilateral in as many as 13% of patients. It is often associated with skeletal immaturity (decreased bone age). Radiographs are usually positive, even early in the disease. Early findings include an asymmetric, small, ossified femoral epiphysis, widening of the joint space as a result of either joint effusion or synovial hypertrophy, and a subchondral linear lucency. The subchondral linear lucency (crescent sign) is best seen on frog-leg views and

represents a fracture through the necrotic bone (Fig. 7-86). When the diagnosis is suspected and radiographs are nondiagnostic, the diagnosis of LCP can be made on MRI (high T2-weighted signal marrow edema, loss of fatty marrow signal on T1-weighted images, asymmetric decreased enhancement with gadolinium) or bone scintigraphy (asymmetric lack of uptake). Later changes in LCP include changes in the femoral epiphysis, such as fragmentation, areas of increased sclerosis and lucency, and loss of height (collapse; see Fig. 7-86). Lucencies may be seen in the adjacent metaphysis in as many as one third of patients. Chronic LCP may result in a broad, overgrown femoral head (coxa magna); a short, broadened femoral neck; and physeal arrest. Problems arise when the overgrown femoral head is not covered by the acetabulum, and this scenario may require surgical reconstruction of the acetabulum.

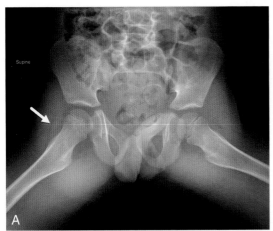

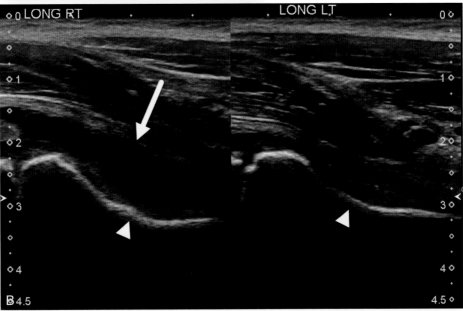

■ **FIGURE 7-84** Hip effusion. **A,** Frog leg lateral radiograph of the pelvis in a five-year-old male shows mild widening of the right hip joint space and bulging of the hip joint capsule (*arrow*) suggesting a joint effusion. **B,** Ultrasound of the hips confirms the right hip effusion (*arrow*). The normal left hip is shown for comparison. The cortical surface of the proximal femur (*arrowhead*) is visible on both the right and left hip.

Meyer dysplasia is a normal variant that simulates LCP (Fig. 7-87). It appears as fragmentation and delayed ossification of the femoral head in children two to three years of age and occurs more commonly in boys. While the femoral head appears fragmented, in reality, it is just incompletely ossified. It is typically differentiated from LCP by the age of presentation.

Slipped Capital Femoral Epiphysis

SCFE is an idiopathic, Salter–Harris type 1 fracture through the proximal physis of the femur that results in displacement (slippage of the femoral epiphysis). It is more common in boys

than in girls (2.5:1), in Black children, and in obese children. Certain conditions, such as patients with renal osteodystrophy, are predisposed. Both hips can be involved in up to one-third of patients. However, both hips do not usually present at the same time. The typical age of diagnosis is 12 to 15 years.

Slippage of the femoral head in SCFE is posterior and to a lesser extent medial. Because of this, findings are more prominent on the frog-leg lateral view than on the frontal AP radiograph. On the frog-leg lateral view, the epiphysis is seen to be displaced in comparison to the metaphysis. The image has been likened to an ice

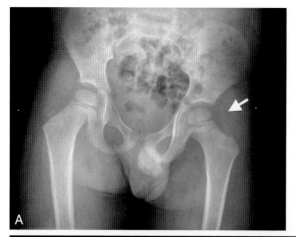

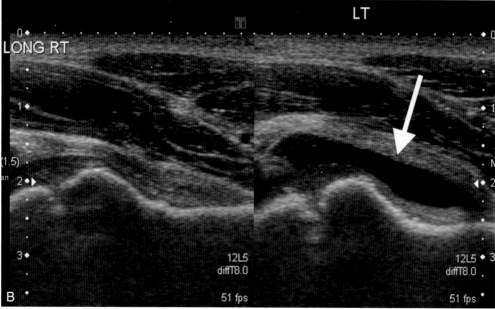

■ **FIGURE 7-85** Toxic synovitis. **A,** Anteroposterior radiograph of the pelvis in a three-year-old male shows pelvic tilt with the left side down and bulging of the fat plane (*arrow*) adjacent to the left greater trochanter. **B,** Ultrasound of the right and left hip shows a moderate left hip effusion (*arrow*).

cream falling off a cone. A line drawn tangential to the lateral cortex of the metaphysis on the frog-leg lateral view should bisect a portion of the ossified epiphysis. If the physis is medial to this line, it has slipped. Findings of SCFE can be very subtle on the frontal view. They include asymmetric widening of the physis and indistinctness of the metaphyseal border of the physis (Fig. 7-88). SCFE is typically treated with pin fixation to prevent further slippage, but the epiphysis is not moved back to its normal position. Potential complications of SCFE include avascular necrosis of the femoral head and chondrolysis.

■ METABOLIC DISORDERS

Rickets

Rickets is the bony manifestations of a heterogeneous group of problems resulting from deficiency of vitamin D or its derivatives. It may result from inadequate dietary consumption, malabsorption, renal disease, or a lack of end-organ response. The lack of vitamin D results in insufficient conversion of growing cartilage into mineralized osteoid and buildup of non-ossified osteoid. Because the radiographic manifestations are most prominent in rapidly growing bones, skeletal surveys to evaluate for rickets can

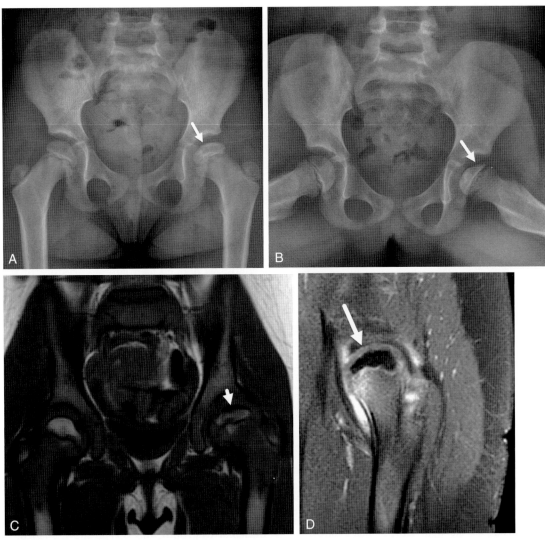

■ **FIGURE 7-86** Legg-Calvé-Perthes disease. Anteroposterior (**A**) and frog leg lateral (**B**) views of the pelvis in a six-year-old female show early changes of left Legg-Calvé-Perthes disease. There is a thin subchondral lucency (*arrow*) in the left femoral head. **C**, Coronal T1-weighted magnetic resonance imaging shows abnormal marrow signal (*arrow*) in the most superior aspect of the left femoral head. **D**, Sagittal fat-saturated T1-weighted postcontrast images shows an abnormal lack of enhancement (*arrow*) of the left femoral head.

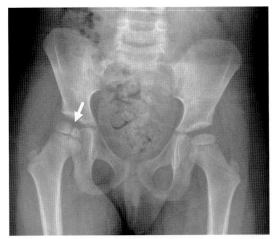

■ **FIGURE 7-87** Meyer dysplasia. Anteroposterior Radiograph of the hip in a four-year-old female shows a vertically oriented cleft (*arrow*) in the right femoral head.

be confined to frontal views of the knees and wrists. Radiographic findings include metaphyseal fraying, cupping, and irregularity along the physeal margin (Fig. 7-89). There is osteomalacia with unsharp, smudged-appearing trabecular markings. One of the more sensitive findings of rickets is loss of the dense zone of provisional calcification. Patients may be predisposed to insufficiency fractures (Looser zones) and slipped capital femoral epiphyses.

Lead Poisoning

Lead poisoning most commonly occurs in children younger than two years of age secondary to consumption of lead-containing substances, such as old paint chips. The incidence of lead poisoning has decreased significantly since 1978, when lead paints were removed from the market.

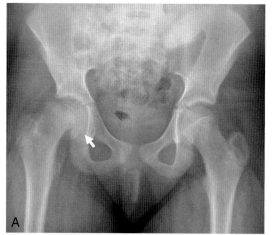

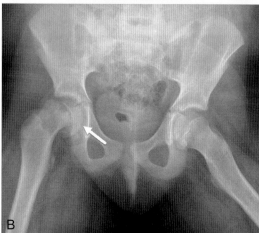

■ **FIGURE 7-88** Slipped capital femoral epiphysis. Anteroposterior (**A**) and frog leg lateral (**B**) views of the pelvis in an 11-year-old female shows asymmetric widening of the proximal femoral physis and medial displacement of the right femoral head (*arrow*) in relation to the femoral neck.

Findings of lead poisoning include broad sclerotic metaphyseal bands (lead lines) in areas of rapid growth, such as the knee (Fig. 7-90). Unfortunately, dense metaphyseal band is also a normal variant. One discriminating factor is that lead lines affect all the metaphyses surrounding the knee, whereas the normal variant type of dense bands spares the proximal fibula. Other common entities that cause dense metaphyseal lines include chronic anemia, chemotherapy, growth arrest lines, treated leukemia, and bisphosphonate therapy.

■ MISCELLANEOUS DISORDERS

Scoliosis

Scoliosis is defined as a lateral curvature of the spine. Most often, scoliosis is idiopathic in origin. This type of scoliosis is typically S-shaped, with the upper (thoracic) curvature convex to the right—a dextrocurvature. Idiopathic scoliosis is usually identified in late childhood or adolescence and is seven times more common in girls. In 80% of cases, diagnosis is made between the ages of 10 years and maturity. The degree of curvature may change quickly during times of rapid growth, such as puberty. Severe scoliosis can be associated with respiratory compromise, neurologic symptoms, and pain. Congenital scoliosis occurs secondary to vertebral segmentation anomalies and is often associated with more abrupt short-segment curves than those found in idiopathic cases. Neuromuscular scoliosis results from neurologic impairment or muscular dystrophy and is typically C-shaped.

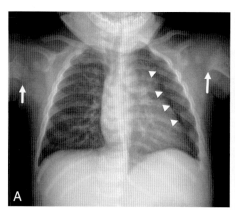

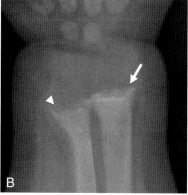

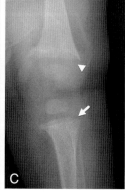

■ **FIGURE 7-89** Rickets. **A,** Anteroposterior (AP) view of the chest in an eight-month-old male shows a bulbous appearance (*arrowheads*) of the anterior ribs at the costochondral junction typical or rachitic rosary. The proximal humeral metaphyses (*arrows*) are irregular with a frayed appearance. **B,** AP radiograph of the wrist shows cupping and fraying of the distal metaphysis of the radius (*arrow*) and ulna (*arrowhead*). **C,** The same changes are found about the knee at the distal femur (*arrowhead*) and proximal tibia (*arrow*).

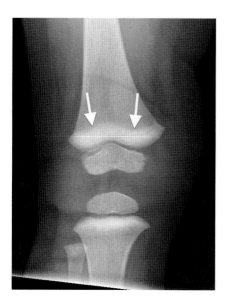

■ FIGURE 7-90 Lead poisoning. Anteroposterior radiograph of the right knee in an 18-month-old female with elevated lead levels shows dense metaphyseal lines of the femur (*arrows*), tibia, and fibula.

Radiographic evaluation is typically performed by means of a frontal view of the thoracolumbar spine. Studies are obtained with the patient standing (when possible) and in the posteroanterior projection to decrease the radiation dose to the breast. Depending on the situation, the frontal view may be complemented by a lateral view, bilateral bending views, or distraction views.

The curvature of the spine is measured by calculating the Cobb angle. Lines are drawn parallel to the end plates of two vertebral bodies, highlighting the greatest curvature (Fig. 7-91). The angle between those two lines represents the angle of curvature. Curves less than 10 degrees are considered normal. Curves less than 25 degrees are often treated by applying an external brace. Rapidly progressive curves or curves greater than 40 degrees are typically treated surgically with posterior spinal fusion.

When reporting findings, it is important to note whether any vertebral anomalies are present, the degree of spinal curvature, any change in curvature compared with previous studies, and the Risser stage. Because the iliac crest apophysis matures in a predictable pattern from the lateral margin to the medial margin, the Risser stage can be used to define skeletal maturity. Risser stage 0 is the least mature and refers to an iliac crest apophysis that has not yet begun to ossify; Risser stages 1, 2, and 3 refer to an iliac crest in which the lateral 25%, 50%, and 75%, respectively, of the iliac crest apophysis have begun to ossify;

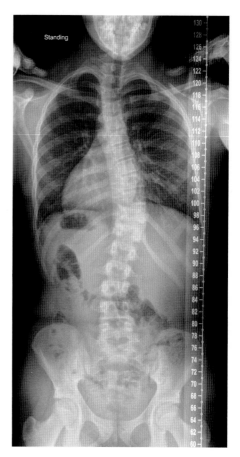

■ FIGURE 7-91 Scoliosis. Anteroposterior radiograph of the spine in a 14-year-old female shows an S-shaped curvature of the spine. The greatest portion of the curve is centered at T11.

Risser stage 4 occurs when the entire iliac crest apophysis ossifies; and finally, the most mature is Risser stage 5, when the iliac crest apophysis has fused to iliac wing. The Risser stage helps surgeons to plan the best time to operate because the more skeletally mature the patient, the less chance there is of further progression of the spinal curvature. In follow-up of postoperative cases, it is important to evaluate the stability of the curve, as well as for fracture or change in position of hardware (Fig. 7-92).

Osteochondral Lesions

Osteochondral lesions, or osteochondritis dissecans, are lesions of adolescence and are typically seen in athletes. They most commonly occur in the lateral aspect of the medial femoral condyle (Fig. 7-93) but can also occur in the elbow (capitellum; Fig. 7-94) or ankle (Fig. 7-95). The defect can vary in size from a few millimeters to 1−2 cm depending on the location.

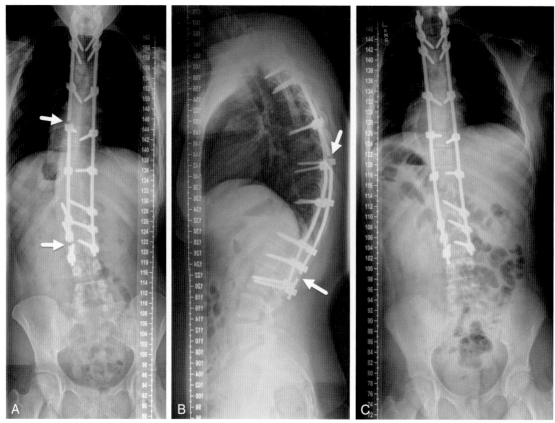

■ **FIGURE 7-92** Fractured scoliosis rods. Anteroposterior (AP) (**A**) and lateral (**B**) view of the spine in a 16-year-old female with a history of scoliosis shows fractures in the mid and inferior aspect of the scoliosis rods (*arrows*). **C,** AP radiograph performed three years earlier shows the intact rods.

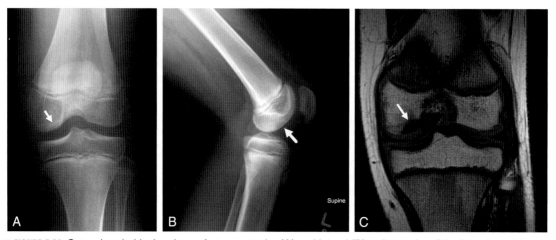

■ **FIGURE 7-93** Osteochondral lesion, knee. Anteroposterior (**A**) and lateral (**B**) radiographs of the knee in an 11-year-old male show an osteochondral lesion (*arrow*) of the lateral aspect of the medial femoral condyle. The lesion has an oval shape and is surrounded by a thin lucent rim and an outer sclerotic border. **C,** Coronal T1-weighted magnetic resonance imaging shows the oval-shaped area of decreased T1 signal (*arrow*) related to the osteochondral lesion. Fluid signal did not extend around the lesion on T2-weighted images (not shown).

Osteochondral lesions are often detected on radiographs obtained for joint pain. The lesions appear as a semicircular area of lucency and can have surrounding sclerosis or fragmentation.

MRI is used to determine stability of the lesion. Determinants of instability vary in children compared with adults but include fluid signal surrounding the lesion, multiple cysts, a large

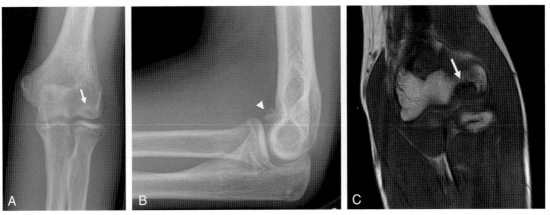

■ **FIGURE 7-94** Osteochondral lesion, capitellum. Anteroposterior (**A**) and lateral (**B**) radiographs of the elbow in a 15-year-old male show a semicircular lucency of the capitellum (*arrow*) with an irregular sclerotic border. A loose fragment (*arrowhead*) is visible on the lateral view. **C,** Coronal T1-weighted magnetic resonance imaging shows the oval-shaped area of decreased T1 signal (*arrow*) within the capitellum related to the osteochondral lesion.

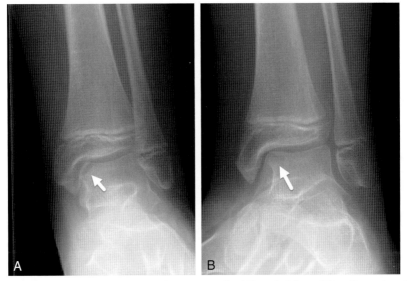

■ **FIGURE 7-95** Osteochondral lesion, talar dome. Anteroposterior (**A**) and oblique (**B**) radiographs of the ankle in a nine-year-old female show an oval lucency (*arrow*) with a sclerotic rim in the medial aspect of the talar dome.

size, thick sclerotic margin, or a loose joint body. Treatment is often conservative because many lesions heal on their own. Surgical therapy is reserved for unstable lesions, lesions that fail to heal with conservative therapy, and lesions in high performance athletes.

Panner Disease

Panner disease is an idiopathic avascular necrosis of the capitellum. It is distinguished from an osteochondral lesion by the patient's age and relation to activity. Panner disease typically occurs in children between 5 and 12 years of age; it is not associated with throwing sports. Osteochondral lesions are more common in patients 13 years of age and older and are usually a result of throwing sports. On radiographs, Panner disease appears as irregularity and fragmentation of the capitellar ossification center, like the appearance of the femoral head in LCP. An elbow effusion is not always present.

Abnormalities of Skeletal Maturity: Bone Age

Clinical indications for evaluating whether a child's skeletal maturity matches the child's true age include short stature, growth hormone deficiency, premature puberty, delayed puberty, and preoperative evaluation for orthopedic surgery (scoliosis, leg length discrepancy).

In such cases, a single frontal view of the left hand is typically obtained and compared with a set of image standards (Greulich and Pyle). The degree of epiphyseal ossification is compared with the standards. The pattern of ossification of the more distal physes of the fingers is considered more accurate than the more proximal finger physes or carpal bones. When reporting such studies, the patient's chronologic age, gender, bone age based on the standards of Greulich and Pyle, calculated standard of deviation of bone age for chronologic age, and whether the bone age falls outside of two standard deviations (i.e., whether it is abnormal) should be included. Other methods of determining the bone age exist and may be useful for certain populations. For example, in the Sontag method, the number of ossification centers of the entire left upper and lower extremity are counted and compared to a standard. This method is useful in determining the bone age of infants and toddlers.

Juvenile Idiopathic Arthritis

Juvenile idiopathic arthritis (JIA) is an idiopathic systemic disease that primarily affects the musculoskeletal system. It differs from adult rheumatoid arthritis in many ways. In JIA, most cases are seronegative, and the diagnosis is made clinically. In addition, while small joint involvement predominates in rheumatoid arthritis, large joint involvement is more common in children with JIA. The joints most frequently involved in JIA include the knee, ankle, wrist, hand, elbow, and hip (Fig. 7-96). In most cases, the disease is pauciarticular, with between two and four joints involved. Before development of radiologic findings, MRI with gadolinium enhancement may show abnormally enhancing thickened synovium, tenosynovitis, and a complex effusion (containing rice bodies or other debris) in involved joints (Fig. 7-97). This may be used to aid in diagnosis and monitor therapy. Initial radiographs may be normal or may show only soft tissue swelling or joint effusion. With more advanced disease in the knee, there may be joint effusion, epiphyseal overgrowth, widening of the intracondylar notch, and accelerated bony maturation. In the cervical spine, there is often ankylosis of the apophyseal joints. When the hands and wrists are involved, the disease is typically most severe in the carpal bones (see Fig. 7-96). Findings include small, square-appearing carpal bones, and narrowing of the intercarpal joint spaces. Later changes include erosions, ankylosis, or subluxation. Children may also have splenomegaly or pleural effusions. Still

disease is an acute form of JIA in which children present with fever, rash, hepatosplenomegaly, and lymphadenopathy. Skeletal involvement is rare in these children.

Hemophilia

With hemophilia, recurrent bleeding into a joint can result in a debilitating arthropathy. The joints most commonly involved include (in decreasing order of frequency of occurrence) the knee, elbow, and ankle. The recurrent hemorrhage deposits hemosiderin within the synovium, and there is associated hypertrophy of the synovium and destruction of the underlying articular cartilage. On radiography, epiphyseal overgrowth may be seen, particularly in the head of the radius (Fig. 7-98). In the knee, there is often squaring of the margin of the patella and widening of the intracondylar notch. In more advanced disease, cartilage destruction, erosions, and subchondral cysts may be present. These findings can appear like those in JIA. On MRI, there is destruction of articular cartilage and hypertrophy of the synovium. The hypertrophied synovium may be dark on T2-weighted images, secondary to the hemosiderin deposition (see Fig. 7-98), giving rise to an appearance similar to pigmented villonodular synovitis. Recurrent hematoma formation can also lead to the formation of pseudotumors, which usually occur in the soft tissues but can cause pressure necrosis and lucency of adjacent bone.

Sickle Cell Anemia and Thalassemia

With severe causes of anemia, such as sickle cell anemia or thalassemia, skeletal changes related to marrow expansion may be seen on radiography. Findings include thinning of the cortex, coarsening of the trabeculae, and bony remodeling (Fig. 7-99). The ribs appear widened. In the skull, the diploic space can become widened and has a hair-on-end appearance, particularly with thalassemia. In sickle cell anemia, there are often areas of bone infarction that may appear as either sclerotic or lucent areas. The vertebral bodies in sickle cell anemia often demonstrate indented and flat portions of the superior and inferior end plates, giving the vertebral bodies a "Lincoln log" or H-shaped appearance (see Fig. 7-99).

With severe anemia, other imaging findings may include cardiomegaly, gallstones, and splenomegaly (or conversely, in sickle cell anemia, there may be autoinfarction of the spleen and a small, calcified spleen). Extramedullary hematopoiesis and a predisposition to osteomyelitis may also be noted.

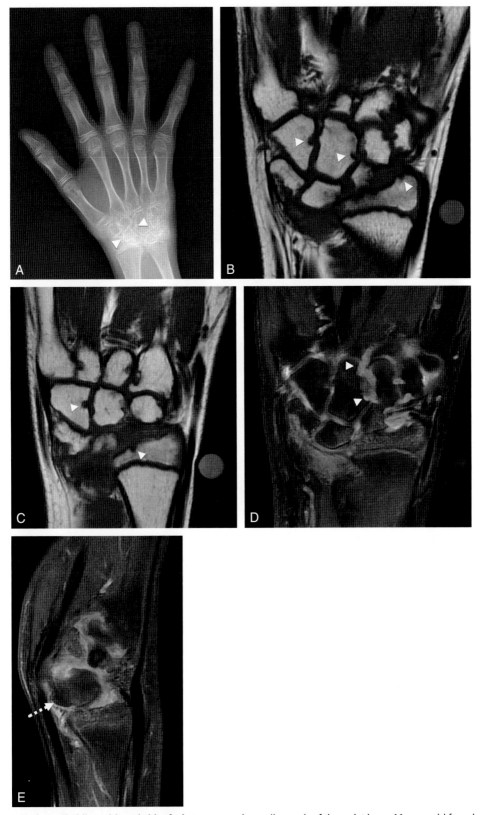

■ **FIGURE 7-96** Juvenile idiopathic arthritis. **A,** Anteroposterior radiograph of the wrist in an 11-year-old female shows erosions (*arrowhead* on some examples) of the carpal bones. The carpal bones have a jumbled appearance, making it difficult to identify all of the bones in proximal and distal carpal rows. Coronal T1-weighted magnetic resonance (MR) images (**B** and **C**) show erosions (*arrowhead*) of every carpal bone as well as the epiphysis of the radius. **D,** Coronal fat-saturated T1-weighted postcontrast MR image shows thickened, enhancing synovium (*arrowhead*) between the carpal bones and extending into erosions. **E,** Sagittal fat-saturated T1-weighted postcontrast MR image shows palmar subluxation of the scaphoid (*dashed arrow*) in relation to the distal radius. The synovium surrounding the carpal bones is thickened and enhancing.

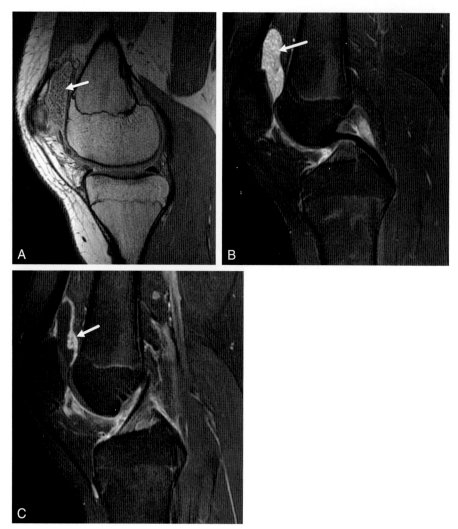

■ **FIGURE 7-97** Juvenile idiopathic arthritis. Sagittal T1-weighted (**A**) and fat-saturated T2-weighted (**B**) magnetic resonance (MR) images of the knee in a 15-year-old female show a moderate effusion (*arrow*) with innumerable rice bodies. **C,** Sagittal fat-saturated T1-weighted postcontrast MR image shows irregular thickening and enhancement of the synovium (*arrow*).

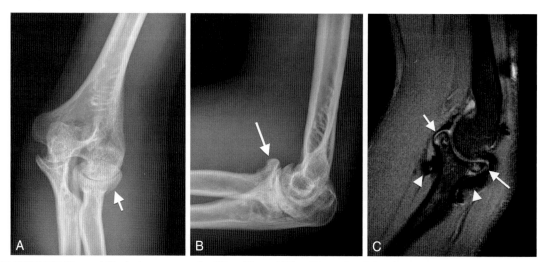

■ **FIGURE 7-98** Hemophilia A. Anteroposterior (**A**) and lateral (**B**) radiographs of the elbow in a 21-year-old male show overgrowth of bones about the elbow. This is most pronounced in the head of the radius (*arrow*). In addition, the joint space is narrowed, the intercondylar notch is widened and deepened, and there are erosions and subchondral cysts of the capitellum. **C,** Sagittal proton density magnetic resonance imaging with fat saturation shows overgrowth of the head of the radius (*arrows*), darkened, hypertrophied synovium (*arrowhead*), and marrow signal abnormality.

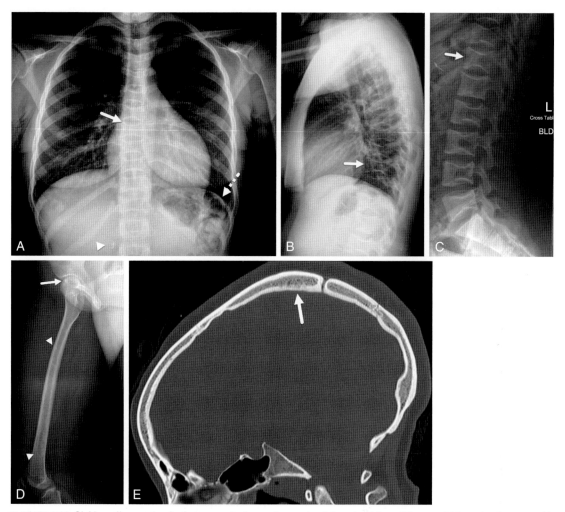

■ **FIGURE 7-99** Sickle cell anemia. **A,** Anteroposterior radiograph of the chest in a 17-year-old female shows an H-shaped configuration of the vertebral bodies (*arrow*), cholecystectomy clips (*arrowhead*), and absence of the splenic shadow with the splenic flexure of the colon extending just below the left hemidiaphragm (*dashed arrow*). The H-shaped vertebral bodies (*arrow*) are better seen on the lateral view of the chest (**B**) and lumbar spine (**C**). **D,** Lateral view of the femur shows chronic changes of avascular necrosis with sclerosis (*arrow*) of the femoral head and a large femoral infarct (*arrowhead*). **E,** Sagittal computed tomography image of the skull shows thickening of the diploic space (*arrow*) from chronic anemia.

Radial Dysplasia

Radial dysplasia, often referred to as radial ray syndrome, refers to a variable degree of hypoplasia or aplasia of the radius (Fig. 7-100). Often the first metatarsal or thumb may be hypoplastic or absent as well. Radial ray syndrome may be seen in association with VATER complex, Holt–Oram syndrome, Fanconi anemia, and thrombocytopenia-absent radius syndrome.

Blount Disease

Blount disease is excessive medial bowing of the tibias (tibia vara), most commonly occurring during infancy. It is an idiopathic disease but is thought to be related to excessive pressure on the medial metaphysis of the tibia, resulting in delayed endochondral ossification. It can be differentiated from physiologic bowing of the tibias by both the degree of angulation and the appearance of the medial metaphysis of the tibia. With Blount disease, there is irregularity, fragmentation, and beaking of the medial tibial metaphysis (Fig. 7-101). Severe cases may require tibial osteotomy.

Neurofibromatosis

The nonmusculoskeletal aspects of neurofibromatosis type 1 are discussed in Chapter 8. Many changes can occur in the bones of patients with

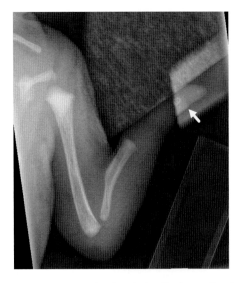

■ **FIGURE 7-100** Radial dysplasia. Radiograph of the arm in a one-day-old male shows an absent radius and a shortened irregular ulnar. Only a single digit (*arrow*) is present at the hand.

this disorder, and most of them are thought to be related to mesodermal dysplasia. The bones may demonstrate overgrowth, bowing, areas of sclerosis, and numerous cortical defects. Characteristic findings include anterolateral tibial bowing (Fig. 7-102), pseudoarthrosis formation (commonly within the tibia and/or fibula), and twisted-appearing (ribbonlike) ribs. The vertebral bodies may demonstrate posterior scalloping because of either dural ectasia or multiple neurofibromas. There is often kyphoscoliosis.

Clubfoot (Talipes Equinovarus)

Talipes equinovarus, or clubfoot, refers to a common congenital abnormality of the foot. To understand both clubfoot and other congenital abnormalities of the foot, it is important to understand the descriptive terminology. The terms *valgus* and *varus* refer to the bowing of the shaft of a bone and bowing at a joint. The name given to the bowing is determined by whether the distal part is more lateral or medial than normal. *Valgus* refers to lateral (think the L in valgus stands for lateral) and *varus* refers to medial. In hindfoot varus, the distal bone of the hindfoot (calcaneus) is angled too far medially in relationship to the more proximal bone of the hindfoot (talus), as seen on the AP view of the foot (Figs. 7-103 and 7-104). Normally this angle is approximately 30 degrees. With clubfoot, this angle is decreased. In addition, on the lateral view of the foot, the lateral talocalcaneal angle is normally approximately 30 degrees. With

clubfoot, there is a decrease in the lateral talocalcaneal angle, with the talus and calcaneus being closer to parallel to each other. This same terminology is used to describe other parts of the body as well. Therefore, genu varum is the bowing of the knee, with the distal part (tibia) being more medial than normal, and coxa valgus is bowing at the hip, with the distal part (femur) being more lateral than normal. Coxa vara and coxa valga can also be membered by the shape of the proximal femur. In coxa vara, the femoral head, neck, and proximal diaphysis have a shape like a lowercase r, like the r in varus. In coxa valga, the femoral head, neck, and proximal diaphysis have a shape like a lowercase l, like the l in valgus.

The terms *equinus* and *calcaneus* refer to the relationship between the ankle (tibia) and hindfoot (calcaneus) as viewed on a lateral radiograph. Equinus is fixed plantar flexion of the calcaneus (distal end pointing down, as a deer walks), and calcaneus is fixed dorsiflexion (distal end of the calcaneus pointing up). With clubfoot, or talipes equinovarus, there is hindfoot varus, hindfoot equinus, and forefoot varus. Normally a line drawn through the long axis of the talus on an AP view of the foot passes through the midsection to the medial section of the metatarsal bones. With forefoot varus, the distal bones (the metatarsals) are located more medial to this drawn line.

Tarsal Coalition

Tarsal coalition is an abnormal fibrous or bony connection between two of the tarsal bones of the feet. Patients with tarsal coalition can present with chronic foot pain or a propensity for ankle injury. It is a common abnormality affecting approximately 1% of the population and usually presents during adolescence. Although there is debate concerning which of the tarsal coalitions is the most common, talocalcaneal and calcaneonavicular coalitions are by far more common than other types. More than half of cases are bilateral. Calcaneonavicular coalition is easily demonstrated on radiographs of the foot. It is best visualized on the oblique view, in which the direct connection (bony coalition) or close proximity and irregularity of the joint margins (fibrous coalition) of the calcaneus and navicular bones (Fig. 7-105) is best depicted. On the lateral view, the anterior superior calcaneus appears longer than normal as it extends toward the navicular bone. The appearance has been likened to an anteater's nose. Rarely, cross-sectional imaging may be needed to confirm the diagnosis. In contrast, findings of talocalcaneal

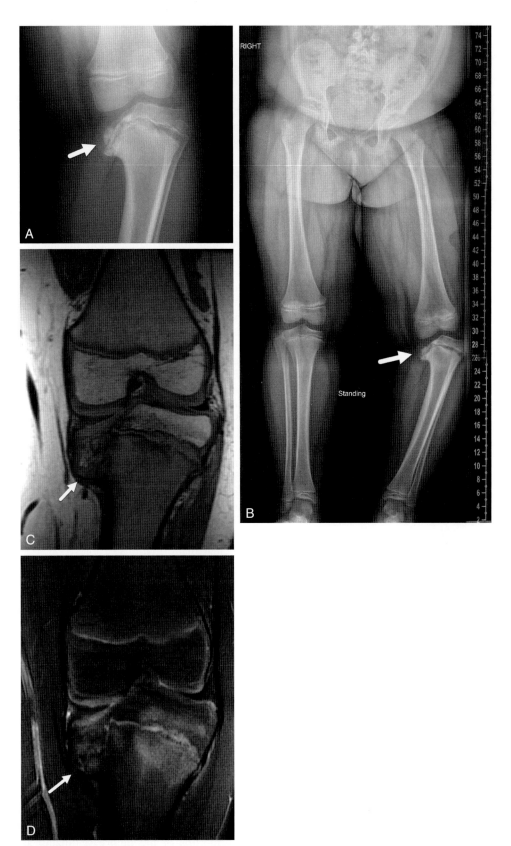

■ FIGURE 7-101 Blount disease. **A,** Anteroposterior (AP) radiograph of the knee in a six-year-old female shows excessive medial bowing of the tibia, fragmentation and beaking (*arrow*) of the medial tibial metaphyses, and widening of the lateral proximal tibia physis. **B,** AP radiograph of the lower extremities shows highlights the severe varus configuration of the left knee. The fragmentation and beaking (*arrow*) of the left medial tibial metaphyses can be compared to the normal appearance on the right. Coronal T1-weighted (**C**) and fat-saturated coronal T2-weighted (**D**) magnetic resonance images show medial down-sloping, fragmentation, and beaking (*arrow*) of the medial tibial epiphysis.

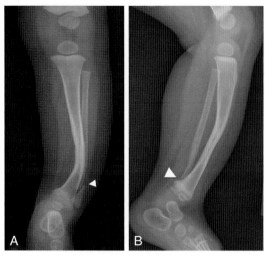

■ **FIGURE 7-102** Neurofibromatosis type 1. Anteroposterior (**A**) and lateral (**B**) radiographs of the left tibia and fibula in a 10-month-old male show anterolateral tibial bowing characteristic of neurofibromatosis type 1. A pseudoarticulation is also present at the distal fibula (*arrowhead*).

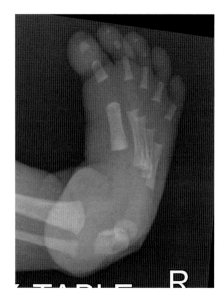

■ **FIGURE 7-103** Clubfoot. Anteroposterior radiograph of the foot in a two-day-old-female shows severe hindfoot varus.

coalition can be subtle on radiography, and CT is performed to make the diagnosis. Radiographic findings include secondary signs, such as talar beaking, poor visualization of the space within the talocalcaneal joint, and a prominent C-shaped band of overlapping bone overlying the calcaneus (Fig. 7-106). On the lateral view, if space can be seen within the talocalcaneal joint, talocalcaneal coalition is not present. However, this space may not be seen within a normal joint

on an oblique film. On coronal (short axis) CT images, talocalcaneal coalition is visualized as bony fusion or irregularity and close proximity (fibrous coalition) between the middle facet of the talus and the sustentaculum tali of the calcaneus. Painful tarsal coalition is treated with surgical excision of the coalition.

■ DISORDERS AFFECTING PRIMARILY SOFT TISSUES

Vascular Anomalies

Vascular malformations and hemangiomas can cause significant morbidity and even mortality in both children and adults. The classification and nomenclature used to describe endothelial malformations have been a source of confusion. Historically, lesions were named according to the sizes of channels within the lesions and the type of fluid the lesion contained. Blood-containing lesions were called hemangiomas, and lymph-containing lesions were referred to as lymphangiomas or cystic hygromas. This classification system was replaced by one described in 1982 by Mulliken and Glowacki, which separated endothelial malformations into two large groups, hemangiomas and vascular malformations, based on their natural history, cellular turnover, and histology. More recently, the International Society for the Study of Vascular Anomalies published a revised classification system. This classification scheme recognizes two main classes of vascular anomalies: vascular tumors and vascular malformations (Tables 7-7).

VASCULAR TUMORS

Vascular tumors can be split into three categories: benign and reactive, locally aggressive, and overtly malignant. The locally aggressive and overtly malignant tumors are rare and will not be discussed further; however, examples of these lesions are provided in Tables 7-7. Benign tumors are quite common. The two most common variants of benign tumors are infantile hemangiomas and congenital hemangiomas. Infantile hemangiomas are the most common tumor of infancy, affecting anywhere between 4% and 10% of all infants (Fig. 7-107). These tumors are more common in girls and in the craniofacial region. These tumors are not present at birth but appear within the first few weeks of life. After appearing, they progressively grow over the first few months of life before stabilizing and then regressing. Most infantile hemangiomas resolve by school age. Infantile hemangiomas are classified by their morphology, extent, distribution,

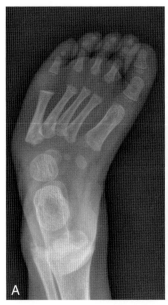
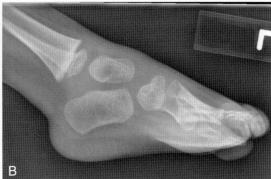

■ **FIGURE 7-104** Clubfoot. **A,** Anteroposterior radiograph of the foot in a three-year-old-male shows severe hindfoot varus. **B,** Lateral radiograph of the foot shows a near parallel configuration of the talus and calcaneus.

and depth of involvement. Infantile hemangiomas can be associated with syndromes such as PHACES (posterior fossa anomaly, hemangioma, arterial anomaly, cardiovascular anomalies, eye anomalies, and sternal clefting).

Congenital hemangiomas are less common (Fig. 7-108). They differ from infantile hemangiomas in that they are present and fully grown at birth. They often regress rapidly, resolving before one year of age. However, they can be subclassified based on the rapidity of involution. Rapidly involuting congenital hemangiomas (RICHs) resolve, whereas noninvoluting congenital hemangiomas (NICHs) do not. RICH lesions can be associated with transient thrombocytopenia or consumptive coagulopathy (Kasabach-Merritt syndrome).

Ultrasound, MRI, or CT can be used to evaluate lesions. Imaging of a hemangioma typically shows a discrete lobulated mass. On MRI, the lesions are hyperintense on T2-weighted images and isointense to muscle on T1-weighted images. Typically, prominent draining veins are identified. Hemangiomas enhance diffusely with contrast and show increased flow on Doppler ultrasound. Involuting hemangiomas can demonstrate areas of fibrofatty tissue with an associated high signal on T1-weighted images and demonstrate less contrast enhancement than proliferating hemangiomas. Unfortunately, many of the soft tissue malignancies of infancy, such as fibrosarcoma and rhabdomyosarcoma, can appear similar to proliferating hemangiomas. Therefore, cases that

do not exhibit the typical appearance and growth patterns of hemangioma are often biopsied to exclude malignancy.

VASCULAR MALFORMATIONS

Vascular malformations are divided into four groups based on their complexity and associated vessels: simple malformations, combined malformations, malformations of named vessels, and malformations associated with other anomalies. Simple malformations are usually composed of one type of vessel, although arteriovenous malformations (AVMs) and nontraumatic arteriovenous fistulas are included in this group. In general, the vascular malformations are present at birth and enlarge in proportion to the growth of the child. They remain present throughout the patient's life. MRI can be used to classify vascular malformations into either low-flow or high-flow lesions because their treatment options differ. Malformations with arterial components are considered high-flow lesions, and those without arterial components are considered low-flow lesions. Low-flow vascular malformations include primarily venous, lymphatic, and mixed malformations. A characteristic imaging finding in vascular malformations is that they tend to be infiltrative, without respecting fascial planes, and they often involve multiple tissue types, such as muscle and subcutaneous fat.

Capillary malformations affect the skin, appearing as pink to red macules (port-wine stain). Many times, the small, superficial lesions

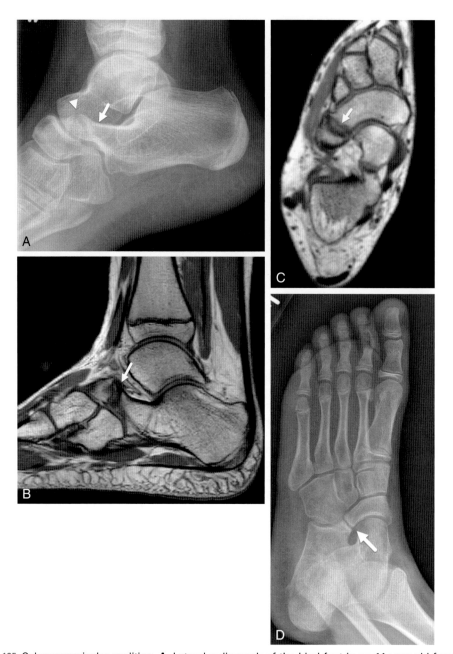

■ **FIGURE 7-105** Calcaneonavicular coalition. **A,** Lateral radiograph of the hind foot in an 11-year-old female shows elongation of the anterior process of the calcaneus (*arrow*) and irregularity (*arrowhead*) of the calcaneonavicular joint. **B,** Sagittal T1-weighted magnetic resonance imaging (MRI) shows elongation of the anterior process of the calcaneus and irregularity and sclerosis (*arrow*) of the calcaneonavicular joint. **C,** Axial T1-weighted MRI shows irregularity and sclerosis (*arrow*) of the calcaneonavicular joint. **D,** Oblique radiograph of the contralateral foot shows close proximity, irregularity, and sclerosis (*arrow*) of the joint margins of the calcaneus and navicular bones.

at midline near the forehead or on the back of the neck fade over time. The remainder of the lesions darken with time and persist. Lesions can be associated with soft tissue or bony overgrowth.

Lymphatic malformations are composed of variously sized lymphatic channels. They are classified according to the size of the channels as microcystic, macrocystic, or mixed. Macrocystic lesions have discrete cystic areas of various sizes. Macrocysts can be aspirated or sclerosed via interventional radiology. Lymphatic malformations are most common in the craniofacial and neck or axillary regions. Lymphatic malformations can be distinguished on physical exam by their normal overlying skin color. On MRI,

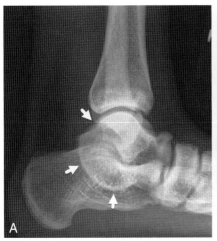
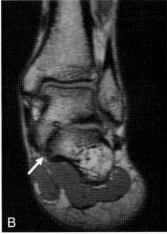
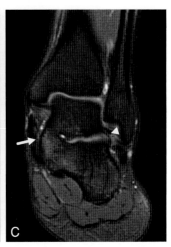

■ **FIGURE 7-106** Talocalcaneal coalition. **A,** Lateral view of the hind foot in a 17-year-old male shows the C sign (*arrows*) with no visible talocalcaneal joint. Coronal T1-weighted (**B**) and fat saturated T2-weighted (**C**) magnetic resonance images show elongation, irregularity, and sclerosis (*arrow*) of the subtalar joint. The T2-weighted image highlights the bone edema adjacent to the coalition. The more normal joint (*arrowhead*) is visible.

✳ **TABLE 7-7** Classification of Vascular Anomalies With Common Examples

Vascular Tumors

1. Benign and/or reactive
   a. Infantile hemangioma
   b. Rapidly involuting congenital hemangioma
   c. Noninvoluting congenital hemangioma
2. Locally aggressive
   a. Kaposiform hemangioendothelioma
   b. Retiform hemangioendothelioma
   c. Kaposi sarcoma
3. Overtly malignant
   a. Angiosarcoma
   b. Epithelioid hemangioendothelioma

Vascular Malformations

1. Simple malformations
   a. Capillary malformation
   b. Lymphatic malformation
   c. Venous malformation
   d. Arteriovenous malformation
2. Combined malformations
3. Malformations of named vessels
4. Malformations associated with other anomalies
   a. Klippel-Trénaunay syndrome
   b. Parkes Weber syndrome
   c. Sturge-Weber syndrome
   d. CLOVES syndrome
   e. Proteus syndrome

lymphatic malformations may contain cystic structures of various sizes, ranging from macrocystic to microcystic (Fig. 7-109). These cystic structures typically appear as high in signal intensity on T2-weighted MRI and do not exhibit central enhancement with gadolinium. Fluid-fluid levels are often present. Gorham-Stout disease, also known as vanishing bone disease, is a special variant of a lymphatic malformation. It is characterized by lymphatic malformations

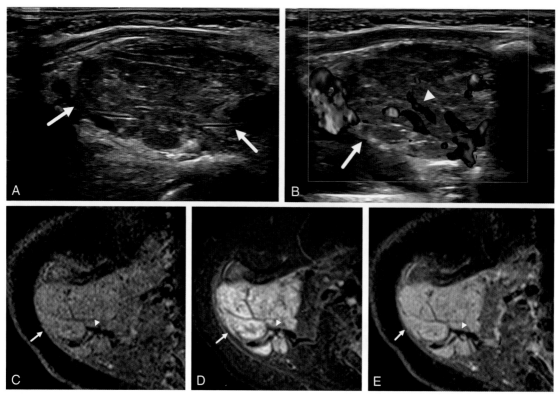

■ **FIGURE 7-107** Infantile hemangioma. **A,** Ultrasound of the soft tissues of the shoulder in a two-month-old female with a palpable mass shows a slightly hypoechoic soft tissue mass (*arrows*). **B,** Color Doppler highlights the increased vascularity of the mass (*arrow*). Fat-saturated axial T1-weighted (**C**), T2-weighted (**D**), and postcontrast T1-weighted (**E**) magnetic resonance images of the shoulder show the soft tissue mass (*arrow*) at the top of the shoulder just posterior to the scapula. A large vessel (*arrowhead*) extends through the mass. There is avid, homogeneous enhancement of the pass on the postcontrast images.

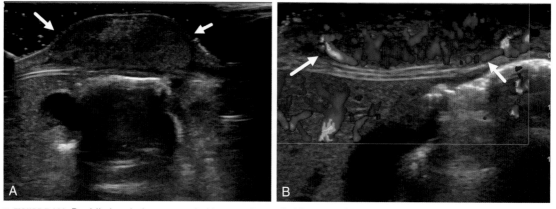

■ **FIGURE 7-108** Rapidly involuting congenital hemangioma. **A,** Ultrasound image of the abdominal wall in a newborn male shows a round, slightly heterogeneous mass (*arrows*) in the subcutaneous skin. **B,** Color Doppler interrogation shows that the mass (*arrows*) is hyperemic.

affecting one or multiple bones with associated progressive osteolysis (Fig. 7-110). Therapy for lymphatic malformations includes percutaneous sclerotherapy or surgical excision.

Venous malformations appear as blue skin lesions that are soft and compressible on palpation. Many venous malformations cause pain; they may also cause decreased range of motion and deformity. Symptoms tend to increase in late childhood or early adulthood. Venous malformations are classified by their distribution as focal, multifocal, or diffuse.

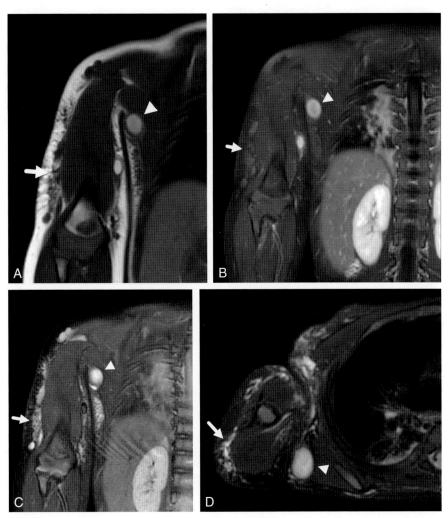

■ **FIGURE 7-109** Lymphatic malformation. Coronal T1-weighted (**A**), short-tau inversion recovery (STIR) (**B**), fat saturated T1-weighted postcontrast (**C**), and axial fat-saturated T2-weighted (**D**) magnetic resonance images of the axilla and upper extremity in a 12-month-old female shows a lymphatic malformation of the axilla, lateral chest wall, and upper extremity. The malformation is made up of large (*arrowhead*) and small (*arrow*) cystic spaces.

Treatment options for venous malformations include elastic compression garments, percutaneous sclerosis, and surgical excision. On MRI, venous malformations appear as a collection of serpentine structures separated by septations (Fig. 7-111). These serpentine structures represent slow-flowing blood within the venous channels and appear as high signal structures on T2-weighted images and intermediate signal structures on T1-weighted images. Phleboliths may be present; they appear as round, low-signal-intensity lesions on MRI. Gadolinium-enhanced T1-weighted images show enhancement of the slow-flowing venous channels.

AVMs are composed of a tangle of vessels with a central nidus and a direct arteriovenous communication. The lesions may present in childhood or adulthood and are often exacerbated during puberty or pregnancy. Presenting symptoms include congestive heart failure, embolism, pain, bleeding, and ulceration. High-flow vascular malformations are much less common than low-flow vascular malformations. On MRI, the lesions appear as a tangle of multiple-flow voids (Fig. 7-112) that demonstrate high flow on gradient echo images. Although the lesions can be associated with surrounding edema or fibrofatty stroma, there is usually no focal, discrete, soft tissue mass. Color Doppler ultrasound demonstrates arterial waveforms in the adjacent venous structures. The most effective treatment for AVMs is transarterial embolization.

Combined vascular malformations are said to be present if two or more simple components are present within a lesion. MRI is an important tool

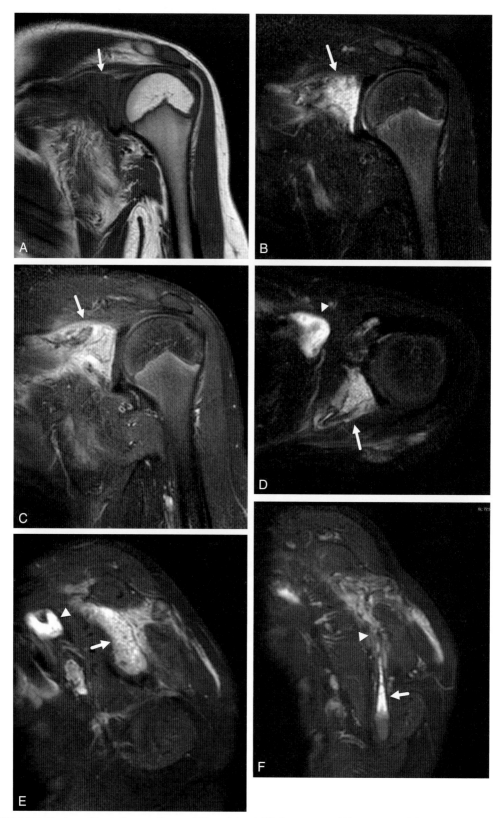

■ **FIGURE 7-110** Gorham-Stout disease. Coronal T1-weighted (**A**), fat-saturated T2-weighted (**B**), and fat-saturated T1-weighted postcontrast (**C**) in a nine-year-old male show expansion of the medullary cavity of the scapula near the glenoid (*arrow*). The mass enhances avidly. Sagittal (**D** and **E**) fat-saturated T2-weighted magnetic resonance image shows expansion of the medullary cavity (*arrow*) and abnormal signal of the scapula. An extra-osseous portion of the lymphatic malformation (*arrowhead*) is also present. **F,** Sagittal fat-saturated T1-weighted postcontrast image shows abnormal marrow signal (*arrow*) and fragmentation (*arrowhead*) of the scapula. Sagittal (**G**) and axial (**H**) computed tomography image obtained five years later shows worsening fragmentation (*arrowhead*) and irregularity (*arrow*) of the scapula.

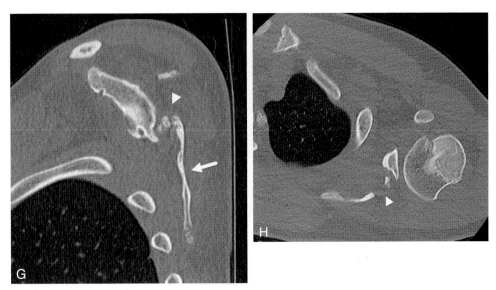

■ FIGURE 7-110 cont'd

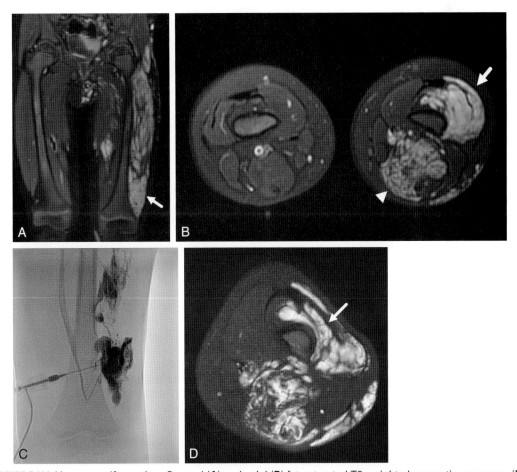

■ FIGURE 7-111 Venous malformation. Coronal (**A**) and axial (**B**) fat-saturated T2-weighted magnetic resonance (MR) images of the thighs show abnormal T2 signal in the anterior (*arrow*) and posterior (*arrowhead*) compartments of the thigh. The anterior compartment collection is made up of larger vascular spaces, while the posterior component is more infiltrative within the muscle. **C,** Contrast injection during sclerotherapy shows the large vascular spaces communicate with a draining vein. **D,** Axial fat-saturated T2-weighted MR image of the left thigh obtained five years later, after multiple sclerotherapies shows a decrease in the size of the venous malformation (*arrow*).

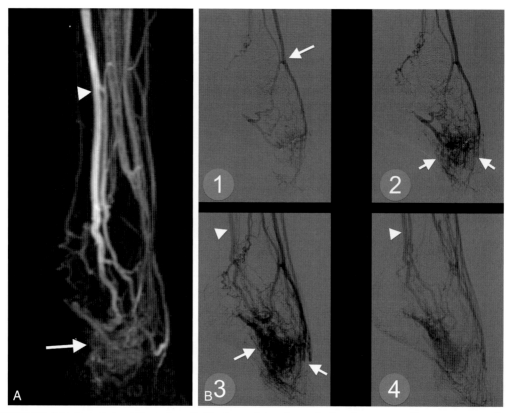

■ **FIGURE 7-112** Arteriovenous malformation. **A,** Maximum intensity projection from magnetic resonance angiogram with intravenous contrast large vessels extending toward the foot. Once in the foot, there is a tangle of small vessels (*arrow*). There is then brisk outflow into a large, bright vein (*arrowhead*). **B,** Sequential images from catheter angiogram (left to right, top to bottom) show inflow of contrast from large arteries extending to the foot (*arrow* in 1). Once in the foot, there is a tangle of small vessels that gradually fills (*arrows* in 2 and 3). On the third image, there is early drainage into a large vein (*arrowhead*). This progresses by the fourth image.

to help to define the combination of components, as well as the extent of the lesion. Malformations of major named vessels affect larger-caliber veins, arteries, or lymphatics. Again, imaging is important to define the extent of involvement, as well as the severity of disease. Finally, vascular malformations associated with other anomalies represent many named syndromes, such as Klippel-Trénaunay syndrome, Parkes Weber syndrome, Sturge-Weber syndrome, Maffucci syndrome, CLOVES (congenital, lipomatous, overgrowth, vascular malformations, epidermal nevi, and spinal or skeletal anomalies) syndrome, and Proteus syndrome.

Dermatomyositis

Dermatomyositis is an autoimmune disease that involves the skeletal muscle and skin. Children typically present with weakness and rash. MRI has been used to aid in making the diagnosis, directing biopsies to high-yield areas, and monitoring the response to therapy. On T2-weighted fat-saturated images, there is dramatically increased signal intensity in the involved muscles, myofascial planes, and subcutaneous tissues (Fig. 7-113). The most commonly involved muscles are those within the anterior compartment of the thigh and those surrounding the hip. There is typically rapid resolution of the abnormal high signal after therapy has been instituted. In patients with chronic dermatomyositis, calcifications may be seen in the soft tissues on radiography (Fig. 7-114).

Soft Tissue Malignancies

Primary malignancies of the soft tissues are uncommon in children. While ultrasound may be used to confirm the presence of a mass, MRI is the imaging modality of choice for evaluating soft tissue masses. The ultimate diagnosis of the mass is related to the patient's age. In infants, fibrosarcoma is the most common soft tissue malignancy, whereas rhabdomyosarcoma is the most common in children (Fig. 7-115).

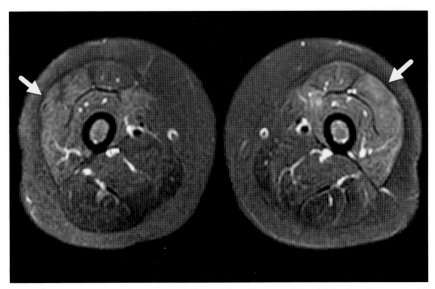

■ FIGURE 7-113 Dermatomyositis. Axial fat-saturated T2-weighted image of the thighs in a five-year-old female shows mild diffuse abnormal hyperintense T2-signal within the anterior compartment (*arrows*).

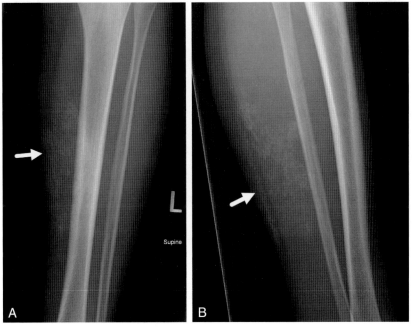

■ FIGURE 7-114 Dermatomyositis. Anteroposterior (**A**) and lateral (**B**) radiographs of the left tibia and fibula in a14-year-old male show amorphous subcutaneous soft tissue calcifications.

Rhabdomyosarcoma is most common in children between two and six years of age. Although it can arise from any muscle, it is most common in the head and neck region and pelvis. When rhabdomyosarcomas arise in the extremities, they are more likely to represent the alveolar subtype and present later in adolescence. Metastases are most common in the lungs, lymph nodes, and bones.

Other potential malignancies include primitive neuroectodermal tumors and synovial sarcomas. Synovial sarcomas tend to occur around joints and are deceptively benign appearing on imaging studies, with smooth, well-defined borders.

Desmoid tumor is a fibroproliferative disorder that is locally aggressive but does not metastasize. The lesions usually involve older children and

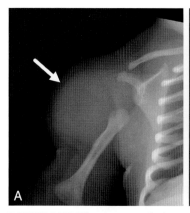
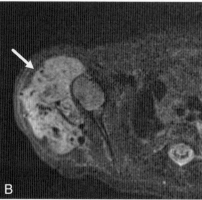
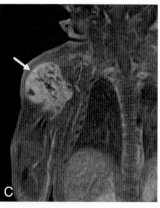

■ **FIGURE 7-115** Fibrosarcoma. **A,** Anteroposterior radiograph of the shoulder in an eight-day-old male shows a large soft tissue mass (*arrow*) with mild scalloping of the adjacent humerus. Axial (**B**) and coronal (**C**) fat-saturated T1-weighted postcontrast magnetic resonance images show the large, homogeneously enhancing soft tissue mass (*arrow*). Multiple vascular flow voids are present within the mass.

occur in the deep soft tissues. On MRI, a desmoid tumor has high signal on T2-weighted images despite its fibrous nature. It has a tendency to recur along the proximal resection margin.

Mimickers of Soft Tissue Malignancies

There are several benign entities that can present as palpable masses on physical examination and may lead to a request for imaging to rule out a malignant soft tissue mass. Knowledge of these entities will lead to accurate diagnosis and avoid potentially unnecessary procedures. Such entities include myositis ossificans, chronic foreign body, posttraumatic fat necrosis, and fibromatosis colli.

MYOSITIS OSSIFICANS

Myositis ossificans typically presents as a tender soft tissue mass. It is thought to be related to an organizing hematoma, but a history of trauma may be difficult to elicit. Eventually (two to six weeks after the event), calcifications within the soft tissues become evident and progress into a sharply circumscribed eggshell appearance. Initial radiographs may fail to show calcifications, and MRI performed at that time may show a nonspecific soft tissue mass. A low-signal ring may be seen on MRI on gradient echo sequences. CT may show calcifications before they are seen on radiography.

CHRONIC FOREIGN BODY

A child may experience a penetrating trauma that introduces a small foreign body, but the trauma may not be remembered. Such a child may

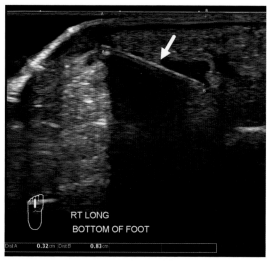

■ **FIGURE 7-116** Foreign body. Ultrasound of the foot in a six-year-old female with a wooden splinter shows a linear hyperechoic foreign body (*arrow*) with posterior acoustic shadowing.

present months later with a palpable soft tissue mass related to formation of granulation tissue around the foreign body and be imaged for work-up of a soft tissue mass. Like acute foreign bodies (Fig. 7-116), typical locations for chronic foreign bodies are those predisposed to trauma, including the plantar aspect of the foot, anterior portion of the knee, and buttocks. Ultrasound is a useful modality to evaluate the soft tissue mass in both the acute and chronic phases. Often ultrasound will reveal the underlying foreign body as an echogenic structure with the center of soft tissue thickening, edema, and hyperemia. When MRI is performed to evaluate a soft tissue mass, the foreign body may appear as a low-signal structure surrounded by soft tissue mass.

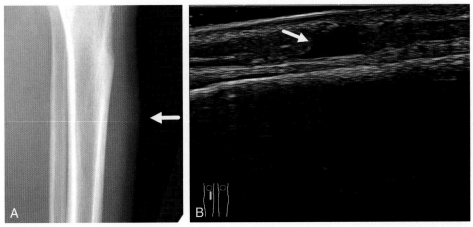

■ **FIGURE 7-117** Subcutaneous granuloma annulare. **A,** Lateral radiograph of the tibia and fibula in a three-year-old female shows a poorly defined soft tissue mass (*arrow*) along the anterior aspect of the tibia. **B,** Ultrasound of the tibia shows that the mass (*arrows*) is elongated, confined to the soft tissue, and has no effect on the underlying bone.

POSTTRAUMATIC FAT NECROSIS

As a result of minor trauma, children may develop fat necrosis in the area of the injured subcutaneous tissue. Months after the event, there may be scar formation in the area of fat necrosis, and it may present as a firm mass on physical examination. At the time of presentation, the traumatic event is usually not remembered. The most common locations for posttraumatic fat necrosis are in the thin layer of subcutaneous tissue anterior to the tibia and the buttocks. On MRI, posttraumatic fat necrosis appears as a linear area of high T2-weighted signal and enhancement. It is confined to the subcutaneous tissues, associated with volume loss in the involved subcutaneous tissues, and not associated with a discrete soft tissue mass. There is a similar condition known as subcutaneous granuloma annulare that also involves the subcutaneous tissues anterior to the tibia and is thought to be related to trauma but does have soft tissue mass related to granulation tissue (Fig. 7-117).

FIBROMATOSIS COLLI

Fibromatosis colli is a term that should not be confused with the more aggressive fibrotic processes of childhood. It is a benign mass in the sternocleidomastoid muscle in neonates who present with torticollis. The cause is poorly understood. Typically, ultrasound is performed to confirm the diagnosis. Ultrasound shows asymmetric fusiform thickening of the sternocleidomastoid muscle (Fig. 7-118), the echogenicity of which is typically heterogeneous and asymmetric but may be increased or decreased compared to

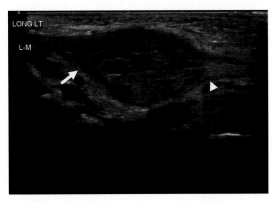

■ **FIGURE 7-118** Fibromatosis colli. Longitudinal ultrasound image of the neck in a 15-day-old female shows fusiform enlargement of the sternocleidomastoid muscle (*arrows*).

the contralateral normal muscle. Most symptoms resolve over time with stretching exercises, and surgical intervention is rarely required.

SUGGESTED READING

Barbuto L, Di Serafino M, Della Vecchia N, et al.: Pediatric musculoskeletal ultrasound: a pictorial essay, *J Ultrasound* 22(4):491–502, 2019.

Barrera CA, Cohen SA, Sankar WN, Ho-Fung VM, Sze RW, Nguyen JC: Imaging of developmental dysplasia of the hip: ultrasound, radiography and magnetic resonance imaging, *Pediatr Radiol* 49(12):1652–1668, 2019.

Bartoloni A, Aparisi Gómez MP, Cirillo M, et al.: Imaging of the limping child, *Eur J Radiol* 109:155–170, 2018.

Delgado J, Jaramillo D, Chauvin NA: Imaging the injured pediatric athlete: upper extremity, *Radiographics* 36(6):1672–1687, 2016.

Gemescu IN, Thierfelder KM, Rehnitz C, Weber MA: Imaging features of bone tumors: conventional radiographs and MR imaging correlation, *Magn Reson Imag Clin N Am* 27(4):753−767, 2019.

Helms CA: *Fundamentals of skeletal radiology*, 5th ed., Amsterdam, Netherlands, 2019, Elsevier.

Kahn SL, Gaskin CM, Sharp VL, et al.: *Radiographic Atlas of skeletal maturation*, Stuttgart, 2011, Thieme.

Keats TE, Anderson MW: *Atlas of normal roentgen variants that may simulate disease*, 9th ed., Philadelphia, PA, 2012, Saunders.

Laor T, Cornwall R: Describing pediatric fractures in the era of ICD-10, *Pediatr Radiol* 50(6):761−775, 2020 May.

Merrow AC, Gupta A, Patel MN, Adams DM: Revised classification of vascular lesions from the international society for the study of vascular anomalies: radiologic-pathologic update, *Radiographics* 36(5):1494−1516, 2014, 2016 Sep-Oct.

Merrow AC, Reiter MP, Zbojniewicz AM, Laor T: Avulsion fractures of the pediatric knee, *Pediatr Radiol* 44(11):1436, 2014.

Messer DL, Adler BH, Brink FW, Xiang H, Agnew AM: Radiographic timelines for pediatric healing fractures: a systematic review, *Pediatr Radiol* 50(8):1041−1048, 2020.

Ngo AV, Thapa M, Otjen J, Kamps SE: Skeletal dysplasias: radiologic approach with common and notable entities, *Semin Muscoskel Radiol* 22(1):66−80, 2018.

O'Dell MC, Jaramillo D, Bancroft L, Varich L, Logsdon G, Servaes S: Imaging of sports-related injuries of the lower extremity in pediatric patients, *Radiographics* 36(6):1807−1827, 2016.

Paddock M, Sprigg A, Offiah AC: Imaging and reporting considerations for suspected physical abuse (non-accidental injury) in infants and young children. Part 1: initial considerations and appendicular skeleton, *Clin Radiol* 72(3):179−188, 2017.

Paddock M, Sprigg A, Offiah AC: Imaging and reporting considerations for suspected physical abuse (non-accidental injury) in infants and young children. Part 2: axial skeleton and differential diagnoses, *Clin Radiol* 72(3):189−201, 2017.

Shah JN, Cohen HL, Choudhri AF, Gupta S, Miller SF: Pediatric benign bone tumors: what does the radiologist need to know?: pediatric imaging, *Radiographics* 37(3):1001−1002, 2017.

Silva MS, Fernandes ARC, Cardoso FN, Longo CH, Aihara AY: Radiography, CT, and MRI of hip and lower limb disorders in children and adolescents [published correction appears in *radiographics, Radiographics* 39(3):779−794, 2019, 2019 Jul-Aug;39(4):1232].

Singer G, Eberl R, Wegmann H, Marterer R, Kraus T, Sorantin E: Diagnosis and treatment of apophyseal injuries of the pelvis in adolescents, *Semin Muscoskel Radiol* 18(5):498−504, 2014.

Taybi H, Lachman RS: *Radiology of syndromes, metabolic disorders, and skeletal dysplasias*, 5th ed., St. Louis, MO, 2006, Mosby.

Voss SD: Staging and following common pediatric malignancies: MRI versus CT versus functional imaging, *Pediatr Radiol* 48(9):1324−1336, 2018.

Wassef M, Blei F, Adamas D, et al.: Vascular anomalies classification: recommendations from the international society for the study of vascular anomalies, *Pediatrics* 136:e203−e214, 2015.

CHAPTER 8

NEURO

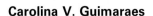

Carolina V. Guimaraes

Pediatric neuroimaging is a distinct subspecialty. Anatomic areas in neuroimaging include the skull, brain, orbits, face and sinuses, neck, and spine. At many children's hospitals, dedicated neuroradiologists perform and interpret all of the neuroimaging. The large amount of information included in pediatric neuroradiology is beyond the scope of this textbook. Specifically, diseases affecting both the pediatric and the adult population and presenting with similar imaging findings such as stroke and vascular anomalies will not be covered. Therefore, this chapter is a review of the commonly encountered entities in pediatric neuroimaging that are unique to the pediatric population or have unique pediatric features.

■ PEDIATRIC NEUROIMAGING MODALITIES: MAGNETIC RESONANCE, COMPUTED TOMOGRAPHY, AND ULTRASOUND

In pediatric neuroimaging, magnetic resonance imaging (MRI), computed tomography (CT), and ultrasound are all used, with some overlap. In general, MRI has become the definitive test in evaluating intracranial abnormalities. It is the test of choice for evaluating brain involvement for neoplasms, vascular lesions, inflammatory processes, demyelinating disorders, metabolic diseases, and developmental abnormalities, as well as for the evaluation of neurodegenerative disorders, focal seizures, unexplained hydrocephalus, and neuroendocrine disorders. CT is typically reserved for the evaluation of trauma and acute neurologic symptoms when MRI cannot be performed due to availability constraints or the patient's inability to lay still. CT has been historically the exam of choice for trauma and shunt malfunction; however, this has changed recently with fast MRI techniques being now widely used for shunt malfunction and recently instituted for trauma at some

institutions. Sinus disease, orbital cellulitis, temporal bones, and neck abnormalities remain often evaluated by CT. The use of MRI for the evaluation of temporal bone, face, and neck abnormalities is rapidly increasing and at many times may either substitute or complement CT evaluation. Neck ultrasound is used for thyroid evaluation and superficial masses. Head ultrasound is reserved for evaluating premature infants and newborns, prior to closure of the anterior fontanelle.

■ BASIC REVIEW OF ADVANCED MAGNETIC RESONANCE IMAGING TECHNIQUES IN PEDIATRIC NEUROIMAGING

A number of advanced MRI techniques are playing an increasing role in the neuroimaging of children. Such techniques and associated basic vocabulary are summarized here. Applications in pediatric patients are also discussed.

Diffusion-Weighted Imaging

Diffusion-weighted imaging (DWI) is determined by the variability in the diffusivity of water molecules in tissues. The random movement of water molecules is known as Brownian motion. In tissues, there is variable restriction of the movement of water molecules relative to tissue structure. Pathologic states may alter the diffusion characteristics of water molecules in the brain and therefore affect the appearance of the DWI images. Images on DWI are influenced not only by diffusion of water molecules but also by other tissue properties, such as T2. To eliminate the influences on imaging appearance of factors unrelated to diffusion of water molecules, the data are processed, most commonly by using a technique called an *apparent diffusion coefficient (ADC) map*. For each DWI sequence, at least two sets of images are created: the DWI images and

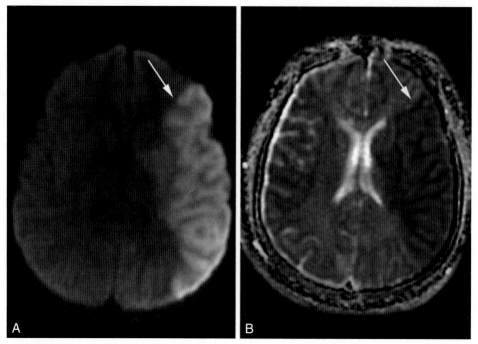

■ **FIGURE 8-1 Diffusion restriction with left middle cerebral artery stroke. A,** Increased signal on DWI sequence at the left middle cerebral artery territory (*arrow*). **B,** ADC map demonstrates low signal corresponding to the area of increase DWI signal (*arrow*), confirming diffusion restriction.

the ADC map. In a pathologic process in which there is true restricted diffusion, the involved area appears high in signal on the DWI images and low in signal on the ADC map (Fig. 8-1A and B). Conversely, in pathologic processes in which there is facilitated diffusion, signal will be low on DWI images and high on the ADC map. Due to the influences of T2 tissue properties on DWI imaging, an area of increased signal on T2-weighted sequences (including T2 fluid-attenuated inversion recovery sequences) may show as increased DWI signal and not represent true diffusion restriction. In this case, signal will be normal or increased on ADC map, instead of decreased. This phenomenon is known as T2 shine-through (Fig. 8-2A—C) and should not be confused with restricted diffusion.

Restricted diffusion is seen in pathologic processes that present with cytotoxic edema including brain infarct and/or ischemia, non-hemorrhagic traumatic injury, seizure-related edema, and encephalitis. Other causes of diffusion restriction include purulent fluid collections (Fig. 8-3A—C), epidermoid cysts, subacute hematoma, and hypercellular tumors. Processes that show facilitated diffusion include

vasogenic edema and cerebrospinal fluid (CSF) collections, such as an arachnoid cyst.

DWI has become an extremely important tool in neuroimaging. One of its major advantages is its high sensitivity for ischemia and infarction—often revealing findings not yet evident on conventional magnetic resonance (MR) sequences. It is also helpful in differentiating among posterior fossa tumors. Hypercellular medulloblastomas have restricted diffusion, whereas low-grade astrocytomas typically do not. Restricted diffusion is also rare in ependymomas. Table 8-1 shows a glossary of terms related to DWI and diffusion tensor imaging (DTI).

Diffusion Tensor Imaging and Tractography

Diffusion is anisotropic in white matter fibers, as axonal membranes and myelin sheaths act as barriers to the motion of water molecules in directions not parallel to their own orientation. By applying diffusion gradients in multiple directions during a diffusion MRI sequence, DTI technique enables the identification of the direction of maximum diffusivity in a voxel and

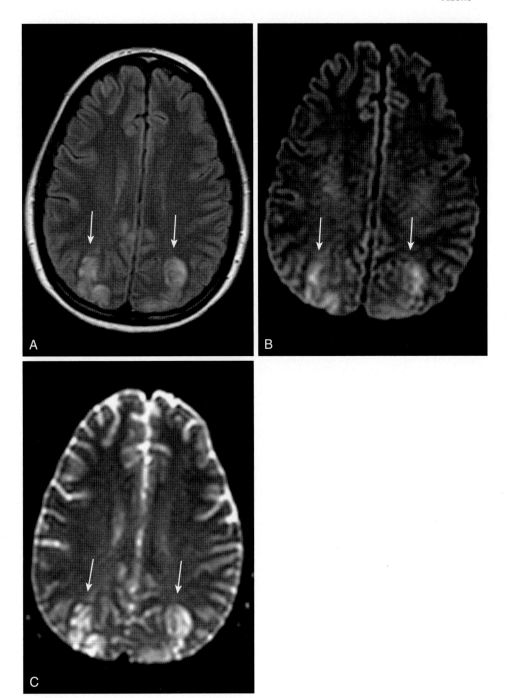

■ **FIGURE 8-2** "T2 Shine-through" in a case of posterior reversed encephalopathy syndrome. **A,** Abnormal increased FLAIR signal within the bilateral occipital cortex and subcortical white matter (*arrows*) in a child presenting with an acute episode of hypertension and new neurologic signs. Corresponding increased signal on DWI (*arrows*) (**B**) and increased signal on ADC map (*arrows*) (**C**) compatible with T2 shine-through rather than diffusion restriction.

therefore the identification of location, orientation, and directionality of the white matter tracts. DTI provides several capabilities not previously possible. (1) Large, individual white matter tracts can be depicted as discrete anatomic structures. The three-dimensional postprocessing technique used to create such images is tractography. (2) Metrics describing the microarchitecture of tissue can be calculated. They include fractional anisotropy, mean diffusivity, radial diffusivity, and axial diffusivity.

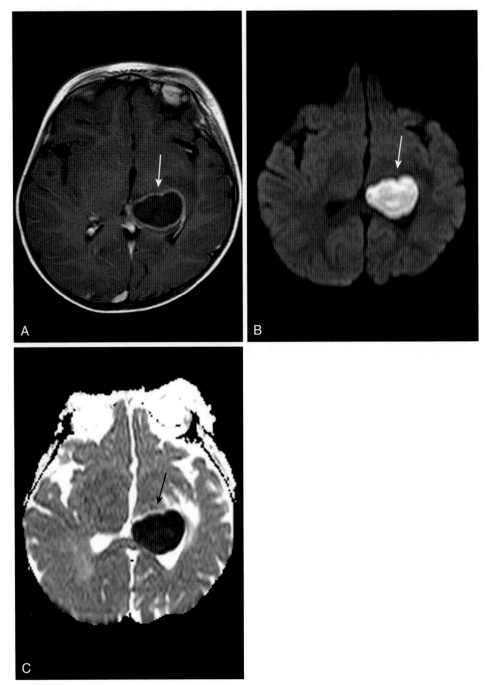

■ **FIGURE 8-3 Diffusion-weighted imaging in a brain abscess. A,** Axial T1-weighted sequence postcontrast shows a ring-enhancing fluid collection causing mass effect over the atrium of the left lateral ventricle (*arrow*). **B,** DWI sequence demonstrates high signal within the abscess cavity (*arrow*). **C,** ADC map demonstrates low signal (*arrow*), consistent with restricted diffusion from purulent material.

Tractography images are typically shown in color. By convention, white matter tracts oriented left to right are shown as red, cephalocaudad as blue, and anteroposterior as green (Fig. 8-4).

DTI and tractography can be used to evaluate myelination. Increased myelination increases anisotropy. Therefore, in normal infants, anisotropy increases with age. Most disease states that affect white matter decrease anisotropy.

Term	Definition
Isotropy	Uniformity of physical properties of a molecule in all directions; in other words, the absence of any kind of polarity
Anisotropy	The opposite of isotropy; having polarity or directionality
Eigenvalue	The mathematical property of a tensor (vector) related to magnitude and direction
Fractional anisotropy	A metric measuring the degree of anisotropy (0 for isotropy and 1 for full anisotropy)
ADC	A measure of the freedom of water diffusion in a particular tissue; increased ADC = increased diffusivity
Tractography	A postprocessing method of creating images representing axonal fiber tracts from diffusion tensor data
Tensor	The magnitude and direction of diffusion; is used similarly to the term *vector*. A 3 × 3 matrix is used to calculate a tensor

TABLE 8-1 Glossary of Terms in Diffusion-Weighted and Diffusion Tensor Imaging

ADC, Apparent diffusion coefficient.

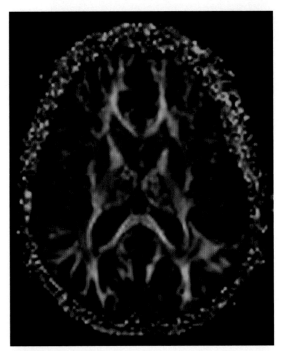

■ **FIGURE 8-4 Tractography color map (eigenvalue map) showing white matter tracts**. Note that *red* denotes tracts oriented left to right, *blue* denotes cephalocaudad, and *green* denotes anteroposterior.

DTI has been used to evaluate stroke, hydrocephalus, trauma, and demyelinating disorders. DTI and tractography have also been used to study and depict the white matter tract abnormalities associated with congenital brain anomalies and in the presurgical evaluation of brain tumors (Fig. 8-5). One important limitation of DTI-based tractography is that it underestimates the white matter tracts in parenchymal locations where there are crossing fibers. This is because a single tensor can resolve only a single fiber direction within a voxel. Recent studies have described new diffusion-based nontensor tractography techniques that demonstrate fiber tracts more accurately, but these are not yet being used in the routine clinical practices.

Perfusion

Perfusion MRI evaluates cerebral microvascular parameters, including cerebral blood volume, mean transit time, and cerebral blood flow. It relies on the use of a tracer that may be exogenous (gadolinium) in dynamic susceptibility contrast-enhanced and dynamic contrast-enhanced techniques or endogenous as in noncontrast arterial spin labeling technique. The main applications of perfusion MRI are evaluation of vascular pathologies (ischemic strokes, vasculopathies, vasospasm) and tumors. In the evaluation of brain tumors, perfusion may help with preoperative tumor grading and biopsy guidance by identifying high perfusion areas suspicious to represent higher grade portions of the tumor. Perfusion also plays a role in the evaluation of tumor treatment response and in the attempt to answer the always difficult question of tumor recurrence versus radiation necrosis.

Magnetic Resonance Spectroscopy

Proton (hydrogen) MR spectroscopy (MRS) is a tool that is used to help to characterize a number of pediatric neurologic conditions. Most often, single-voxel spectroscopy is created using a 1-cubic centimeter sample area. The results of spectroscopy are typically depicted as a spectrum, with each metabolic peak characterized by resonance frequency, height, width, and area (Fig. 8-6). Metabolic profiles depicted on MRS have been much less specific than originally hoped. However, the information obtained can provide useful information that complements the information derived from conventional MRI in many pediatric disorders, including neoplasms, hypoxic ischemic insult, and metabolic diseases.

The most commonly evaluated brain metabolites include *N*-acetylaspartate (NAA), creatine

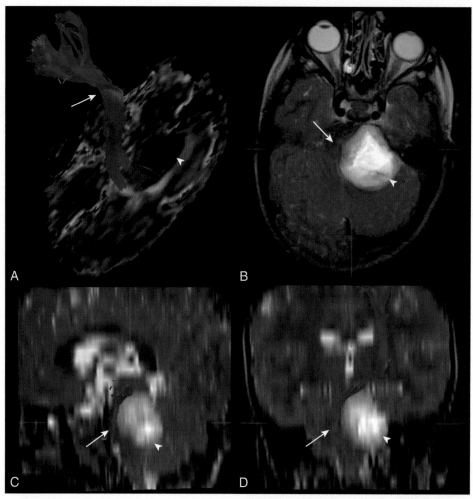

■ **FIGURE 8-5 Diffusion tensor imaging.** Left brainstem glioblastoma multiforme in a 5-year-old male extending into the brachium pontis. Tractography (**A**) and three-dimensional fiber representation of the left corticospinal tract (**B,** axial; **C,** sagittal; **D,** coronal) obtained for surgical planning. Left corticospinal tract (*arrow*) overlaid on anatomic images. Note the corticospinal tract (*arrow*) displaced medially by the large brainstem mass (*arrowhead*). *Images courtesy of James L. Leach, MD.*

(Cr), choline (Cho), myoinositol (mI), and lactate (Lac) (see Fig. 8-6). NAA is a neuronal marker and is decreased in most disorders that decrease neuronal viability and density, such as neoplasms (Fig. 8-7), infarcts, radiation injuries, and many white matter diseases. NAA is markedly elevated in Canavan disease and may also be elevated in Salla disease and Pelizaeus–Merzbacher disease. Cho compounds reflect the synthesis and degradation of cell membranes; therefore, increased Cho is seen when there is high cellular

turnover, as occurs with most tumors (see Fig. 8-7). Lac is a product of anaerobic glycolysis, typically elevated in the setting of acute ischemia (Fig. 8-8), infarction, abscess, many high-grade tumors, and some metabolic diseases, such as mitochondrial disorders. mI is considered a glial marker, elevated in gliosis and astrocytosis in pediatrics. Cr is relatively constant; therefore, it is used as an internal reference for calculation of metabolite ratios. Cr deficiency syndromes are rare causes of decreased Cr levels. Taurine (Tau)

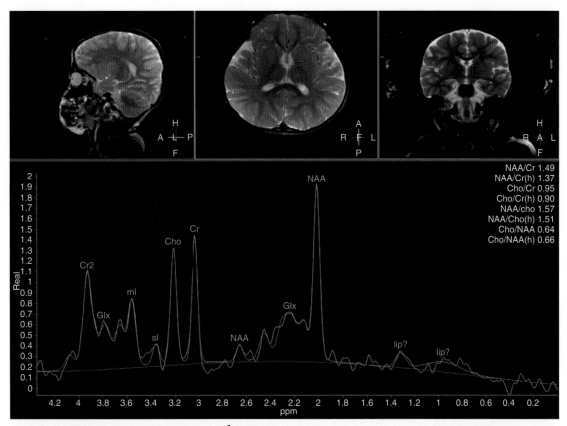

NAA/Cr 1.49
NAA/Cr(h) 1.37
Cho/Cr 0.95
Cho/Cr(h) 0.90
NAA/cho 1.57
NAA/Cho(h) 1.51
Cho/NAA 0.64
Cho/NAA(h) 0.66

■ FIGURE 8-6 **Normal short echo single voxel ¹H-MR Spectroscopy.** Voxel placed at the left basal. Note the normal stair-step relationship of choline (Cho; 3.2 ppm), creatine (Cr; 3.0 ppm), and NAA (NAA; 2.0 ppm) peaks. A peak related to myoinositol is also noted (ml; 3.6 ppm). Location of pathologic lactate peak (not present in this normal example) is at 1.3 ppm.

is not a commonly seen metabolite in clinical MRS; however, it has been shown to be elevated in medulloblastoma and therefore is an important metabolite to recognize in pediatric posterior fossa tumors (at 3.3 ppm, above baseline on short TE 30–35 and below baseline on TE 144).

There are differences in metabolite levels in the gray and white matter. The concentration of NAA in gray matter is higher than in white matter, and Cho concentration is typically higher in white matter. There are also differences in metabolite levels in the developing brain, especially during the first year of life. In the newborn period, NAA levels are low and mI and Cho levels are high (Fig. 8-9). Small Lac peak can also be found in healthy newborns.

Functional Magnetic Resonance Imaging

Functional MRI (fMRI) is a noninvasive method of evaluating regional neuronal activity within the brain. Neuronal activity increases metabolic activity, which results in increased blood flow to that region and a relative increase in the ratio of oxygenated hemoglobin to deoxygenated hemoglobin. Deoxyhemoglobin is paramagnetic; therefore, a change in the ratio affects the magnetic state of the tissue and, as a result, changes the local MRI signal. This phenomenon is called the *blood oxygenation level–dependent (BOLD) effect*. fMRI techniques show these changes superimposed on anatomic information. fMRI is used to document regional neuronal activity during a specific task. The most validated

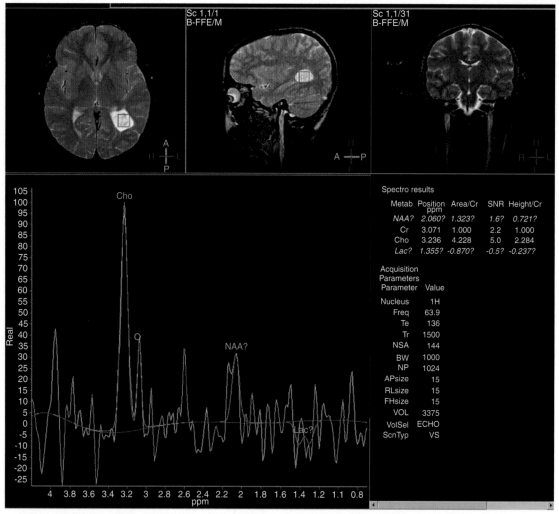

Spectro results

Metab	Position ppm	Area/Cr	SNR	Height/Cr
NAA?	2.060?	1.323?	1.6?	0.721?
Cr	3.071	1.000	2.2	1.000
Cho	3.236	4.228	5.0	2.284
Lac?	1.355?	-0.870?	-0.5?	-0.237?

Acquisition Parameters

Parameter	Value
Nucleus	1H
Freq	63.9
Te	136
Tr	1500
NSA	144
BW	1000
NP	1024
APsize	15
RLsize	15
FHsize	15
VOL	3375
VolSel	ECHO
ScnTyp	VS

■ **FIGURE 8-7** **Abnormal spectroscopy (TE:135) in a child with a supratentorial pilocytic astrocytoma.** Note a large Cho peak and diminished NAA, typical of neoplasms. There is also some elevation of lactate, depicted as an inverted doublet at 1.3 ppm. Although pilocytic astrocytoma is a low-grade tumor, spectra may mimic a more aggressive lesion.

use is for localization of different body representations in the primary motor and somatosensory cortex, as well as language lateralization (Fig. 8-10A–F). Clinically, fMRI has been used in the evaluation of patients with seizures and planning of surgical approaches to brain tumors. It also has been a very useful research tool in increasing our understanding of brain function. Current research is mostly focused on resting state techniques (R-fMRI), which measure BOLD fluctuations of spontaneous neuronal activity without the performance of a specific task.

■ NEONATAL HEAD ULTRASOUND

Neonatal head ultrasound is performed through the open fontanels of neonates and infants using high-frequency transducers. Images are commonly obtained in the sagittal and coronal planes via the anterior fontanel using a sector transducer (Fig. 8-11A and B). Linear high-resolution transducers are used to assess the extraaxial spaces (Fig. 8-12A and B) and superficial cortex. Additional images via the mastoid fontanel enable the detection of posterior fossa hemorrhages (Fig. 8-13A and B) and congenital

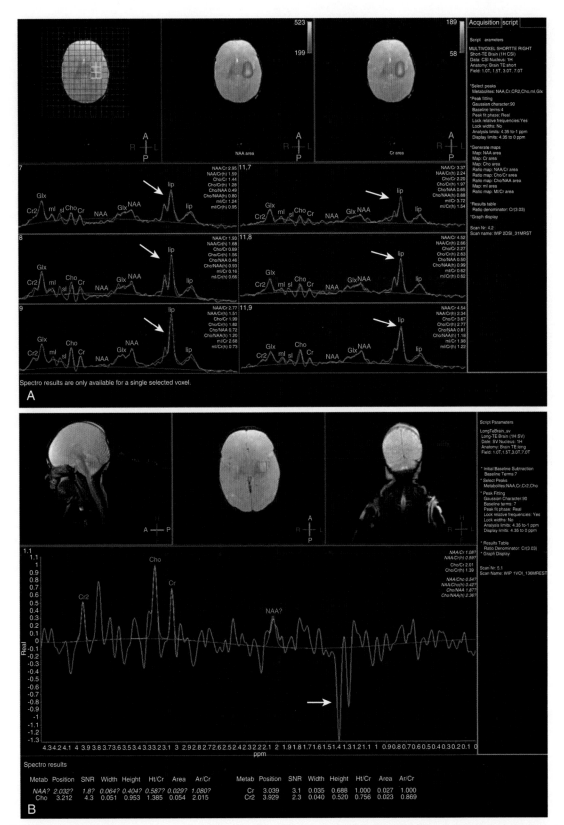

■ **FIGURE 8-8** **Abnormal spectroscopy in a neonate with history of hypoxic ischemic injury. A,** Multivoxel short echo spectroscopy (TE:35) at the left basal ganglia. Note large doublet at 1.3 bpm (*arrows*), likely a combination of lipids and lactate. **B,** Intermediate echo single-voxel spectroscopy (TE:135) confirmed the presence of lactate, seen as an inverted doublet at 1.3 bpm (*arrow*).

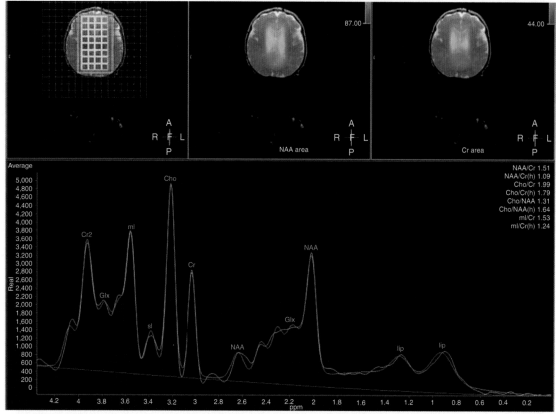

■ **FIGURE 8-9 Normal neonate spectroscopy.** Multivoxel short echo spectroscopy of the deep gray matter structures in a normal neonate demonstrating low NAA peak relative to Cho and mI levels. This is typical in the neonatal period and should not be confused with an abnormal decrease in NAA.

anomalies. Evaluation via the posterior fontanel can be used for differentiation of white matter injury versus anisotropy artifact in cases of abnormally increased posterior periventricular white matter echogenicity. In premature infants, head ultrasound is most commonly used to diagnose and follow up intracranial complications, such as germinal matrix hemorrhage and white matter injury of prematurity (periventricular leukomalacia). It can also be used to screen for congenital abnormalities and hydrocephalus. Another common indication is evaluation of an infant with a large head circumference.

Germinal Matrix Hemorrhage

The germinal matrix is a fetal structure that is a stem source for neuroblasts. It typically involutes by term but is still present in premature infants, mostly within the caudothalamic groove (the space between the caudate head and the thalamus). The germinal matrix is highly vascular and is subject to hemorrhaging with fluctuation in cerebral blood pressure. Germinal matrix hemorrhage most commonly occurs in premature infants during the first days after birth. Potential complications include destruction of the precursor cells within the germinal matrix, hydrocephalus, and hemorrhagic infarction of the surrounding periventricular tissues. Cerebellar hemorrhage can also be seen in very premature patients (Fig. 8-13A and B).

On ultrasound, germinal matrix hemorrhage is seen as an ovoid echogenic mass within the caudothalamic groove (Figs. 8-14A and B). For those not well acquainted with head ultrasound, there may be confusion in differentiating germinal matrix hemorrhage from the normally echogenic choroid plexus. In contrast to germinal matrix hemorrhage, normal choroid plexus should never extend as anterior as the caudothalamic groove on a parasagittal view

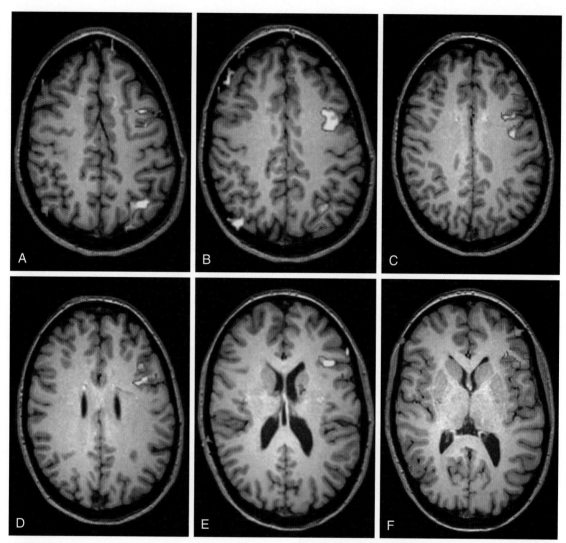

■ FIGURE 8-10 **Functional magnetic resonance imaging.** Right-handed child with chronic seizures and right frontal cortical dysplasia (not shown). Preoperative evaluation for hemispheric language dominance—verb generation task. **A–F,** Areas of significant BOLD-related signal change (*orange-yellow areas*) during silent verb production are noted to be predominately left sided, including left inferior frontal, consistent with left hemispheric language dominance.

(Fig. 8-11B). Hemorrhage may extend into the ventricular system and lead to hydrocephalus. Germinal matrix hemorrhage is categorized into one of four grades (Table 8-2). Intraparenchymal hemorrhage (grade IV) is secondary to venous infarction of the deep medullary veins (Fig. 8-15A and B and Fig. 8-16) rather than a direct extension of hemorrhage. Grades I and II hemorrhages tend to have good prognosis. In contrast, grades III and IV hemorrhages tend to have poor prognosis, including high incidences of neurologic impairment, hydrocephalus, and death.

Benign Enlargement of Extraaxial Spaces

Benign enlargement of extraaxial spaces (benign macrocrania) is a diagnosis of exclusion. The term refers to children with large heads (head circumference greater than 97% for age), prominent subarachnoid spaces, and normal development. Typically, such children present between 6 months and 2 years of age. After 2 years of age, the head size usually normalizes, and the children have no long-term consequences. The parents of such children often have

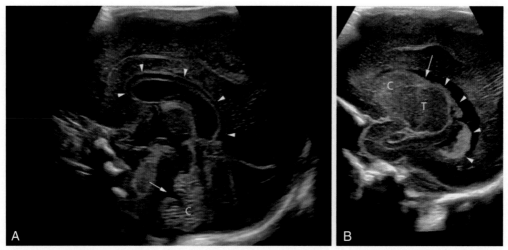

■ FIGURE 8-11 **Normal findings in a premature neonate on sagittal ultrasound of the head. A,** Midline sagittal view demonstrates normal midline structures, including corpus callosum (*arrowheads*), cerebellar vermis (*C*), and fourth ventricle (*arrow*). Note the normally increased echogenicity of cerebellar vermis. **B,** Off-midline sagittal view demonstrates normal caudothalamic groove (*arrow*), between the caudate nucleus (*C*) and thalamus (*T*). Note choroid plexus (*arrowheads*).

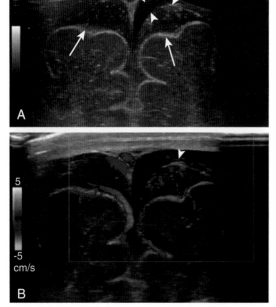

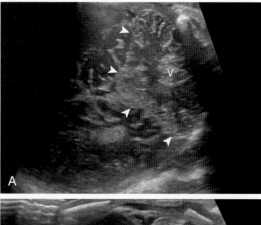

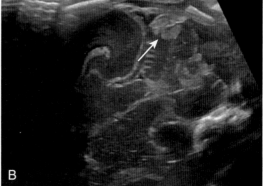

■ FIGURE 8-12 **Ultrasound of the extraaxial spaces. A,** Ultrasound via the anterior fontanel using high-resolution transducer demonstrates the subarachnoid spaces bilaterally (between *arrows*). Small subdural collection is seen on the left (between *arrowheads*). **B,** Doppler interrogation shows normal abundant vasculature within subarachnoid spaces. Note that a few bridging veins can be seen within a pathological subdural collection (*arrowhead*).

■ FIGURE 8-13 **Ultrasound of the posterior fossa via mastoid window in two different patients.** Note that images are oriented with patient anterior to left and posterior to right. **A,** Normal cerebellar hemispheres (*arrowheads*) and cerebellar vermis (*V*). **B,** Different patient showing focal area of hemorrhage along the lateral inferior aspect of the right cerebellar hemisphere (*arrow*) compatible with cerebellar hemorrhage, depicted only with mastoid window views.

large heads or had large heads as infants. On imaging, there is a prominent size of subarachnoid spaces and normal to borderline prominent ventricular system (Fig. 8-17A–C). Imaging is

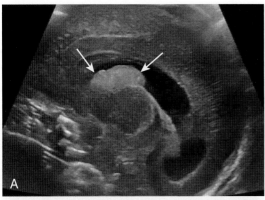

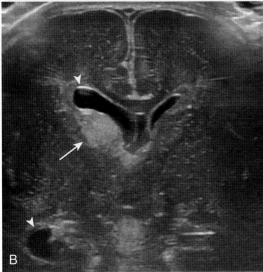

■ **FIGURE 8-14 Grade III germinal matrix hemorrhage. A,** Off-midline sagittal ultrasound demonstrates echogenic mass (*arrows*) in the caudothalamic groove, compatible with germinal matrix hemorrhage. **B,** Coronal view again demonstrates germinal matrix hemorrhage within the right caudothalamic grove (*arrow*) with associated enlargement of right lateral ventricle (*arrowheads*) compatible with grade III hemorrhage. Note the smooth-appearing brain with markedly diminished sulcation, consistent with prematurity.

TABLE 8-2 Grades of Germinal Matrix Hemorrhage	
Grade	**Morphologic Findings**
I	Hemorrhage confined to germinal matrix
II	Intraventricular hemorrhage without ventricular dilatation
III	Intraventricular hemorrhage with ventricular dilatation
IV	Intraparenchymal hemorrhage

otherwise normal. Clinical follow-up is necessary to exclude loss of milestones or continued increase in head circumference that may indicate communicating hydrocephalus.

■ NORMAL MYELINATION

Significant changes in brain myelination occur during the first 24 months of life. Before myelination, white matter is hydrophilic and, because it contains water, appears high in signal on T2-weighted images and low in signal on T1-weighted images (Figs. 8-18A and B and 8-19). With myelination, the white matter becomes hydrophobic and, because it contains less water, appears low in signal on T2-weighted images and high in signal on T1-weighted images (Fig. 8-18C and D). Myelination starts in utero and progresses from caudal to cranial, central to peripheral, and dorsal to ventral, paralleling neurologic development. In myelinating white matter, T1 shortening precedes T2 shortening. Therefore, T1-weighted sequence is the preferred sequence for the evaluation of normal myelination from birth until 6 months of age, whereas T2-weighted sequence is more frequently used after 6 months, especially after 1 year of age. Myelination in a term infant on T1-weighted sequence is seen along the vermis, dentate nucleus, dorsal brainstem, cerebellar peduncles, globus pallidi, ventrolateral thalami, posterior aspect of the posterior limb of internal capsule (PLIC), central corona radiata, perirolandic regions, and optic tracts (Fig. 8-20A–D). During the first 3 months of life, there is progressive myelination of the spinal cord and brainstem, followed by myelination of the cerebellar white matter. The corpus callosum begins to myelinate in the splenium (posterior part) at 2–3 months of age, proceeds anteriorly, and is completely myelinated through the rostrum (anterior part) by 6–8 months of age. Table 8-3 summarizes the expected myelination milestones in T1 and T2 sequences, with key milestones highlighted in bold. Myelination becomes similar to adult patterns on T2-weighted sequence by 24–36 months of age, with the exception of few terminal zones. Terminal zones of myelination can be seen in the frontotemporal subcortical white matter until the age of 36–40 months, whereas the commonly identified posterior periventricular terminal zones of myelination can be seen as late as teenage years (Fig. 8-21A and B).

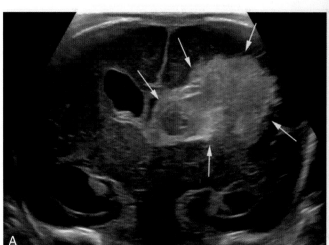

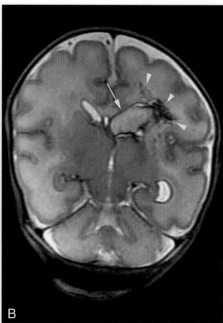

■ FIGURE 8-15 **Left grade IV germinal matrix hemorrhage. A,** On coronal ultrasound, there is a large echogenic area of hemorrhage (*arrows*) occupying the left lateral ventricle and adjacent brain parenchyma. **B,** Coronal T2-weighted sequence of the same patient's MRI a few weeks later demonstrating evolving blood products within the lateral ventricle (*arrow*) and adjacent brain parenchyma (*arrowheads*) in the distribution of the deep medullary veins.

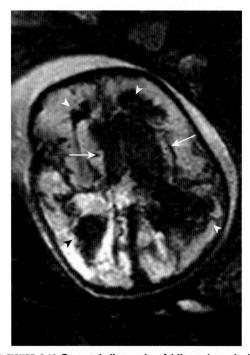

■ FIGURE 8-16 **Prenatal diagnosis of bilateral grade IV hemorrhage on fetal MRI.** Echo planar imaging (EPI) sequence demonstrates susceptibility artifact compatible with blood within the enlarged lateral ventricles (*arrows*) and at the periventricular white matter in the expected location of the deep medullary veins (*arrowheads*).

Assessing myelination has become a key component in the evaluation of children with developmental delay. Abnormal myelination is a nonspecific finding and can be secondary to a number of causes, including metabolic disease, infection, trauma, hypoxia–ischemia, and genetic or malformative syndromes.

White Matter Injury of Prematurity and Hypoxic Ischemic Insult

Perinatal partial asphyxia in premature neonates can result in damage to the periventricular white matter, the watershed zone of the premature infant, and result in white matter injury of prematurity (periventricular leukomalacia). It most commonly affects the white matter adjacent to the atria, frontal horns, and corona radiata along the lateral ventricles (Fig. 8-22). On ultrasound, increased heterogeneous echogenicity is seen within the periventricular white matter (Fig. 8-23A and B). It is associated with neurologic sequelae, such as movement disorders, seizures, and spasticity. In severe cases, there may be cystic necrosis and development of periventricular cysts during the subacute and chronic phases (Fig. 8-24). With time, there is often volume loss of the involved white matter (Fig. 8-25A and B). Doppler interrogation of the circle of Willis may add value in the evaluation of acute ischemia and

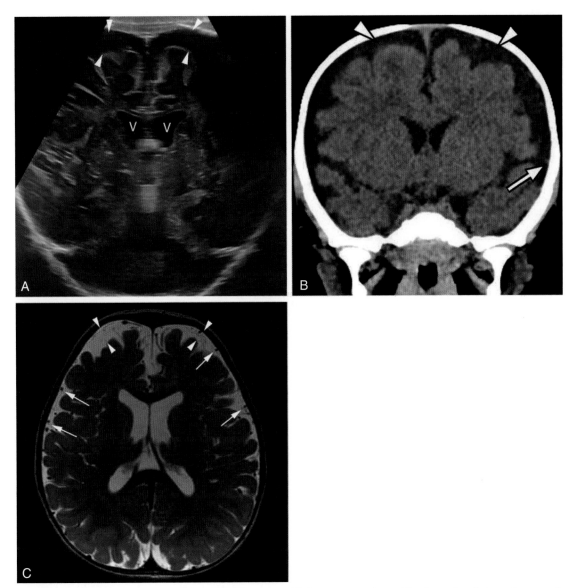

■ FIGURE 8-17 **Benign enlargement of extraaxial spaces of infancy presenting with a large head circumference. A,** Image from coronal ultrasound shows prominent subarachnoid spaces (*arrowheads*) and borderline prominence of the lateral ventricles (*V*). **B,** Coronal reformat from CT study and **C,** Axial T2-weighted sequence from MRI also showing bilateral symmetric enlargement of subarachnoid spaces (*arrowheads*). Note the peripherally located cortical vessel away from the brain parenchyma (*arrow*), helping in the differentiation from chronic subdural collections, which are known to cause medial (toward the brain) displacement of these vessels.

increase intracranial pressure. Premature and full-term infants exhibit a generally accepted resistive index range of approximately 0.6−0.9, in the absence of cardiac disease or peripheral vascular disease. Lower values may indicate acute hypoxia or ischemia, as a result of increased diastolic flow through cerebral vasodilation. Higher values may suggest cerebral swelling where intracranial pressures rise higher than

systemic pressures, leading to decreased diastolic flow.

Partial asphyxia in term neonates and older children will affect the border zones (watershed zones) between the anterior and middle and/or middle and posterior circulations (see Fig. 8-31A and B).

Profound prolonged asphyxia affects the most metabolic active areas of the brain, especially the

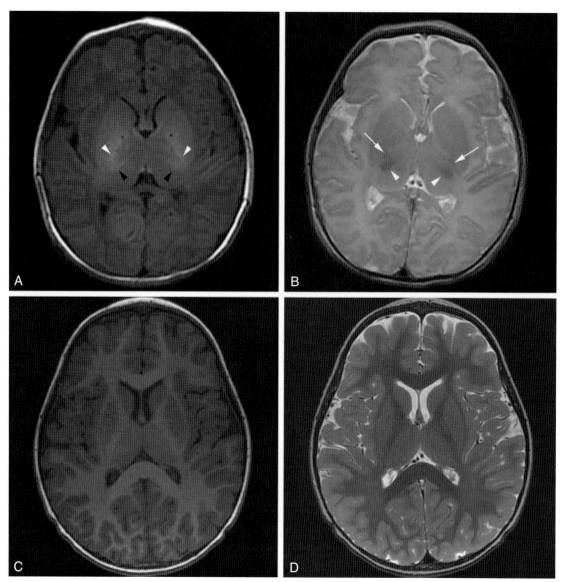

■ FIGURE 8-18 **Normal brain magnetic resonance imaging at term and 24 Months.** Axial T1- (**A**) and axial T2-weighted (**B**) sequences of a term neonate demonstrating normal low T1 signal and high T2 signal of unmyelinated white matter. **A,** Normal myelination of the posterior aspect of the PLIC (*white arrowheads*), ventrolateral thalami (*black arrowheads*), and globus pallidi (*) seen as T1 hyperintense signal. **B,** T2 hypointense signal within the myelinated PLIC (*arrows*) and ventrolateral thalami (*white arrowheads*). Axial T1- (**C**) and axial T2-weighted (**D**) sequences of a 24-month-old child demonstrating normal myelination characterized by increased T1 and decrease T2 white matter signal compared with neonatal MRI.

basal ganglia and perirolandic regions, in both preterm and term neonates. Findings on MRI include symmetric increase T1 and T2 signal, especially along the posterior lentiform nuclei (putamen and globus pallidi) and the ventrolateral thalami. Diffusion restriction is often present if the patient is imaged after 24 h and prior to 10–14 days after the insult. In term neonates (above 36 weeks of gestation), another early

finding of profound hypoxic ischemic insult includes absent visualization of the T1 hyperintense signal of the myelinated posterior limb of the internal capsule (Fig. 8-26A and B). The recent use of hypothermia to treat neonates with hypoxic ischemic insult has led to a decreased number of positive MRI cases and, when positive, the resultant imaging findings may be delayed. A mixed pattern involving both the basal

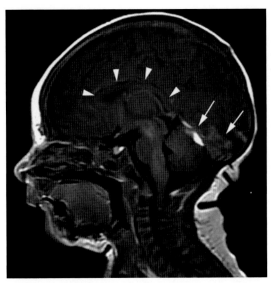

■ FIGURE 8-19 **Normal neonate.** Sagittal T1-weighted sequence shows low signal and mild thinning of the corpus callosum, normal in the neonatal period due to lack of myelination (*white arrowheads*). The pituitary gland demonstrates increased T1 signal throughout (*black arrowhead*), normal in neonates. Note small amount of hemorrhage along the tentorium near the straight sinus and posterior occipital convexity (*arrows*). This is a common and clinically not significant finding related to recent delivery.

ganglia and white matter can also be present. Head ultrasound may identify early signs of hypoxic ischemic insult, such as accentuated gray–white matter differentiation, slit-like ventricles secondary to edema, and blurring of interhemispheric fissure (Fig. 8-27). Chronic changes of profound hypoxic ischemic insult include signal abnormality and volume loss of the posterior lentiform nuclei and ventrolateral thalami (Fig. 8-28) with or without associated white matter volume loss.

Imaging mimickers of hypoxic ischemic insult in encephalopathic neonates include neonatal hypoglycemia and metabolic diseases such as molybdenum cofactor deficiency (Fig. 8-29A and B), pyruvate dehydrogenase deficiency, nonketotic hyperglycinemia (will have elevated glycine peak 3.55 ppm), urea cycle disorders, and aminoacidurias. Neonatal hypoglycemia presents with diffusion restriction along the posterior parieto-occipital regions and can be confirmed clinically with glucose levels (Fig. 8-29A). Metabolic diseases mimicking hypoxic ischemic insult tend to present after a week or more of life, different from perinatal hypoxic ischemic insult, which usually presents during the first 24 h of life.

■ NEURODEVELOPMENTAL ABNORMALITIES

Neurodevelopmental abnormalities are the result of in utero disruption in central nervous system (CNS) formation. Causes include genetic, environmental, infectious, vascular, or metabolic etiologies. Classification can be made based on the stage of developmental insult (Table 8-4) including abnormalities of dorsal induction, ventral induction, and cortical development. Malformations of cortical development (MCDs) can be categorized as disorders of cell proliferation and apoptosis; cell migration; and postmigrational neuronal development. The type of developmental lesion often reflects the timing of the in utero disturbance. Multiple distinct developmental abnormalities may be present simultaneously.

Neurodevelopmental abnormalities can also result from destruction of already formed structures (encephaloclastic insult). Most commonly they are related to a vascular injury that can be the result of a number of underlying causes. The most commonly encountered sequelae of encephaloclastic insults are porencephaly, encephalomalacia, and hydranencephaly. Encephaloclastic insults can also result in MCDs such as schizencephaly and polymicrogyria if occurred during the late migration/postmigration phases of brain development.

Porencephaly and Encephalomalacia

Before the end of the second trimester, parenchymal injury does not result in glial scar formation. During this early time period, focal injury results in the development of a fluid-filled space called a *porencephalic cyst*. On imaging, this appears as a thin-walled, CSF-containing cyst that may communicate with the ventricles (Fig. 8-30). During the third trimester and neonatal period, parenchymal injury incites some glial scar formation, resulting in softening of the brain parenchyma (encephalomalacia) and tissue loss with or without reactive gliosis. Encephalomalacia appears as areas of high T2-weighted signal frequently with associated septations in the region of injury (Fig. 8-31A and B).

Hydranencephaly

Hydranencephaly is the result of significant injury to the majority of the cerebral hemispheres secondary to an in utero destructive process. The cause is thought to be vascular in origin with involvement of both internal carotid

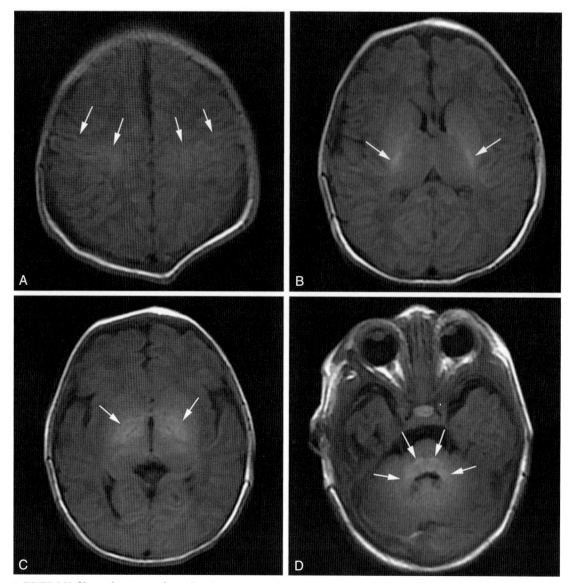

■ FIGURE 8-20 **Normal pattern of myelination at term.** From superior to inferior, axial T1-weighted images of the brain parenchyma in a normal term neonate. Increased T1 signal compatible with myelinated white matter (*arrows*) is seen along the perirolandic regions and central corona radiata (**A**), posterior limb of internal capsules (**B**), inferior globus pallidi and subthalamic nucleus (**C**), posterior brainstem, and cerebellar peduncles (**D**). See Table 8-3 for detailed list of myelinated structures at term and myelination milestones.

arteries. Infectious vasculitis has been identified as a potential cause. The supratentorial compartment is almost entirely filled with CSF. A few areas of preserved parenchyma may be seen along the convexities and thalami (Fig. 8-32A–C). The brainstem is usually hypoplastic due to decreased descending white matter tracts, and the cerebellum is typically intact. These structures remain because they are supplied by the vertebrobasilar arterial system. The presence of the falx cerebri and the separation of the thalami seen in hydranencephaly (see Fig. 8-32B) help to differentiate this

disorder from severe (alobar) holoprosencephaly. It is sometimes very difficult and impossible to differentiate hydranencephaly from severe hydrocephalus (Fig. 8-33).

Chiari

CHIARI TYPE 1

Chiari type 1 is the presence of an abnormal inferior location of the cerebellar tonsils, at least 5 mm below the foramen magnum (Fig. 8-34). The cerebellar tonsils are typically elongated in morphology rather than round, and there are

✳ **TABLE 8-3** Myelination Milestones		
Age	**T1 High Signal**	**T2 Low Signal**
Term	**Rolandic or perirolandic gyri** (up to 2 mo) **Central CR** **PLIC** **Globus pallidi** **Lateral thalamus** **Optic radiations** **Dorsal brainstem** **Cerebellar peduncles** **Dentate nucleus** **Vermis**	Central CR Posterior $^1/_3$ of PLIC Dorsal pons Vermis
By 3–4 mo	**Splenium of corpus callosum** Cerebellar white matter **ALIC** Anterior pons Hippocampus Central occipital white matter	$^1/_2$ PLIC Optic radiations Middle cerebellar peduncle Dentate nucleus
By 6 mo	**Genu of corpus callosum** Deep frontal white matter	**Splenium of corpus callosum** **Entire PLIC** Cerebellar white matter Anterior pons
By 8 mo	Near adult, except for most peripheral temporal and frontal subcortical branches	**Genu of corpus callosum** **ALIC (at least partially)** Increasing myelination of CR
By 12 mo	Temporal white matter	CR ALIC Deep occipital white matter
By 14–18 mo	Subcortical U-fibers	Deep frontal white matter Branching occipital white matter
18–24 mo	Fully myelinated	Near adult, except for most peripheral temporal and frontal subcortical branches
24–36 mo		Fully myelinated

ALIC, Anterior limb of internal capsule; *CR*, corona radiata; *PLIC*, posterior limb of internal capsule.

different degrees of CSF effacement at the craniocervical junction. The medulla and fourth ventricle are commonly in normal positions although low position of the cervicomedullary junction may be seen in cases of complex Chiari 1 (also known as Chiari 1.5) which are often associated with a posteriorly tilted dens of C2 and sometimes with a hypoplastic clivus and basilar invagination. Complications of Chiari type 1 include hydrocephalus and hydromyelia (see Fig. 8-34). It may be suspected on CT when the foramen magnum appears "full" with soft tissue (Fig. 8-35). It is best visualized on sagittal MR images. Phase-contrast CSF flow MR sequence may be used to show CSF space effacement and pistoning movement of the cerebellar tonsils. Chiari 1 may be acquired with increase intracranial pressure and may also resolve with child growth, therefore not always a true malformation.

CHIARI TYPE 2

Chiari type 2 is a true malformation of hindbrain and is almost always associated with spinal myelomeningoceles. Conversely, almost all patients with myelomeningoceles have Chiari type 2 malformation. Patients with this abnormality have small posterior fossa and associated inferior displacement of the cerebellum, medulla, and fourth ventricle into the upper cervical canal (Fig. 8-36). Associated imaging findings include a kinked appearance of the medulla, colpocephaly (disproportionate enlargement of the occipital horns of the lateral ventricles), fenestration of the falx associated with interdigitating gyri across the midline, enlargement of the massa intermedia, inferior pointing of the lateral ventricles, and tectal beaking (a pointed appearance of the quadrigeminal plate). Chiari type 2

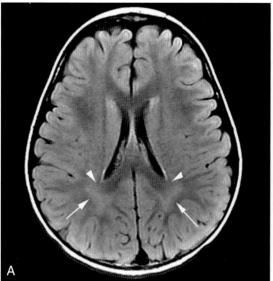
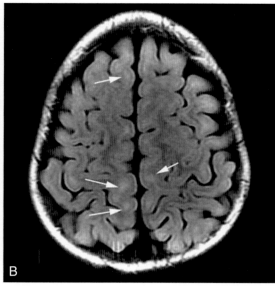

■ FIGURE 8-21 **Terminal zones of myelination in a normal 40-month-old child. A,** Axial T2 FLAIR sequence shows focal increased FLAIR signal within the bilateral posterior periventricular white matter compatible with terminal zones of myelination (*arrows*). Note the thin band of normal myelinated white matter between the terminal zones and the lateral ventricles (*arrowheads*). This helps in the differentiation from periventricular gliosis seen in white matter injury of prematurity. **B,** Axial T2 FLAIR sequence shows hyperintense T2 signal within the high fronto-parietal subcortical white matter (*arrows*) compatible with terminal zones of myelination. This can also be seen along the anterior temporal lobes (not shown).

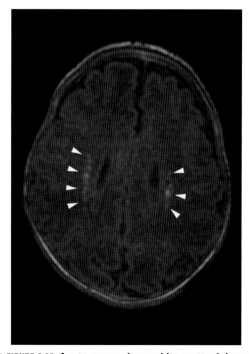

■ FIGURE 8-22 **Acute, noncavitary white matter injury of prematurity.** Axial T1-weighted sequence demonstrates multiple punctate foci of increased T1 signal within the periventricular white matter bilaterally (*arrowheads*). This is compatible with early changes of white matter injury of prematurity and is often not depicted by ultrasound. DWI may demonstrate corresponding foci of restricted diffusion (not seen in this case).

malformations are usually associated with hydrocephalus, often diagnosed prenatally (Fig. 8-37A and B).

Prenatal correction of myelomeningocele can be performed in a subset of fetuses, following specific inclusion criteria. The aim is to decrease the degree of hindbrain herniation and the postnatal need of ventricular shunting, as well as to improve lower extremity function (Fig. 8-38A and B).

Chiari type 3 is very rare and includes an occipital encephalocele or upper cervical dysraphism instead of a lower spinal myelomeningocele.

Holoprosencephaly

Holoprosencephaly results from lack of complete cleavage of the brain into two hemispheres. Although there is a continuous spectrum of severity, holoprosencephaly is classically classified into one of three distinct groups: alobar, semilobar, or lobar. The severity of the brain abnormality is usually reflected in the severity of the associated midline facial abnormality.

Alobar holoprosencephaly (Fig. 8-39A and B) is the most severe form and is characterized by a monoventricle. The thalami are fused and there is no attempt at cleavage of the cerebral hemispheres. There is no falx cerebri or corpus callosum. There is a single anterior cerebral artery

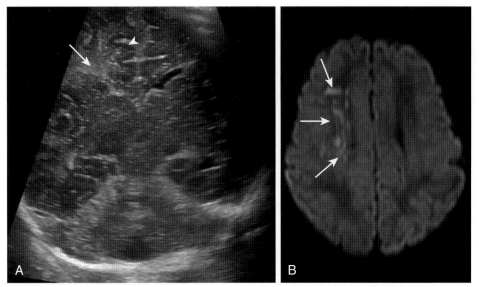

■ **FIGURE 8-23 Ischemic Insult by Ultrasound. A,** Coronal ultrasound demonstrating increased right periventricular white matter echogenicity (*arrow*) and accentuated gray–white matter differentiation (*arrowhead*). There is also decreased size of ipsilateral lateral ventricle due to edema. **B,** Diffusion-weighted sequence MRI confirmed area of diffusion restriction (*arrows*).

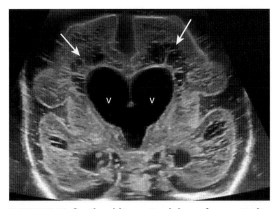

■ **FIGURE 8-24 Cystic white matter injury of prematurity.** Coronal ultrasound shows heterogeneous echogenicity in the frontal periventricular white matter with multiple cystic changes compatible with cavitary evolution of white matter injury of prematurity (*arrows*). There are similar lesions in the temporal lobes. There is associated enlargement of ventricular system (*V*). Note the markedly diminished sulcation consistent with prematurity.

(azygous artery). These infants are commonly stillborn or have a very short life span.

With the intermediate form, semilobar holoprosencephaly (Fig. 8-40A and B), the cerebral hemispheres are partially cleaved from each other posteriorly. The temporal horns of the lateral ventricles may be formed, but there is a single ventricle anteriorly. There is at least partial separation of the thalami. Midline structures, such as the falx and corpus callosum, may be present posteriorly but not anteriorly.

Lobar holoprosencephaly is a milder form in which the occipital and temporal horns are well formed, but there is failure of cleavage of the frontal lobes. The septum pellucidum is absent, and the corpus callosum may be absent or dysplastic.

A less severe form of holoprosencephaly is syntelencephaly or middle interhemispheric variant, and may be seen as fusion only of the midline posterior frontal lobes and/or parietal lobes (Fig. 8-41). Different degrees of septum pellucidum and corpus callosum agenesis/dysgenesis can be present.

Another milder form of lobar holoprosencephaly is septopreoptic holoprosencephaly. In this variant, the midline fusion is limited to the septal and preoptic regions. The fornices are commonly thick or fused and the anterior commissure may be hypoplastic or absent.

Septo-optic Dysplasia

Septo-optic dysplasia is another type of ventral induction malformation, analogous to mild holoprosencephaly. It was originally described as

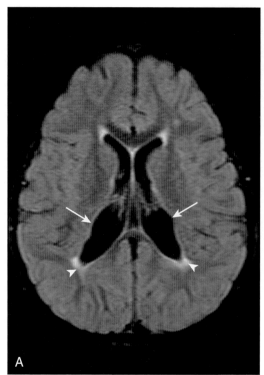

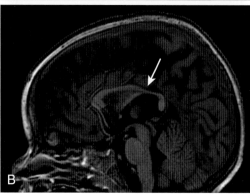

■ **FIGURE 8-25 Chronic changes of white matter injury of prematurity. A,** Axial FLAIR image demonstrates periventricular white matter volume loss with mildly enlarged and dysmorphic lateral ventricles (*arrows*). There is also mildly increased periventricular white matter signal adjacent to the lateral ventricles, compatible with gliosis (*arrowheads*). **B,** Sagittal T1-weighted sequence shows mild thinning of the corpus callosum, especially at its posterior body (*arrow*), as a result of white matter volume loss.

absence of the septum pellucidum and hypoplasia of the optic nerves (diagnosed most often by ophthalmological evaluation) (Fig. 8-42A and B). It was later discovered that there are often associated pituitary abnormalities and

dysfunction (in approximately two thirds of patients). Currently, several authors believe that a combination of any two of the three findings is part of the disease spectrum. Pituitary abnormalities may include absent visualization of T1 bright posterior pituitary gland, ectopic posterior pituitary gland (Fig. 8-43), interrupted or hypoplastic pituitary stalk, or hormonal abnormalities with no obvious imaging finding. Septo-optic dysplasia may also present with schizencephaly, heterotopia, and incomplete hippocampi inversion. In septo-optic dysplasia, the frontal horns of the lateral ventricles have a squared appearance on coronal MR images. The septum pellucidum may also be completely or partially absent in cases of congenital hydrocephalus due to increase ventricular pressure (see Figs. 8-53A and 8-121A), an important differential diagnosis, as not all cases of absent septum pellucidum are related to septo-optic dysplasia.

Dysgenesis of Corpus Callosum

Dysgenesis of the corpus callosum includes complete absence (agenesis), partial absence, and changes in morphology and size. The corpus callosum is the largest brain commissure (white matter tract connecting the left and right cerebral hemispheres). It normally develops from two independent portions, anterior and posterior, and the anterior corpus callosum enlarges and becomes visible earlier. When a portion of the corpus callosum is absent or dysgenic, it is most commonly the posterior portion that is absent, although this is not always true (Fig. 8-44A–D). Absence of the corpus callosum can occur in isolation or in conjunction with many of the other developmental (Fig. 8-45A–D) and genetic abnormalities. On coronal MR images, the lateral ventricles are separated, and the third ventricle extends more superiorly than normal, positioned between the lateral ventricles. The white matter tracts, which normally would cross the midline via the corpus callosum, run along the medial surface of the lateral ventricles and form the bundles of Probst (see Fig. 8-44C). Lateral ventricles assume a parallel configuration on axial views, and colpocephaly (see Fig. 8-44B) is often present (dilatation of atrium and occipital horns of the lateral ventricles). Midline masses, such as lipomas and interhemipheric cysts (see Figs. 8-44B and 8-45A and B), can also be associated.

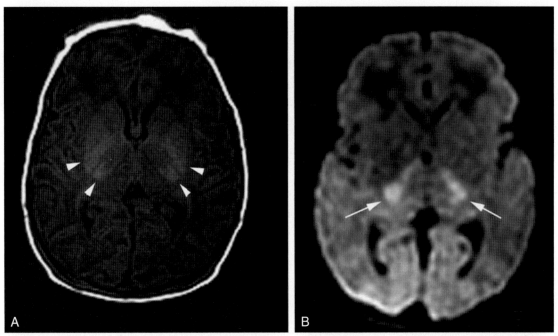

■ **FIGURE 8-26 Acute findings of profound hypoxic ischemic insult. A,** Axial T1-weighted sequence of a term neonate demonstrates absence of the T1 hyperintense PLIC signal and increased signal within the ventrolateral thalami and posterior lentiform nucleus (*arrowheads*). **B,** Axial DWI demonstrating diffusion restriction within the ventrolateral thalami and PLIC.

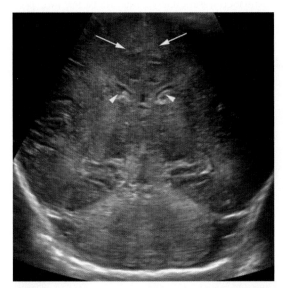

■ **FIGURE 8-27 Ultrasound findings of hypoxic ischemic insult.** Coronal head ultrasound of a neonate with history of hypoxic ischemic insult demonstrates small size of the lateral ventricles (*arrowheads*) due to parenchymal edema and blurring of the gray–white matter differentiation (*arrows*).

Posterior Fossa Anomalies with Enlarged Cerebrospinal Fluid Spaces

Causes of enlarged posterior fossa fluid spaces include a spectrum of etiologies that vary from normal developmental variants (mega cisterna magna) to more significant malformations. They can be divided into five major groups: Dandy–Walker malformation, cerebellar vermian hypoplasia, Blake pouch cyst, mega cisterna magna, and arachnoid cyst.

Dandy–Walker malformation is characterized by complete or partial agenesis of the cerebellar vermis in conjunction with the presence of a large posterior fossa. The CSF spaces are enlarged, and the torcula is elevated (Fig. 8-46). The falx cerebelli is absent. Often there are also supratentorial abnormalities that may include holoprosencephaly, agenesis of the corpus callosum, polymicrogyria, and heterotopias. Hydrocephalus is also not uncommon. The patient outcome depends on severity of vermian hypoplasia and associated supratentorial abnormalities.

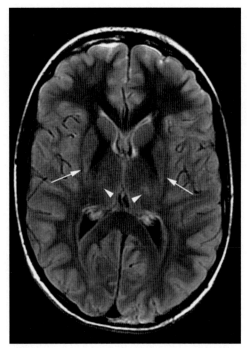

■ FIGURE 8-28 **Chronic findings of profound hypoxic ischemic insult.** Axial FLAIR sequence demonstrating volume loss and increased signal within the ventrolateral thalami (*arrowheads*) and the posterior lentiform nucleus (*arrows*).

Cerebellar vermian hypoplasia (formerly known as Dandy–Walker variant or continuum) is characterized by mild, moderate, or severe hypoplasia of the cerebellar vermis. As a result, there is enlargement of the normal communication between the fourth ventricle and posterior fossa extra axial spaces. The overall size of the posterior fossa is not enlarged, and there is a normally positioned torcula Fig. 8-47.

Blake pouch cyst is more commonly seen in the prenatal scenario, when fetal MRI is performed to evaluate for Dandy–Walker malformation versus vermian hypoplasia. Blake pouch is a normal embryological CSF-filled structure. It is seen during the development of the posterior fossa as a CSF outpouching that extends posteriorly from the inferior aspect of the developing fourth ventricle. When there is absent, incomplete, or late fenestration of this pouch (future foramens of Luschka and Magendie), a persistent cystic structure causing enlarged communications of the fourth ventricle and retrocerebellar extraaxial spaces is seen and referred to as Blake pouch cyst. The cerebellar vermis is usually uplifted but normally formed.

When enlarged posterior fossa CSF spaces are present with a fully developed and normally positioned cerebellar vermis, there are two possibilities. If the CSF spaces exhibit no mass effect

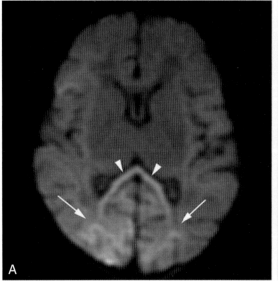
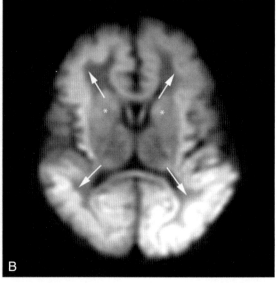

■ FIGURE 8-29 **Mimickers of neonatal hypoxic ischemic Insult. A, Neonatal Hypoglycemia.** Encephalopathic term neonate during the first 24 h of life. Axial DWI sequence demonstrating diffusion restriction within the posterior parieto-occipital lobes (*arrows*) and splenium of the corpus callosum (*arrowheads*) in a term neonate with history of hypoglycemia. This distribution of parenchymal injury could be seen in partial asphyxia; however, it is also characteristic for neonatal hypoglycemia, and resolution with normal glucose levels is key for the correct diagnosis. **B, Molybdenum Cofactor Deficiency.** Term neonate with history of seizures 10 days after delivery. Axial DWI sequence demonstrating diffuse subcortical white matter diffusion restriction (*arrows*) and mild involvement of the basal ganglia (***), a finding that can be seen in hypoxic ischemic insult or metabolic diseases. The clinical presentation 10 days after delivery is the most important clue raising the suspicion for a metabolic disease in this case.

	Mechanism		
Abnormality	**(Abnormality of)**	**Description**	**Imaging Findings**
Chiari type 2	Dorsal induction and complex hindbrain malformation	Small posterior fossa with inferior displacement of cerebellum, fourth ventricle, and brainstem into cervical canal; associated with myelomeningocele	Colpocephaly Fenestrated falx Large massa intermedia Tectal beaking Cervicomedullary kink Hydrocephalus
Holoprosencephaly	Ventral induction	Failure in cleavage of brain into two cerebral hemispheres	Alobar type: Single ventricle Fused thalami Absent corpus callosum and falx
Dandy–Walker malformation	Defect in rhombencephalon formation and/or abnormal fenestration of foramens of Magendie and Luschka	Complete or partial agenesis of the cerebellar vermis in conjunction with an enlarged retrocerebellar CSF spaces and/or cyst	Posterior fossa is enlarged (elevated torcula) May be an isolated posterior fossa anomaly or present with multiple associated supratentorial abnormalities
Molar tooth malformation	Neuronal progenitor cell Ciliary dysfunction (ciliopathy)	Absent decussation of superior cerebellar peduncles giving the appearance of a molar tooth on axial plane	Deep interpeduncular fossa and marked vermian hypoplasia May have associated encephalocele, kidney, eye, and limb abnormalities Clinical presentation with cognitive deficits and intellectual disabilities
Rhombencephalosynapsis	Defect in rhombencephalon formation of unknown etiology	Complete or partial cerebellar vermian agenesis with fusion of the cerebellar hemispheres	Fusion of cerebellar hemispheres with midline continuation of cerebellar folia Posterior convex margins of the cerebellum on axial plane Absent primary fissure and rounded fastigial point on sagittal plane. Common association with congenital hydrocephalus due to aqueduct stenosis
Microlissencephaly	Neuronal proliferation and cell apoptosis	Arrest neuronal proliferation resulting in decreased number of neurons	Microcephaly and simplified pattern of gyration
Megalencephaly	Neuronal proliferation and cell apoptosis	Increase neuronal proliferation arrests apoptosis resulting in overgrow of cerebral parenchyma	Enlarged and dysplastic cerebral hemisphere (hemimegaloencephaly) with enlarged ipsilateral ventricle Enlarged dysplastic bilateral cerebral hemispheres (dysplastic megalencephaly) Sporadic or part of megalencephaly syndromes Intractable epilepsy

TABLE 8-4 Common Developmental Abnormalities of the Brain

Continued

	TABLE 8-4			

Abnormality	Mechanism (Abnormality of)	Description	Imaging Findings
Gray matter heterotopia	Neuronal migration	Arrested migration of neurons, resulting in heterotopic areas of gray matter within the subependymal regions or white matter	Sporadic or part of megalencephaly syndromes Intractable epilepsy Nodular or laminar appearance Isointense to gray matter Other migration abnormalities, hippocampal, and callosal anomalies may be seen
Lissencephaly	Neuronal migration	Arrest neuronal migration causing failure of development of gyri and sulci	Smooth cortical surface ("Figure eight" appearance of the brain) Cortical thickening Other migration abnormalities are common Part of many genetic disorders
Cobblestone malformation	Neuronal migration	Overmigration of neurons with lack of normal laminar organization of the cortex	Smooth external cortical surface Pebbled appearance of the cortex Hypoplastic and kinked brainstem Often associated with aqueductal stenosis, eye abnormalities, and congenital muscular dystrophies
Cortical dysplasia	Neuronal proliferation (FCD type II and glioneuronal tumors) postmigration (FCD type I and III)	Abnormality of neuronal proliferation and/or postmigration leading to dysplastic cortex	Imaging commonly normal Type II FCD may show focal cortical thickening, blurring of gray–white matter, and triangular-shaped white matter signal changes May have associated glioneuronal tumor (dual pathology)
Polymicrogyria	Late migration/ postmigration	Cortex showing multiple small gyri and sulci	Predilection to perisylvian region Small gyri may appear fused, given appearance similar to pachygyria Encephaloclastic or genetic syndromes
Schizencephaly	Postmigration	Gray matter–lined cleft extending from lateral ventricle to cerebral surface	Absent septum pellucidum—common Other migration abnormalities, hippocampal, and callosal anomalies may be seen Results from encephaloclastic insult

TABLE 8-4

Abnormality	Mechanism (Abnormality of)	Description	Imaging Findings
Dysgenesis of the corpus callosum	Commissure formation	Complete or partial absence of the corpus callosum	Parallel lateral ventricles Bundles of Probst Colpocephaly High-riding third ventricle
Vein of Galen malformation	Disorder of vascular differentiation	Arteriovenous fistula to embryonic precursor of the vein of Galen resulting in large posterior midline venous varix	May cause brain ischemia or infarct from "steal phenomenon" May present with hydrocephalus Congestive heart failure may be the first identified symptom
Hydranencephaly	Encephaloclastic	Destruction of the cerebrum secondary to insult affecting the bilateral internal carotid arteries	Cerebrum replaced by CSF Falx is present Thalami separated Normal or enlarged head circumference
Porencephaly	Encephaloclastic	Cyst formation from injury to brain parenchyma during first or second trimester	Thin-walled CSF cyst May communicate with lateral ventricle (no cortical lining) No septations

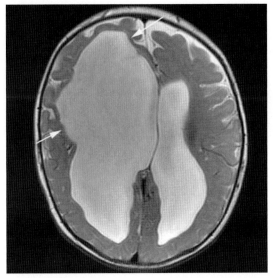

■ **FIGURE 8-30** Porencephalic cyst shown on axial T2-weighted MRI as a large CSF cyst (*arrows*) that is contiguous with the right lateral ventricle. The communication is not lined by gray matter.

on the cerebellum and the falx cerebelli is present, a mega cisterna magna is considered to be present. A mega cisterna magna may be in the spectrum of a persistent Blake's pouch cyst, as proposed by recent articles, and is considered a developmental variant. If the CSF spaces appear cystic and exhibit mass effect on the cerebellum, an arachnoid cyst is considered more likely (Fig. 8-48). The differentiation between a mega cisterna magna and an arachnoid cyst may be difficult. However, regardless of the name chosen, if there is minimal or no mass effect on the cerebellum, the finding is considered incidental and of no clinical significance.

Molar Tooth Malformation

Molar tooth malformation is the main intracranial imaging finding in patients with Joubert syndrome and related disorders. Joubert syndrome and related disorders are a group of genetic disorders resulting in dysfunction of the neuronal progenitor cells cilia (ciliopathy).

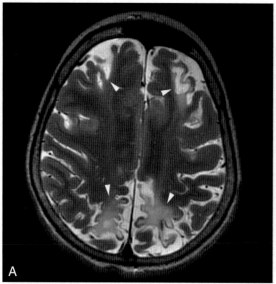
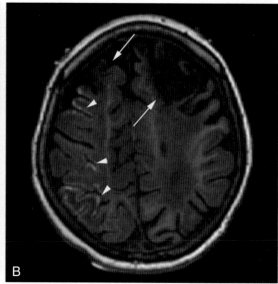

■ FIGURE 8-31 **Encephalomalacia. A,** Axial T2-weighted sequence shows bilateral frontal and parieto-occipital para-sagittal areas of increased T2 signal, with central areas of CSF signal, and focal volume loss compatible with encephalomalacia (*arrowheads*) in the border zones distribution. Findings are compatible with sequela of prior partial asphyxia. **B,** Axial T1-weighted sequence again demonstrating areas of encephalomalacia (*arrows*). Note also increase in T1 signal within cortical ribbon of involved parenchyma (*arrowheads*) compatible with mineralization seen as result of laminar necrosis.

Imaging findings include elongated horizontally oriented superior cerebellar peduncles and deep interpeduncular fossa resembling a molar tooth on axial imaging (Fig. 8-49A). Additionally, a marked hypoplastic cerebellar vermis is characteristic (Fig. 8-49B). This may be confused with Dandy–Walker malformation on prenatal ultrasound.

Rhombencephalosynapsis

Rhombencephalosynapsis is a malformation of the rhombencephalon with complete or partial absence of the cerebellar vermis and midline fusion of the cerebellar hemispheres (Fig. 8-50A and B). Additional imaging findings include a small transverse cerebellar diameter (see Fig.8-121C) and convex posterior cerebellar margins at the expected level of the vermis on axial plane as well as a rounded fastigial point and absent primary fissure on sagittal plane (see Fig. 8-45B). This malformation is frequently associated with aqueduct stenosis diagnosed prenatally (see Fig. 8-121B-C). Additional malformations/syndromes associated with rhombencephalosynapsis include VACTERL, holoprosencephaly, and Gomez–Lopez–Hernandez syndrome (rhombencephalosynapsis, focal alopecia, craniosynostosis, and trigeminal nerve abnormalities).

Microlissencephaly

Microlissencephaly is the result of an arrest in cell proliferation resulting in both microcephaly and a simplified pattern of gyration (Fig. 8-51).

Lissencephaly (Agyria-Pachygyria)

Lissencephaly is the result of migrational abnormality resulting in a smooth appearance of the brain secondary to absent sulcation and gyration (agyria) (Fig. 8-52) or markedly decreased sulcation and gyration (oligogyria). Pachygyria is another overlapping term defined as abnormally broad and flat gyri with shallow sulci. Findings are best visualized with MRI, usually with patchy areas of both agyria and oligogyria/pachygyria. These abnormalities are commonly associated with other migrational abnormalities. They also occur as part of a number of genetic syndromes. Two malformations often associated with agyria and pachygyria are classic lissencephaly and cobblestone malformations. Classic lissencephaly is due to arrest of neuronal migration and is formally known as lissencephaly type I. MRI demonstrates a smooth brain with a thickened cortex and a band of hyperintense T2 signal within the cortex (sparse cell zone). The brain may demonstrate the classic "Figure eight"

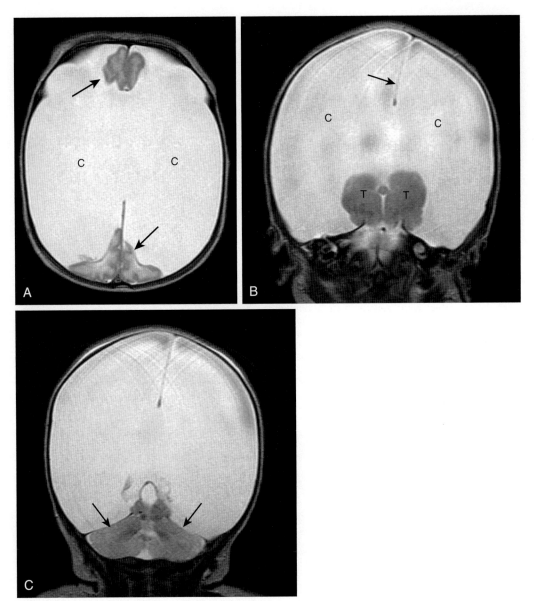

■ **FIGURE 8-32 Hydranencephaly A,** Axial T2-weighted sequence shows most of cerebrum replaced by CSF (*C*). Note only a small portion of preserved cerebral parenchyma along the anterior and posterior parasagittal regions (*arrows*). **B,** The thalami (*T*) are present bilaterally and are not fused. A falx cerebri (*arrow*) is present. **C,** Note normal cerebellar structures within the posterior fossa (*arrows*).

morphology (see Fig. 8.52). Cobblestone malformations are due to overmigration of neurons into the subarachnoid space via defects in the pial limitans membrane. These were formally known as cobblestone lissencephalies or lissencephalies type II. They are commonly associated with congenital muscular dystrophy. On imaging, there is markedly decreased sulcation with a pebbled appearance of the cortex (Fig. 8-53A). Other findings may include vermian hypoplasia,

cerebellar dysplasia (Fig. 8-53C), brainstem hypoplasia, kinked pontomesencephalic junction, pontine cleft, ocular anomalies, and aqueduct stenosis leading to ventriculomegaly (Fig. 8-53A and B).

Gray Matter Heterotopias

Heterotopias are abnormalities of neuronal migration characterized by arrest in radial

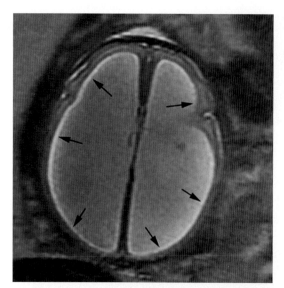

■ FIGURE 8-33 **Severe hydrocephalus.** Axial T2-weighted sequence of a fetus with severe hydrocephalus demonstrating the supratentorial compartment mostly filled by CSF and thinned brain parenchyma displaced laterally (*arrows*). The presence of a complete or near complete band of peripheral parenchyma helps to differentiate marked hydrocephalus from hydranencephaly. Note also the preserved falx helping in the differentiation from holoprosencephaly.

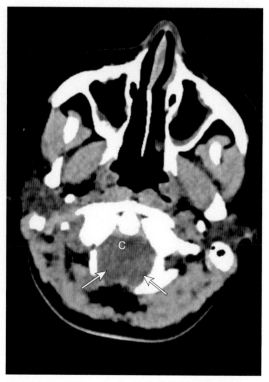

■ FIGURE 8-35 **Chiari 1.** Axial noncontrast CT at the level of the posterior arch of C1, just below the foramen magnum. There is tissue crowding composed of normal upper spinal cord (*C*) and low-lying cerebellar tonsils (*arrows*). Findings compatible with Chiari 1. This can be confirmed on sagittal reconstructions when equivocal on axial images.

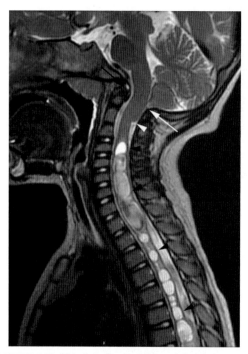

■ FIGURE 8-34 **Chiari 1.** Sagittal T2-weighted sequence showing low-lying, peg-shaped cerebellar tonsils (*white arrow*) and cervicomedullary junction (*white arrowhead*) causing crowding of CSF spaces at the craniocervical junction. There is also a posteriorly tilted C2 dens causing impression upon the anterior cervicomedullary junction (*black arrow*). Note associated extensive septated hydromyelia (*black arrowheads*) within the visualized spinal cord.

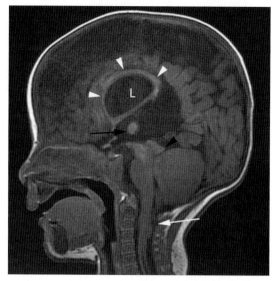

■ FIGURE 8-36 **Chiari 2 malformation.** Sagittal T1-weighted image shows downward displacement of cerebellar tonsils (*white arrow*). The posterior fossa is small, and the fourth ventricle is compressed. There is a prominent massa intermedia (*black arrow*) and beaked tectum (*black arrowhead*). Note enlargement of lateral ventricle (*L*) and consequent superiorly displaced and thinned corpus callosum (*arrowheads*).

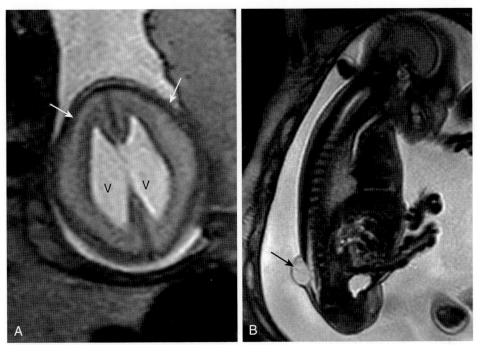

■ FIGURE 8-37 **Chiari 2 malformation on fetal magnetic resonance imaging. A,** Axial, single shot fast spin echo (SSFSE) sequence from fetal MRI of fetal head demonstrates bilateral enlargement of lateral ventricles (*V*) and bifrontal skull concavities compatible with classic lemon head sign (*arrows*). **B,** Sagittal SSFSE sequence of the spine shows lumbosacral myelomeningocele sac (*black arrow*). Note thin band of low T2 signal within myelomeningocele sac, representing neuroelements.

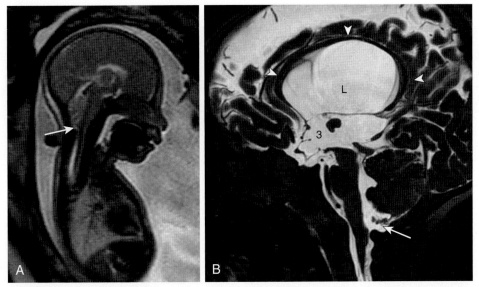

■ FIGURE 8-38 **Chiari 2 myelomeningocele repair in utero. A,** Fetal MRI: small posterior fossa and low-lying cerebellar tonsils (*arrow*) seen in this fetus with known myelomeningocele, compatible with Chiari 2 malformation. Fetus underwent successful in utero repair of myelomeningocele. **B,** Postnatal sagittal T2-balanced steady state free precession (b-FFE) sequence of same patient shows resolution of hindbrain herniation (*arrow*). However, there is persistent dilatation of third (*3*) and lateral ventricles (*L*), a common finding after repair. Thinning of corpus callosum (*arrowheads*) is commonly seen in cases of neonatal hydrocephalus such as this one.

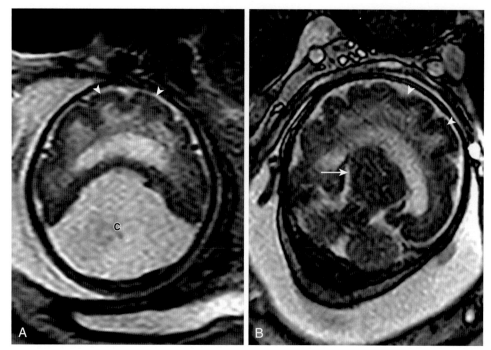

■ FIGURE 8-39 **Alobar Holoprosencephaly. A,** Axial fetal MRI shows complete fusion of cerebral hemispheres (*arrowheads*) and a single ventricle is present. A large CSF-containing structure is seen posterior to the fused parenchyma. This is known as a dorsal cyst (*C*). Note the absence of falx. **B,** Coronal view again demonstrates fused cerebral parenchyma (*arrowheads*) and fused thalami (*arrow*).

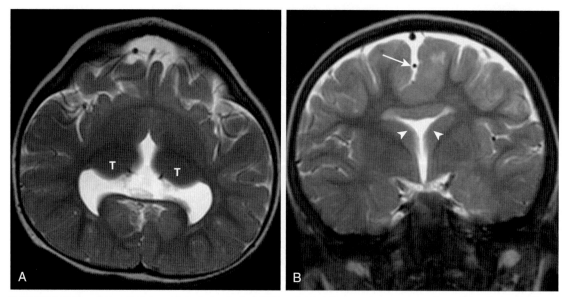

■ FIGURE 8-40 **Semilobar Holoprosencephaly. A,** Axial T2-weighted image shows separation of the thalami (*T*) and separated occipital lobes but fusion of the frontal lobes. There is a single monoventricle and absence of the septum pellucidum. **B,** Coronal T2-weighted image shows monoventricle (*arrowheads*). Note the single anterior cerebral artery (Azygous artery, *arrow*).

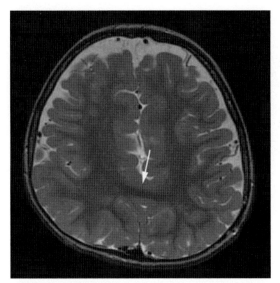

■ FIGURE 8-41 **Middle interhemispheric variant of holoprosencephaly**. Axial T2-weighted sequence shows abnormal midline fusion of brain parenchyma only at the high frontoparietal region (*arrow*).

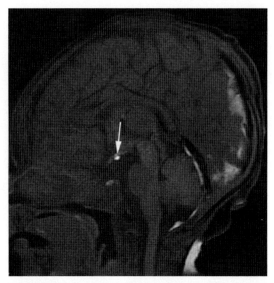

■ FIGURE 8-43 **Ectopic posterior pituitary**. Patient with history of growth hormone deficiency. Sagittal T1-weighted sequence without contrast shows abnormal position of the posterior pituitary bright spot, located posterior to the optic chiasma (*arrow*) instead of within the posterior sella. Note also the absent visualization of the pituitary stalk (interrupted stalk).

migration of the neurons on their route from the subependymal area to the cortex. Heterotopias may be isolated or associated with other migrational disorders. On CT and MRI, the lesions may appear as nodular (Figs. 8-54 and 8-55) or linear/band (Fig. 8-56) areas of gray matter signal within the white matter, most typically in the subependymal and subcortical regions. Bilateral periventricular subependymal nodular heterotopia may be familial with either X-linked or autosomal recessive pattern of inheritance.

Schizencephaly

Schizencephaly is currently considered a disorder of postmigrational development resulting from an encephaloclastic insult. The term refers to a cleft in the cerebral hemisphere lined with dysplastic gray matter (Fig. 8-57). The cleft typically extends from the lateral ventricle to the

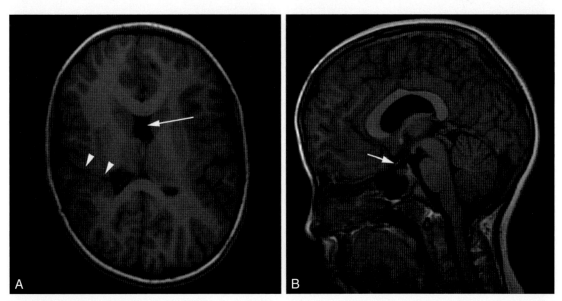

■ FIGURE 8-42 **Septo-optic Dysplasia (SOD)**. **A,** Axial T1-weighted sequence shows absent septum pellucidum (*arrow*). Note also associated closed lip schizencephaly (*arrowheads*). **B,** Sagittal T1-weighted sequence shows small size of the optic chiasm (*arrow*).

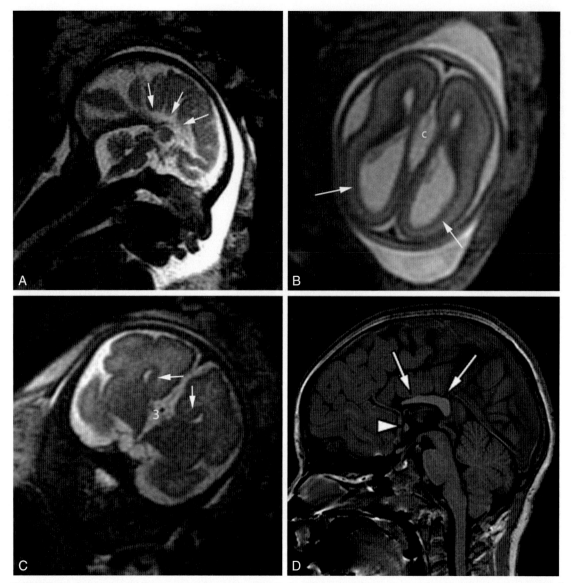

■ FIGURE 8-44 **Agenesis and dysgenesis of corpus callosum in different patients. A,** Sagittal T2-weighted sequence of a fetus shows absent corpus callosum and cingulate gyrus (*arrows*). **B,** Axial T2-weighted sequence of a different fetus shows the typical parallel configuration of the lateral ventricles with associated colpocephaly (*arrows*). **C,** Probst bundles (*arrows*) visualized on coronal T2-weighed sequence. Also note "bull horn" configuration of lateral ventricles and high-riding third ventricle (*3*). **D,** Postnatal sagittal T1-weighted sequence shows an abnormally short corpus callosum (*arrows*) with lack of visualization of its anterior portions. Note the presence of a preserved anterior commissure (*arrowhead*).

surface of the brain. The presence of gray matter lining the entire cleft is the diagnostic feature that separates schizencephaly from other causes of clefts, such as porencephaly. Schizencephaly is often characterized as being open or close lipped (Fig. 8-58). The lesion can be unilateral or bilateral and can occur anywhere in the cerebral hemispheres. In many cases, there may be associated absent septum pellucidum (Fig. 8-58).

Polymicrogyria

Polymicrogyria is a disorder of late neuronal migration/postmigrational development that results from small defects in the pial limitans membrane and therefore demonstrates overlapping phenotypical features with cobblestone malformation. On imaging, multiple small and disorganized gyri are seen (Figs. 8-59 and 8-60).

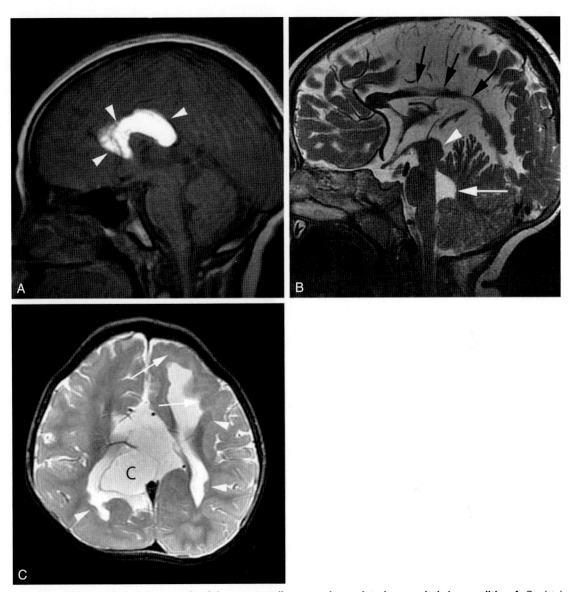

■ FIGURE 8-45 **Agenesis and dysgenesis of the corpus callosum and associated congenital abnormalities. A,** Sagittal T1-weighted sequence shows a large tubulonodular pericallosal lipoma (*arrowheads*) associated with agenesis of the corpus callosum. **B,** Sagittal T2-weighted sequence in a patient with history of congenital hydrocephalus. There is marked thinning of the corpus callosum (*black arrows*) due to abnormal formation secondary to in utero increased intraventricular pressure. Note also thick tectum (*arrowhead*) with aqueductal stenosis and a rounded fastigial point of the fourth ventricle due to associated rhombencephalosynapsis (*white arrow*). **C,** Axial T2-weighted sequence of a female patient with Aicardi syndrome shows multiple associated malformation of cortical development including polymicrogyria (*arrows*) and periventricular nodular heterotopias (*arrowheads*). Note also interhemispheric cyst (*c*).

It is usually associated with other MCDs. It can be the result of an encephaloclastic insult such as prenatal infection (see Fig. 8-91D), ischemia, toxic exposure, metabolic disorder (see Fig. 8-90B), or part of a genetic disorder.

Focal Cortical Dysplasia

Focal cortical dysplasia (FCD) is characterized by abnormal cortical lamination. It is the most common cause of intractable epilepsy in

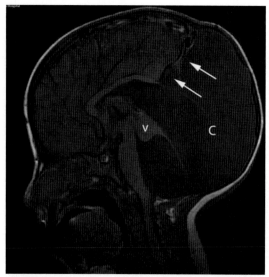

■ FIGURE 8-46 **Dandy–Walker malformation in a newborn infant. A,** Sagittal T1-weighted MR image shows large posterior fossa and posterior fossa CSF spaces (*C*). The cerebellar vermis is markedly hypoplastic (*v*). The torcula (*arrows*) is elevated.

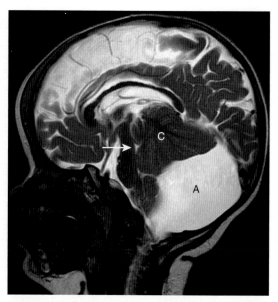

■ FIGURE 8-48 **Posterior fossa arachnoid cyst.** Sagittal T2-weighted MR image shows posterior fossa cyst (*A*) that does not communicate with the fourth ventricle (*arrow*). There is mass effect on the cerebellum (*C*).

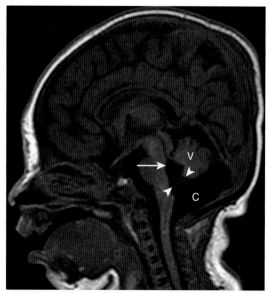

■ FIGURE 8-47 **Cerebellar vermian hypoplasia.** Sagittal T1-weighted MR image shows mild inferior vermian hypoplasia (*V*) and prominent retrocerebellar CSF spaces (*C*). There is an enlarged communication (*arrowheads*) of the posterior fossa CSF spaces with the fourth ventricle (*arrow*), as a result of vermian hypoplasia. There is a normal position of the torcula, the posterior fossa is not enlarged.

children. It is mostly sporadic but can be related to familial genetic causes. There are currently three different types of FCD described: FCD type I, FCD type II, and FCD type III.

FCD type II contains dysmorphic neurons and tends to present earlier in life and with higher incidence of medically refractory seizures. On imaging, FCD type II may demonstrate a focal area of altered cortical thickness, blurring of the gray–white matter differentiation, and increased T2 signal within the underlying white matter. The white matter signal changes are the result of glial proliferation and reduced myelination and frequently extend from the subcortical white matter to the surface of the adjacent lateral ventricle (Fig. 8-61). FCD type II phenotype overlaps with tuberous sclerosis (TS) as both of these entities result from mutations of genes encoding the mTOR pathway.

Type I FCD has more subtle cortical changes with no dysmorphic neurons. As a result, the majority of cases have normal MRI imaging or at most present with subtle changes in cortical thickness and blurring of gray–white matter interface.

Type III FCD is a combination of type I cortical changes and presence of an associated

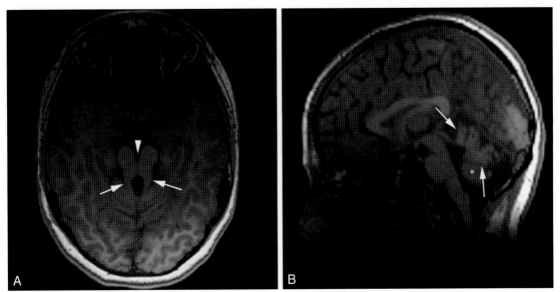

■ FIGURE 8-49 **Molar tooth malformation. A,** Axial T1-weighted sequence of a patient with Joubert syndrome shows molar tooth appearance of the midbrain with horizontal parallel superior cerebellar peduncles (*arrows*) and deep interpeduncular cleft (*arrowhead*). **B,** Sagittal T1-weighted sequence shows a hypoplastic cerebellar vermis (*arrows*). Note pseudovermis (*) made of the medially rotated cerebellar hemispheres.

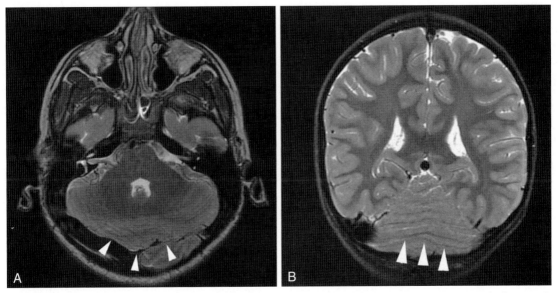

■ FIGURE 8-50 **Rhombencephalosynapsis. A,** Axial T2-weighted sequence shows partially absent cerebellar vermis with posterior convex margins of fused cerebellar hemispheres (*arrowheads*). **B,** Coronal T2-weighted sequence shows continuity of cerebellar hemispheres folia at the midline (*arrowheads*).

abnormality. Associated abnormalities can vary from hippocampal sclerosis (Fig. 8-62A and B), glioneuronal tumors (Fig. 8-63), vascular malformations, or porencephalic changes.

The association of FCD type II with a glioneuronal tumor or hippocampal sclerosis is known as "dual pathology."

Megalencephaly

Megalencephaly disorders are the result of abnormal cell proliferation or apoptosis resulting in parenchymal overgrowth. Hamartomatous overgrowth of one cerebral hemisphere or part of the cerebral hemisphere is known as

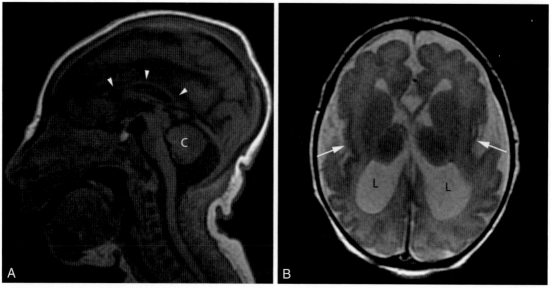

■ **FIGURE 8-51 Microlissencephaly. A,** Sagittal T1-weighted sequence shows microcephaly and diffuse thinning of the corpus callosum (*arrowheads*). Note also dysplastic cerebellar vermis (*c*). **B,** Axial T2-weighted sequence shows small cerebral volume with simplified pattern of gyration. Note underopercularization, characterized by a wide Sylvian fissure bilaterally (*arrows*), and prominent lateral ventricles (*L*).

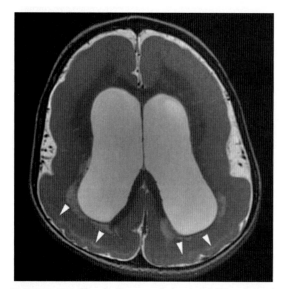

■ **FIGURE 8-52 Classic lissencephaly.** Axial T2-weighted image of a patient with Miller–Dieker syndrome shows the smooth surface of the bilateral cerebral hemispheres and shallow Sylvian fissures (Figure eight configuration). Note the thin band of increased T2 signal within the abnormal cortex (sparse cell zone) (*arrowheads*). This is seen in cases of classic lissencephaly.

hemimegalencephaly (Fig. 8-64). When both cerebral hemispheres are enlarged and dysplastic, this is known as dysplastic megalencephaly (or bilateral hemimegalencephaly) (Fig. 8-65). Megalencephaly disorders can be isolated or be

part of many syndromic genetic conditions, including neurocutaneous and hemihypertrophy syndromes. Imaging findings include enlarged cerebral hemispheres with or without obvious cortical malformations. The most common clinical presentation is early onset intractable seizures. Other symptoms include hemiplegia and developmental delay.

Vein of Galen Malformation

With vein of Galen malformation, or vein of Galen aneurysm, there are arteriovenous connections of cerebral arteries with a persistent embryonic vein (median prosencephalic vein of Markowski). On imaging, there is an enlarged varix at the location of the vein of Galen and straight sinus, which corresponds to the enlarged persistent median prosencephalic vein (Fig. 8-66). The most common type of vein of Galen malformation is the "choroidal type," which presents with multiple abnormal vessel connections (usually thalamoperforating, choroidal, and anterior cerebral arteries) to the anterior wall of the vein, causing significant arteriovenous shunting. These malformations may be depicted prenatally or present during the neonatal period. They often are associated with congestive heart failure due to associated left-to-right shunting. On chest radiography, there is cardiomegaly, signs of congestive heart failure, and widening of the superior mediastinum secondary to vascular enlargement caused by the

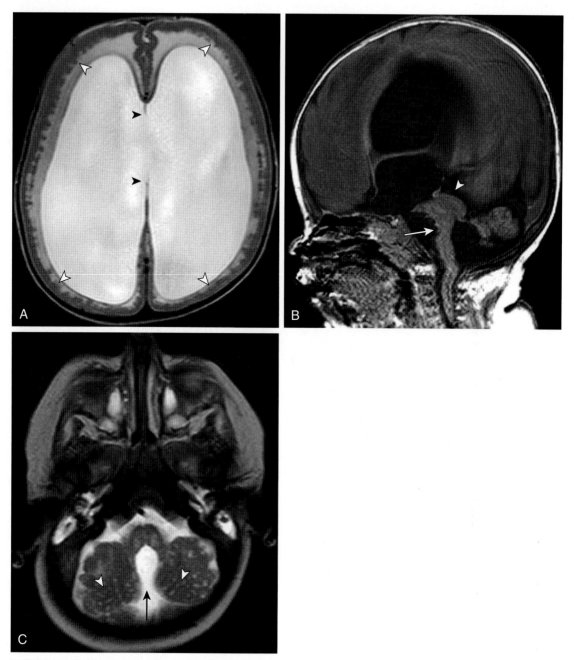

FIGURE 8-53 Cobblestone malformation. A, Axial T2-weighted sequence demonstrates smooth surface of the brain with "pebbled" appearance of the cerebral cortex (*white arrowheads*). There is also marked lateral ventriculomegaly and partial absence of septum pellucidum (*black arrowheads*). **B,** Sagittal T1-weighted sequence shows hypoplastic and kinked brainstem (*arrow*). The cerebellar vermis is also hypoplastic, and the tectum is thickened (*arrowhead*). Note the enlargement of the third and lateral ventricles secondary to tectal thickening resulting in aqueduct stenosis. Fourth ventricle is enlarged due to brainstem and cerebellar hypoplasia. **C,** Axial, T2 sequence of the posterior fossa confirmed hypoplasia of cerebellar vermis depicted here as an enlarged communication of fourth ventricle with extraaxial spaces (*black arrow*). Cerebellar hemispheres are dysplastic with multiple small cystic changes, a few marked by *white arrowheads*.

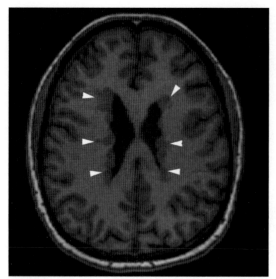

■ FIGURE 8-54 **Heterotopic gray matter**. Axial T1-weighted MRI of a patient with Filamin A mutation shows nodular foci of gray matter (*arrowheads*) lining the lateral ventricles. Nodules have the same signal as gray matter, consistent with heterotopic gray matter.

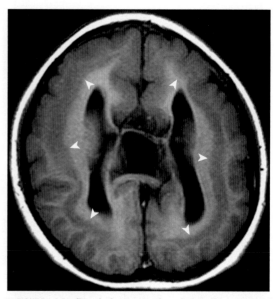

■ FIGURE 8-56 **Band heterotopia**. Axial T1-weighted sequence shows abnormal band of gray matter (*arrowheads*) located medially to the subcortical white matter. There is also an abnormal appearance of the cortex with areas of pachygyria. Note associated findings of callosum agenesis, including parallel lateral ventricles and high-riding third ventricle.

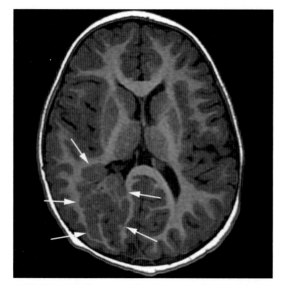

■ FIGURE 8-55 **Transmantle heterotopia**. Axial T1-weighted sequence shows a band of multiple heterotopic gray matter foci extending from the cortex to the lateral ventricle, compatible with transmantle heterotopia (*arrows*).

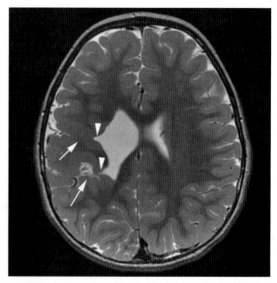

■ FIGURE 8-57 **Closed-lip schizencephaly**. Axial T2-weighted image shows two areas of parenchymal clefts lined by opposing dysplastic cortex (*arrows*) compatible with closed-lip schizencephalic clefts. Note the small outpouching of the lateral ventricles extending into the clefts (*arrowheads*), helping differentiate from transmantle heterotopias.

increased blood flow to and from the head. There may be associated hydrocephalus and brain ischemic changes due to steal phenomenon (Fig. 8-67A and B). A "mural type" vein of Galen malformation is seen when there are fewer larger caliber connections (usually posterior choroidal or collicular arteries). This type of malformation carries a better prognosis—with lower incidence of cardiac heart failure and brain ischemia, as well as better response to treatment. Most vein of

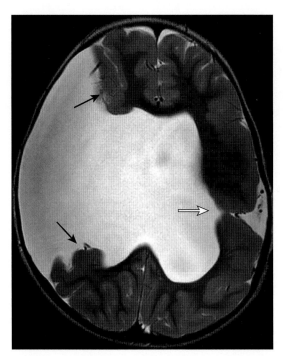

■ FIGURE 8-58 **Open-lip schizencephaly.** Axial T2-weighted image shows large fluid-filled space that is in communication with the right lateral ventricle. The communication is lined by gray matter (*black arrows*), consistent with an open-lip schizencephaly. On the left, a smaller closed lip schizencephalic cleft is seen (*white arrow*). Note common association of absent septum pellucidum.

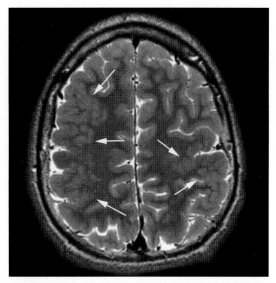

■ FIGURE 8-60 **Postnatal polymicrogyria.** Axial T2-weighted sequence shows extensive bilateral fronto-parietal polymicrogyria (*arrows*).

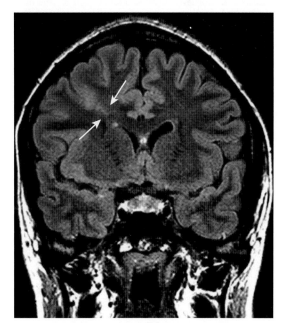

■ FIGURE 8-61 **Cortical dysplasia type IIb.** Coronal FLAIR sequence shows a triangular-shaped area of increased signal (*arrows*) extending from the right frontal cortex into the deep white matter near the surface of the right lateral ventricle. Note also mild thickening of the involved cortex and focal blurring of the gray–white matter differentiation.

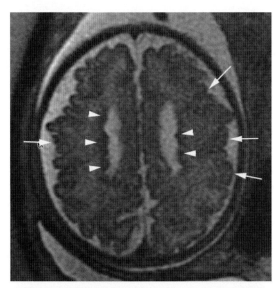

■ FIGURE 8-59 **Fetal polymicrogyria.** Axial T2-weighted sequence of a fetal MRI demonstrates extensive bilateral frontoparietal polymicrogyria (*arrows*). Note also extensive periventricular heterotopias (*arrowheads*).

Galen malformations are treated by arterial embolization. Outcome depends on the severity of the malformation and degree of shunting. Severe cases commonly die in the neonatal period. Mild cases can achieve cure.

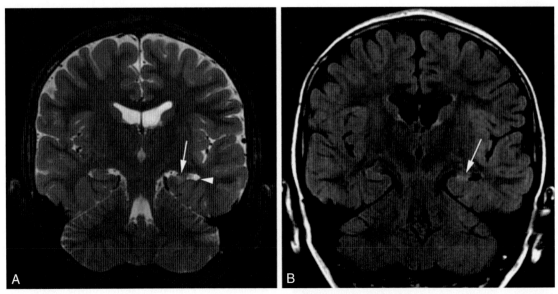

■ FIGURE 8-62 **Mesial temporal lobe sclerosis. A,** Coronal T2-weighted sequence shows decreased size of the left hippocampus (*arrow*) when compared with the normal contralateral side. Note also mild prominence of the left temporal horn of the lateral ventricle (*arrowhead*), which can be a secondary finding in cases of mesial temporal sclerosis. **B,** Coronal FLAIR sequence also shows increased signal within the small left hippocampus (*arrow*).

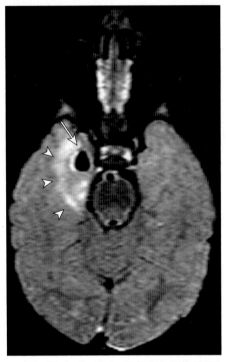

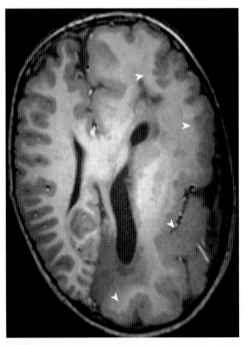

■ FIGURE 8-64 **Hemimegalencephaly.** Axial T1-weighted sequence shows an enlarged and markedly dysplastic left cerebral hemisphere. Note diffuse cortical malformation compatible with polymicrogyria (*arrowheads*) and enlarged left lateral ventricle.

■ FIGURE 8-63 **Dysembryoplastic Neuroepithelial Tumor in a patient presenting with seizures.** Axial FLAIR sequence demonstrates right mesial temporal lobe abnormality, including a focal cyst (*arrow*) with surrounding increased FLAIR signal (*arrowheads*). This was resected surgically and confirmed to represent a DNET and associated cortical dysplasia (dual pathology).

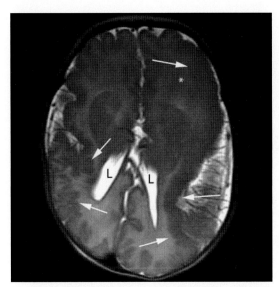

■ FIGURE 8-65 **Dysplastic megalencephaly.** Axial T2-weighted sequence shows bilateral enlarged and markedly dysplastic cerebral hemispheres. Note diffuse cortical malformation (*arrows*) including polymicrogyria and pachygyria and dysmorphic lateral ventricles (*L*).

■ NEUROCUTANEOUS SYNDROMES

The neurocutaneous syndromes (phakomatoses) are a group of related diseases that affect tissues of ectodermal origin, primarily the skin and nervous system. Some of the more common phakomatoses that present in childhood include neurofibromatosis, Tuberous Sclerosis, and Sturge–Weber syndrome.

Neurofibromatosis

Neurofibromatosis is the most common of the phakomatoses and is divided into subcategories, of which neurofibromatosis type 1 (NF-1) and neurofibromatosis type 2 (NF-2) are the most common.

NF-1 is an autosomal dominant disorder. Diagnostic criteria for NF-1 are listed in Table 8-5. The neuroimaging manifestations of NF-1 are multiple. The most common lesions of the CNS are the "NF-1 spots" that appear as high T2-weighted foci in the basal ganglia (especially globus pallidus), thalami, mesial temporal lobes, internal capsule, splenium, brainstem, and cerebellar white matter (Fig. 8-68A and B). The lesions are areas of myelin vacuolization and typically become apparent at around 3 years of age, increase in number and size until approximately 12 years of age, and then regress. Other lesions of NF-1 include optic pathway gliomas (Fig. 8-69A and B), cerebral astrocytomas, hydrocephalus, vascular dysplasia (including aneurysms and moyamoya vasculopathy Fig. 8-70), dural ectasia, and sphenoid wing dysplasia (Fig. 8-71). Patients with NF-1 can develop cranial nerve schwannomas, peripheral neurofibromas, plexiform neurofibromas (Fig. 8-72A and B), and malignant peripheral nerve sheath tumors. Plexiform neurofibromas are locally aggressive masses that are histologically more disorganized than typical neurofibromas. In the head and neck, they often involve

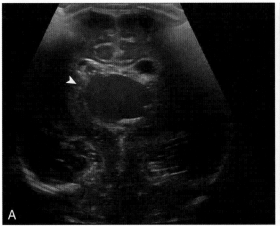
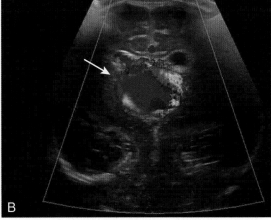

■ FIGURE 8-66 **Vein of Galen malformation in a newborn presenting with signs of heart failure. A,** Coronal, grayscale ultrasound image shows a large midline fluid structure posterior to the third ventricle (*arrowhead*). **B,** Color Doppler demonstrates vascular flow within it compatible with an enlarged median prosencephalic vein (*arrow*).

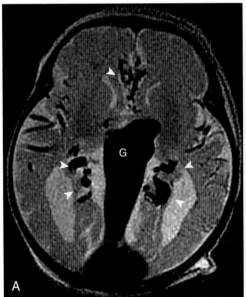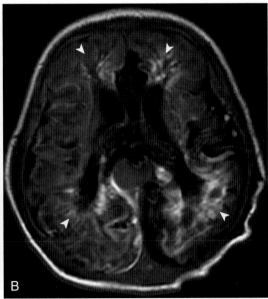

■ FIGURE 8-67 **Vein of Galen malformation. A,** Axial T2-weighted sequence demonstrates a markedly enlarged posterior midline flow void at the expected location of the straight sinus and vein of Galen (*G*) compatible with an enlarged median prosencephalic vein. Note multiple enlarged and tortuous feeding arterial structures from the anterior and posterior circulation (*arrowheads*). **B,** Follow-up, axial T1-weighted sequence demonstrates volume loss and periventricular signal abnormalities (*arrowheads*) compatible with chronic ischemic changes due to steal phenomenon from the malformation.

✳ **TABLE 8-5** Diagnostic Criteria for Neurofibromatosis Type 1
Two or more of the following: 1. Six or more café au lait macules 2. Two or more neurofibromas or one plexiform neurofibroma 3. Axillary or inguinal freckles 4. Visual pathway gliomas 5. Two hamartomas of the iris (Lisch nodules) 6. Distinctive bony lesion (sphenoid wing dysplasia or thin long bones with pseudoarthrosis) 7. Parent, sibling, or child with NF-1

the scalp and orbit. They are often monitored by imaging to evaluate for findings suspicious for malignant degeneration. Spinal manifestations include posterior vertebral scalloping (resulting from dural ectasia or neurofibromas), scoliosis, and lateral meningoceles.

NF-2 is characterized by the presence of bilateral acoustic schwannomas (Fig. 8-73). Other associated lesions include meningiomas, gliomas, neurofibromas, and schwannomas of other cranial nerves. Patients most commonly present in adulthood.

Tuberous Sclerosis

TS is an autosomal dominant syndrome associated with a classic triad of seizures, mental retardation, and adenoma sebaceous (facial angiofibroma of the skin). Although this triad is described as characteristic, the incidence of all three symptoms occurring in conjunction is actually low. The disease may affect the skin, CNS, orbits, skeletal system, lungs, and abdominal organs.

The most common neuroimaging finding is the presence of tubers. These are hamartomatous lesions that appear as subependymal nodules, typically along the walls of the lateral ventricles (Fig. 8-74), or parenchymal lesions within the subcortical white matter and cortex. The signal characteristics of subependymal nodules are variable and are related to age. In older patients, lesions are often calcified. In younger children, the lesions tend to be isointense to gray matter. Enhancement is variable. When a subependymal nodule near the foramen of Monro rapidly enlarges, malignant subependymal giant cell astrocytoma (SEGA) is suspected (Fig. 8-75). Such tumors frequently obstruct CSF flow and can lead to hydrocephalus. Parenchymal tubers are characterized as areas of increased T2 signal,

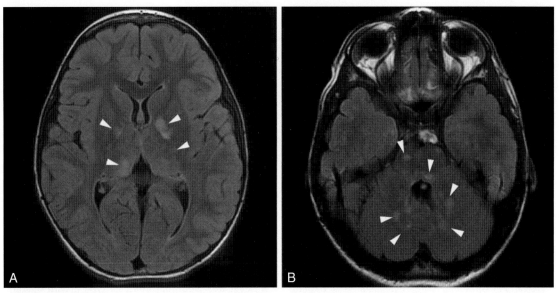

■ FIGURE 8-68 **Neurofibromatosis type 1. A,** Axial FLAIR sequence shows NF-1 spots as abnormal increased signal within the globus pallidi and thalami bilaterally (*arrowheads*). **B,** Myelin vacuolization spots of NF-1 also noted within the brainstem and bilateral cerebellar white matter (*arrowheads*).

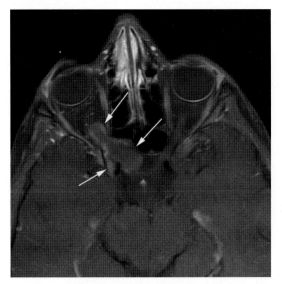

■ FIGURE 8-69 **Optic pathway glioma in a patient with neurofibromatosis type 1. A,** Axial T1-weighted sequence postcontrast shows enlarged right prechiasmatic and intraorbital optic nerve (*arrows*) with abnormal enhancement compatible with optic pathway glioma.

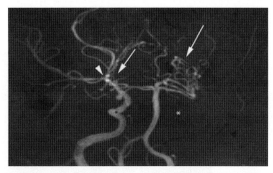

■ FIGURE 8-70 **Moyamoya vasculopathy in a patient with NF-1.** MR angiography shows absent left internal carotid artery (ICA) (*white **) and marked narrowing of the right carotid terminus (*arrowhead*) with multiple bilateral collateral vessels (*arrows*). Note normal right ICA at the skull base level (*black **).

predominantly within the subcortical white matter. Some of these lesions can involve the cortex and rarely may calcify. Parenchymal tubers are a cause of seizures, and determination of which lesion is the epileptogenic focus can be difficult. Other imaging findings include radial migration lines (Fig. 8-76) and gyri expansion associated with cystoid degeneration of parenchymal tubers (Fig. 8-77).

Visceral manifestations of TS are covered elsewhere and include renal cysts, renal angiomyolipomas, cardiac rhabdomyomas, pulmonary lymphangioleiomyomatosis, and hamartomas of other organs.

Sturge—Weber Syndrome

Sturge—Weber syndrome, or encephalotrigeminal angiomatosis, is characterized by low-flow vascular malformation both intracranially and extracranially. The syndrome manifests as

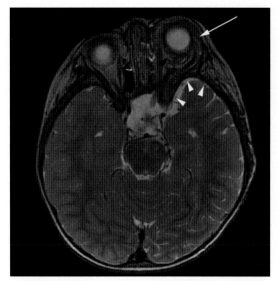

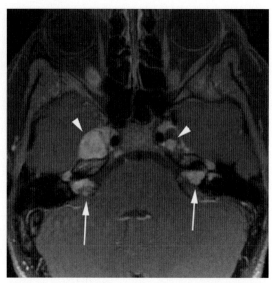

■ FIGURE 8-71 **Sphenoid wing dysplasia in a patient with NF-1.** Axial T2-weighted sequence shows a hypoplastic left sphenoid wing characterized by widening of the middle cranial fossa (*white arrowheads*). Note also associated left eye proptosis (*arrow*), resulting from a combination of sphenoid wind dysplasia and intraorbital plexiform neurofibroma (*black arrowhead*).

■ FIGURE 8-73 **Neurofibromatosis type 2 with bilateral acoustic schwannomas.** Axial T1-weighted sequence postcontrast at the level of the internal auditory canals (IAC) shows enhancing masses at the bilateral IACs (*arrows*) consistent with bilateral acoustic schwannomas. Note also additional masses at the bilateral cavernous sinus, schwannomas versus meningiomas (*arrowheads*).

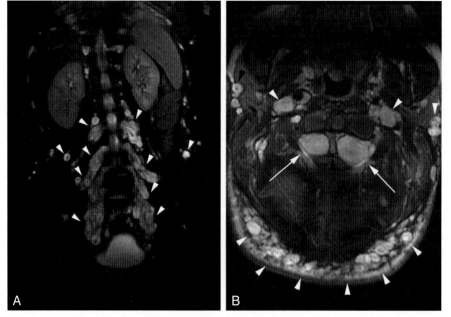

■ FIGURE 8-72 **Spinal neurofibromas in a child with neurofibromatosis type 1. A,** Coronal T2-weighted fat-saturated image shows multiple T2 hyperintense retroperitoneal masses along the spinal nerve roots and paraspinal soft tissues (*arrowheads*) consistent with plexiform neurofibromas. Note focal central low attenuation within many of the nodular masses compatible with characteristic "target" sign. **B,** Axial imaging shows neurofibromas (*arrows*) extending into the spinal canal and causing marked compression over the spinal cord. Note also multiple additional neurofibromas throughout the neck soft tissues (*arrowheads*).

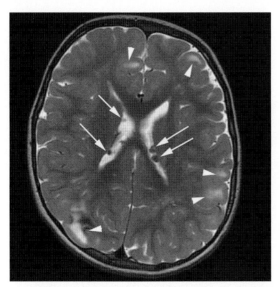

■ FIGURE 8-74 **Tuberous sclerosis in a patient with seizures.** Axial T2-weighted MRI shows bilateral subependymal nodules (*arrows*) consistent with tubers. Note also multiple parenchymal tubes, a few of them marked by *arrowheads*.

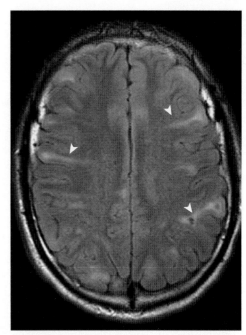

■ FIGURE 8-76 **Tuberous sclerosis.** Axial FLAIR sequence demonstrates radial migration lines seen in TS (*arrowheads*).

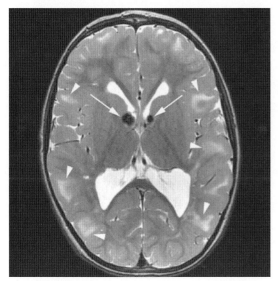

■ FIGURE 8-75 **Tuberous sclerosis.** Axial T2-weighted image demonstrates bilateral calcified subependymal nodules near the foramen of Monro. The nodules (*arrows*) had demonstrated interval increase in size when compared with prior (not shown), suspicious for SEGA. Few parenchymal tubers marked by *arrowheads*.

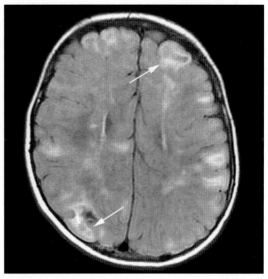

■ FIGURE 8-77 **Tuberous sclerosis.** Axial T2-weighted sequence showing multiple subcortical and cortical parenchyma tubers causing gyri expansion (*arrows*).

abnormalities of the skin (facial port-wine nevus in the distribution of the trigeminal nerve), leptomeninges, and choroid of the eye. The altered leptomeningeal flow secondary to pial vascular malformation (angioma) results in venous stasis and chronic ischemic injury to the affected underlying brain. On neurologic imaging, there is serpiginous calcifications, abnormal enhancement, and atrophy of the involved gyri (Fig. 8-78A–D). Other findings may include prominence of choroid plexus on the involved side and choroidal angiomas of the orbits (Fig. 8-79). The cranium is commonly thickened adjacent to the brain abnormalities. Clinical manifestations include seizures, mental retardation, and hemiparesis.

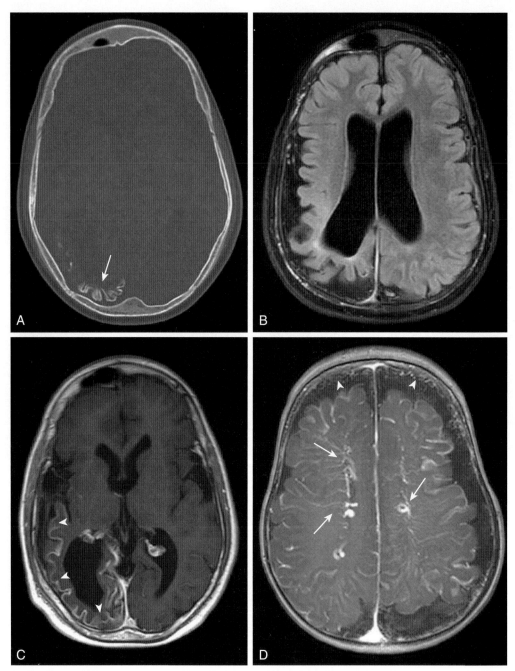

■ **FIGURE 8-78 Sturge–Weber syndrome. A,** Noncontrast CT in bone window shows abnormal gyriform calcifications (*arrow*) within the right parietooccipital region. **B,** Axial FLAIR sequence demonstrates regional parenchymal volume loss. **C,** Abnormal gyriform enhancement (*arrowheads*) is seen on postcontrast T1 sequence. **D,** Axial T1-weighted sequence postcontrast, in a different patient with bilateral involvement, demonstrates prominent and tortuous bilateral deep medullary veins (*arrows*) and peripheral cortical veins within the subarachnoid space (*arrowheads*).

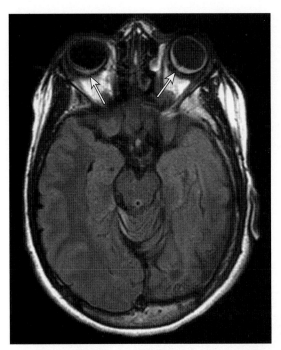

■ FIGURE 8-79 **Orbital involvement of Sturge—Weber syndrome.** Axial FLAIR sequence demonstrates crescentic area of increased signal along the bilateral choroidal surface of the globes (*arrows*), compatible with choroidal angiomas. This is not a very common finding on imaging, even when choroidal involvement is present. The diagnosis is typically made on ophthalmological evaluation.

Von Hippel—Lindau

Patients with von Hippel—Lindau (VHL) most commonly present in early adulthood with multiorgan tumors (especially kidney, adrenal, pancreas, and CNS). Few cases present during pediatric age group. The most common CNS tumor is hemangioblastoma, commonly presenting within the posterior fossa or spine. There are often multiple lesions. On MRI, hemangioblastomas are similar on morphologic characteristic to a pilocytic astrocytoma—cystic with a mural nodule. The mural nodule of hemangioblastomas demonstrates marked increase perfusion, helping the differentiation between these two different tumors. Other head and neck tumors seen in VHL include choroid plexus papilloma and endolymphatic sac tumors.

■ METABOLIC AND DEGENERATIVE DISORDERS

A large number of genetic mutations can manifest as disorders of brain metabolism and structure. Most of these diseases are rare and

untreatable. Clinically, metabolic disorders tend to present with progressive nonspecific symptoms such as seizures, hypotonia, and delayed or loss of achieved milestones. Categories of disease include lysosomal storage disorders, mitochondrial disorders, peroxisomal disorders, urea cycle disorders, and amino acid disorders. On MRI, these disorders typically demonstrate abnormal myelination and increased T2-weighted signal involving portions of white matter, gray matter, or a combination of the two, most often in a bilateral symmetric pattern. There may be associated atrophy of the involved structures. The distribution of the abnormal signal can be helpful in narrowing the differential diagnosis (Figs. 8-80A—C through 8-90A—C). MRS can also provide helpful information. Representative disorders and the associated distribution of abnormalities are listed in Table 8-6.

■ INFECTION

Many of the imaging findings in CNS infections (meningitis, cerebritis, empyema, encephalitis, and parenchymal abscess) are similar in children and adults and are not emphasized here. This section focuses on several of the issues unique to children.

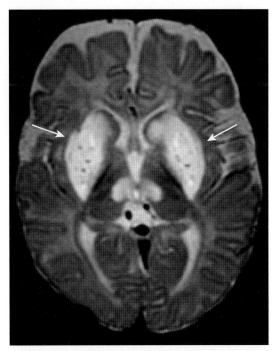

■ FIGURE 8-80 **Leigh disease in a 5-month-old boy.** Axial T2-weighted MR image shows abnormal, increased signal within the basal ganglia (*arrows*) and medial thalami. There is bilateral frontal volume loss.

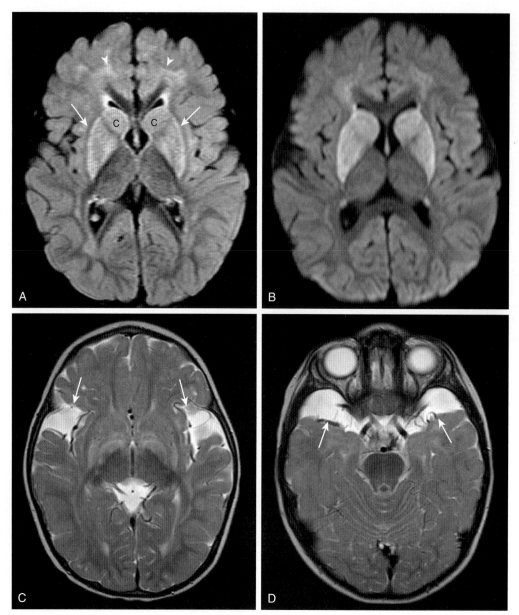

■ **FIGURE 8-81 Glutaric aciduria type 1. A,** Axial FLAIR sequence demonstrates abnormal, bilateral, symmetric, increased signal within the head of caudate nucleus (*C*) and lentiform nucleus (*arrows*), as well as bilateral anterior periventricular white matter (*arrowheads*). **B,** Diffusion sequence shows restricted diffusion in corresponding areas. **C,** T2-weighted sequence demonstrates bilateral widening of sylvian fissures (*arrows*) due to underopercularization. **D,** Note also bilateral prominent CSF at the middle cranial fossa (*arrows*). Glutaric aciduria type 1 can present with nontraumatic subdural collections and is part of the differential diagnosis for child abuse.

Congenital Infections

There are a number of in utero infections (TORCH: toxoplasmosis, other [syphilis, human immunodeficiency virus (HIV), ZIKA], rubella, cytomegalovirus [CMV], herpes; see Chapter 7) that can affect the CNS. These infections demonstrate unique findings as compared with CNS infections that occur later in life because in utero infections affect brain development. The severity of the abnormality commonly reflects the time period during which the infection occurred, more severe when affecting early pregnancy.

CMV is the most common TORCH infection to involve the CNS. Imaging findings include periventricular calcifications, migrational

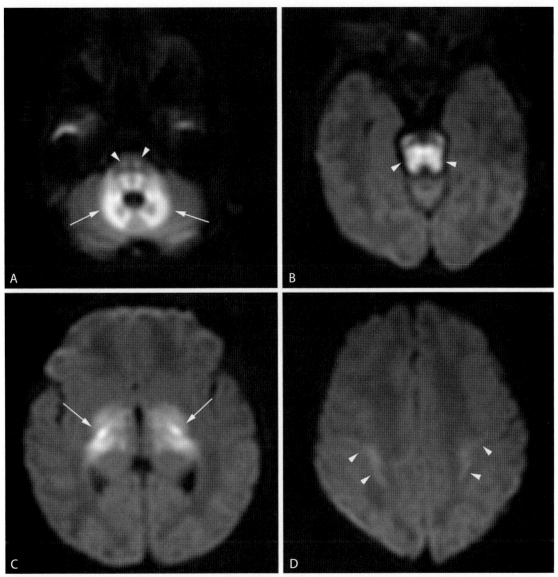

■ **FIGURE 8-82 Maple syrup urine disease. A–D**, Axial DWI sequence shows typical distribution of restricted diffusion in Maple Syrup Urine Disease. **A,** Central corticospinal tracts (*arrowheads*), cerebellar peduncles, and cerebellar white matter (*arrows*). **B,** Dorsal brainstem (*arrowheads*). **C,** Globus pallidi, thalami, and posterior limb of the internal capsule (*arrows*). **D,** Superior aspect of the corticospinal tracts (*arrowheads*).

abnormalities (such as polymicrogyria and lissencephaly), increased white matter T2 signal, cortical cysts (especially at the temporal lobes), cerebellar hypoplasia, and ventricular enlargement (Fig. 8-91A and B). Clinical manifestations include microcephaly, hearing impairment, mental retardation, and developmental delay.

Toxoplasmosis is the second most common TORCH infection to involve the CNS. The parenchymal calcifications seen in toxoplasmosis are more variable in location than those seen

with CMV, with predilection to basal ganglia and periventricular white matter. Other manifestations include hydrocephalus, not a finding commonly seen in other TORCH infections. No migrational abnormalities are seen. Differential diagnosis of periventricular calcifications in the neonatal period also includes more rare entities, such as lymphocytic choriomeningitis infection and pseudo-TORCH syndromes (Aicardi–Goutières syndrome and Baraitser–Reardon syndrome).

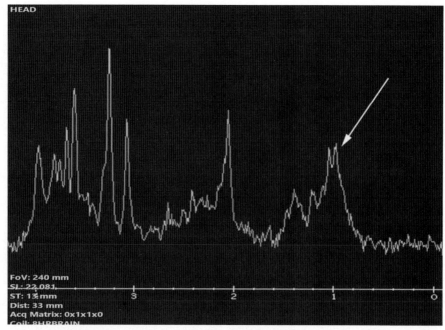

■ FIGURE 8-83 **Spectroscopy in maple syrup urine disease.** Short TE MR spectroscopy shows an abnormal peak at 0.9ppm (*arrow*) compatible with branched-chain amino acids and keto acid.

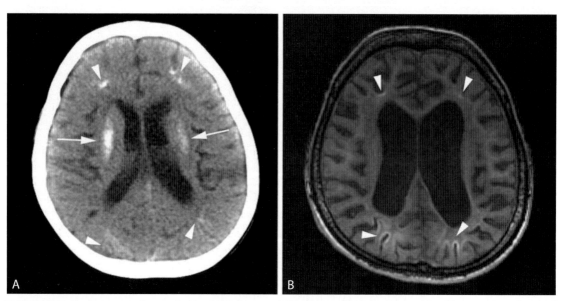

■ FIGURE 8-84 **Cockayne syndrome. A,** Head CT shows calcifications within the bilateral lentiform nucleus (*arrows*) and cortex along the deep sulci (*arrowheads*). **B,** Axial T1 weighted also showing deep sulci cortical calcifications (*arrowheads*).

Recently emerged ZIKA virus can also present with intracranial calcifications, most of which are located at the gray–white matter interface. Periventricular and basal ganglia calcifications are less common. Another prominent feature of congenital ZIKA infection is marked microcephaly.

With congenital infection by HIV, CNS abnormalities are mostly related to primary HIV involvement rather than secondary

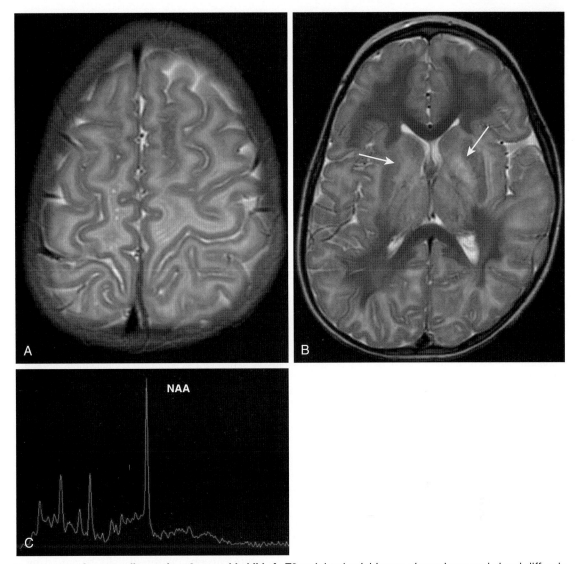

■ **FIGURE 8-85 Canavan disease in a 3-year-old child. A,** T2-weighted axial image shows increased signal diffusely throughout the subcortical white matter. **B,** T2-weighted axial image more inferiorly shows increased signal in globus pallidi bilaterally (*arrows*). Again, there is increased signal in subcortical white matter. **C,** MR spectroscopy shows increased NAA peak.

complications (opportunistic infections and tumors) seen in adults. The majority of children with congenital HIV infection have CNS manifestations, typically progressive encephalopathy. Imaging findings include diffuse atrophy, delayed myelination, and calcifications. The calcifications most commonly occur within the basal ganglia and subcortical white matter of the frontal lobes.

Congenital herpes is secondary to herpes simplex virus type 2 (HSV2). Imaging findings of meningoencephalitis include cortical and white matter signal abnormality, diffusion restriction, and meningeal enhancement. HSV2 infection has no predilection of location as opposed to HSV1, which typically affects the temporal lobes.

Encephalitis

Encephalitis is inflammation of the brain, sometimes seen in conjunction with meningeal inflammation. It can occur secondary to direct

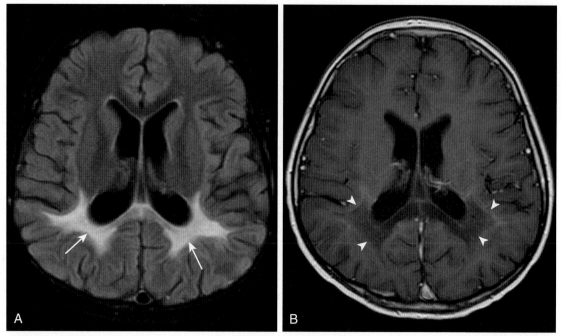

■ FIGURE 8-86 **Adrenoleukodystrophy. A,** Axial FLAIR sequence shows abnormal, increased signal in the posterior periventricular white matter (*arrows*). **B,** Axial postcontrast image demonstrates abnormal enhancement along the outer margins of the signal abnormality (*arrowheads*).

viral infection, can be associated with an auto-immune response to a virus or immunization, or can be the extension of a meningeal infection. Children typically present with seizures, lethargy, or focal neurologic deficits. Several types of encephalitis occur predominantly during childhood.

1. *HSV1* can lead to necrotizing meningoen-cephalitis. When it occurs secondary to the reactivation and migration of a previous latent infection via the branches of the trigeminal nerve, it typically affects one or both temporal lobes (Fig. 8-92A–C). On MRI, high signal is seen within the cortex of one or both temporal lobes, with or without diffusion restriction. There are often areas of hemorrhage within the affected areas.

2. *Subacute sclerosing panencephalitis* is thought to be an encephalitis that occurs secondary to reactivation of latent measles infection. It is a rare disease of childhood. Imaging demonstrates nonspecific atrophy and increased T2-weighted signal within the cerebral cortex and white matter (Fig. 8-93).

3. *Acute disseminated encephalomyelitis (ADEM)* is an immunologic disease that occurs in response to a recent viral infection or

immunization. It typically occurs days to weeks after the preceding stimulus. On MRI, areas of increased T2-weighted signal are typically seen in the white matter (Fig. 8-94), brainstem, and cerebellum. Deep gray matter structures (basal ganglia) can also be affected. Treatment is typically with steroids, and most children completely recover.

4. *Acute Necrotizing Encephalopathy* is a poorly understood entity characterized by severe acute encephalopathy, usually triggered by a prior viral infection. On imaging, there is prominent bilateral symmetric involvement of the thalami with marked signal abnormality and swelling (Fig. 8-95A–C). It may also involve the putamina, internal capsule, and brainstem. Hemorrhage, cavitation, and enhancement within the affected areas may occur. This disease has a high mortality rate and can be sporadic or have a genetic familial predisposition.

5. *Rasmussen Encephalitis* is a rare chronic en-cephalitis of unknown etiology causing intractable epilepsy. Imaging findings are characterized by progressive unilateral brain atrophy and variable degrees of hyperintense signal within the affected hemisphere (Fig. 8-96A and B)

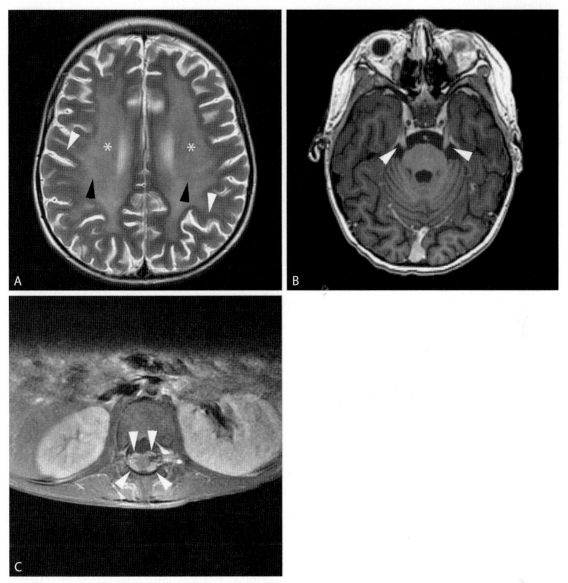

■ FIGURE 8-87 **Metachromatic leukodystrophy (MLD). A,** Axial T2-weighted sequence shows abnormal increased T2 signal within most of the cerebral white matter (*) with preservation of the subcortical U-fibers (*white arrowheads*). Note the dark bands of preserved signal giving the "tigroid" appearance (*black arrowheads*). **B,** Abnormal enhancement within the bilateral cranial nerve V (*arrowheads*). This patient had additional multiple abnormally enhancing cranial nerves which are not shown here. **C,** Abnormal enhancement within lumbar nerve roots (*arrowheads*).

■ TUMORS

Tumors of the CNS are the most common solid malignancies of childhood. On imaging, the differential diagnosis remains mostly based on the categorization of the tumors according to their anatomic location: posterior fossa, supratentorial, intraventricular, sellar–suprasellar, and pineal region. Radiogenomics is a growing field in radiology which attempts to reconcile the recent advances in tumor genetics and molecular phenotyping, which now guide prognosis and treatment. Radiogenomics is a somewhat new and complex topic that is beyond the scope of this book.

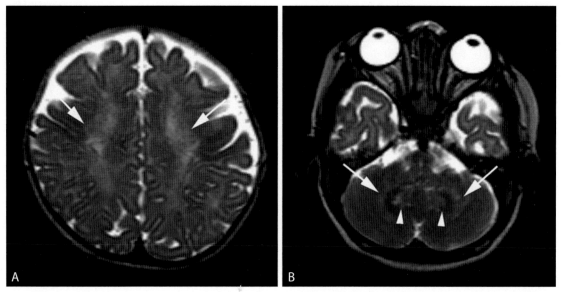

■ **FIGURE 8-88 Krabbe disease. A,** Axial T2-weighted sequence shows abnormal confluent hyperintense signal within the bilateral centrum semiovale (*arrows*). This pattern may be similar to the one seen in MLD. **B,** Axial T2-weighted sequence shows hyperintense signal within the bilateral deep dentate nucleus (*arrowheads*) and surrounding cerebellar white matter (*arrows*).

Posterior Fossa Tumors

Tumors of the posterior fossa are more common in childhood than in adulthood. The most common posterior fossa tumors in children include cerebellar astrocytoma, medulloblastoma, atypical teratoid rhabdoid tumor (ATRT), brainstem glioma, and ependymoma (Table 8-7). Posterior fossa tumors often present with obstructive hydrocephalus secondary to mass effect on the fourth ventricle and sylvian aqueduct.

CEREBELLAR ASTROCYTOMA

Cerebellar astrocytoma (pilocytic subtype) is the most common type of posterior fossa tumor. It is a low-grade malignancy and has the best prognosis of any CNS malignancy. Most require surgical treatment only, if full resection is achieved. The lesions occur most commonly in the cerebellar hemispheres. The classic appearance on imaging is a cystic cerebellar hemisphere mass with a peripheral enhancing nodule (Fig. 8-97). However, cerebellar astrocytomas can be predominantly cystic or completely solid in appearance (Fig. 8-98A and B). The margins of the lesions are usually well defined. The fourth ventricle is displaced, and the margin between

the lesion and the fourth ventricle is typically also well defined (see Figs. 8-97 and 8-98). Unlike medulloblastomas and ependymomas, cerebellar astrocytomas usually do not demonstrate areas of calcification or hemorrhage and do not demonstrate restriction on diffusion-weighted sequence. Differential diagnosis of a well-circumscribed cystic cerebellar mass with mural nodule in children includes medulloblastoma (which will show diffusion restriction within the solid component), rarely ganglioglioma and hemangioblastoma. Ganglioglioma is also a low-grade tumor; however, it is most commonly seen in the supratentorial compartment and may have calcifications. Hemangioblastoma tends to occur most commonly in the adult population but may be seen in older children, especially in the setting of VHL. Hemangioblastoma will show marked increase perfusion within the solid component.

MEDULLOBLASTOMA

Medulloblastoma is the second most common posterior fossa tumor in children and is the most malignant. On imaging, the lesion appears as a hypercellular mass within the posterior fossa demonstrating diffusion restriction on MRI and

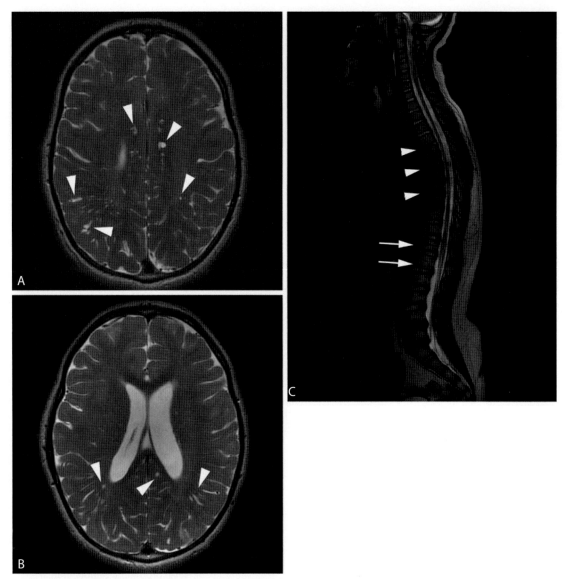

■ **FIGURE 8-89 Mucopolysaccharidosis. A,** Axial T2-we enlarged perivascular spaces, some of the marked by *arrowheads*. **B,** Axial T2-weighted sequence at the level of the lateral ventricles shows prominence of the ventricular system and additional enlarged perivascular spaces (*arrowheads*). **C,** Sagittal T2-weighted sequence of the spine shows multiple endplate deformities (*arrowheads*) and anterior vertebrae beaking (*arrows*). Note also craniocervical and lumbar spinal canal stenosis.

hyperdensity of CT (Fig. 8-99A—D). The most common location is within the fourth ventricle, often originating along the roof of the fourth ventricle, although it may be seen anywhere within the posterior fossa. Medulloblastomas tend to be more homogeneous in signal than cerebellar astrocytomas or ependymomas, but this is also variable. Solid-cystic medulloblastoma

can occur. In these cases, restricted diffusion within the solid component is key to the correct diagnosis. Spectroscopy may show elevated Tau at 3.3 ppm. There is a propensity for seeding within the intracranial and intraspinal CSF spaces (Fig. 8-100 and see Fig. 8-99D). Evaluation of the entire spine with contrast is necessary to rule out drop metastases.

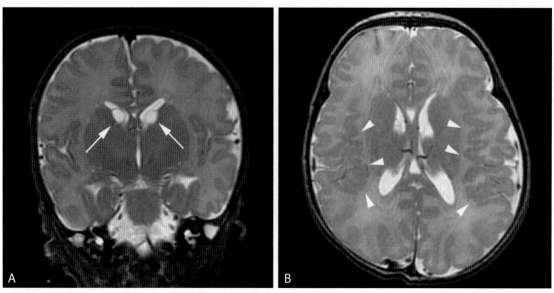

■ FIGURE 8·90 **Zellweger syndrome. A,** Coronal T2-weighted sequence shows bilateral subependymal germinolytic cysts (*arrows*). **B,** Axial T2-weighted sequence shows bilateral polymicrogyria (*arrowheads*).

	TABLE 8-6 Metabolic and Degenerative Disorders of the Central Nervous System			
Disorder	**Category of Disease**	**Primary Distribution of Abnormality**	**Key Imaging Features**
Leigh disease	Mitochondrial disorder	Deep gray matter	Bilateral symmetric signal abnormality involving the striatum (caudate and putamen), periaqueductal gray matter, substantia nigra, subthalamic nuclei, dorsal pons, and cerebellar nuclei
Glutaric aciduria type 1	Mitochondrial disorder	Deep gray matter	Basal ganglia signal abnormality, primarily involving the striatum (caudate and putamen) Enlarged operculum Bilateral prominent middle cranial fossa CSF spaces
Maple syrup urine disease	Amino acid disorder	Deep gray + white matter	Cytotoxic edema (hyperintense T2 signal and DWI restriction) during the first few days of life within the newborn myelinated areas: perirolandic, globus pallidus, thalami, dorsal brainstem, and cerebellar white matter MRS showing 0.9–1 ppm peak due to methyl group branched-chain ketoacids
Kearns–Sayre disease	Mitochondria disorder	Deep gray + white matter	Basal ganglia signal abnormality, primarily globus pallidus Involvement of subcortical U-fibers and cerebellum Sparing deep gray matter May have basal ganglia calcification

	TABLE 8-6		

Disorder	Category of Disease	Primary Distribution of Abnormality	Key Imaging Features
Cockayne	Miscellaneous metabolic disorder—nucleotide excision repair disease	Deep gray + white matter	Abnormal white matter myelination Progressive parenchymal atrophy Basal ganglia and cortical calcifications
MELAS (mitochondria encephalomyopathy with lactic acidosis and stroke)	Mitochondria disorder	Deep gray + white matter	Stroke-like episodes and parenchymal changes not always conforming to an arterial territory Basal ganglia calcifications Parenchymal atrophy
Canavan disease	Amino acid disorder	Deep gray + white matter	Diffuse white matter signal abnormality including peripheral white matter, sparing internal capsule, and corpus callosum Globus pallidi signal abnormality, sparing caudate and putamen Macrocephaly Increase NAA on MRS
Alexander disease	Miscellaneous metabolic disorder	White matter	Frontal predominance of white matter signal changes, including peripheral white matter Macrocephaly May demonstrate parenchymal enhancement
Megalencephaly leukoencephalopathy with subcortical cysts (MLC)	Miscellaneous metabolic disorder	White matter	Diffuse white matter signal changes Subcortical "cysts" (more common on temporal lobes) Macrocephaly
Pelizaeus–Merzbacher	Miscellaneous metabolic disorder—X-linked	White matter	Diffuse white matter hypomyelination due to absent myelin formation, including subcortical fibers and internal capsule
Adrenoleukodystrophy	Peroxisomal disorder	White matter	White matter demyelination, 80% posterior predominance along the peritrigonal regions May show peripheral enhancement surrounding the affected areas (leading edge of enhancement)
Vanishing white matter	Miscellaneous metabolic disorder	White matter	Extensive progressive white matter signal abnormality On later stages, white matter becomes similar to CSF
Metachromatic leukodystrophy	Lysosomal storage disorders	White matter	Confluent periventricular white matter signal changes Spare subcortical U-fibers until late disease Stripped appearance of affected white matter "tigroid" pattern (sparing periventricular myelin) May have enhancement of cranial nerves and cauda equina

Continued

Disorder	Category of Disease	Primary Distribution of Abnormality	Key Imaging Features
Krabbe disease	Lysosomal storage disorders	White matter	Initial involvement of the central white matter sparing subcortical U-fibers Involvement of the cerebellar white matter around dentate nucleus May have hyperintense basal ganglia and thalami on CT Enhancement of lumbar nerve roots occasionally present
Phenylketonuria	Amino acid disorder	White matter	White matter signal changes, initially periventricular and posterior predominance
Mucopolysaccharidosis	Lysosomal storage disorders	White matter	Multiple enlarged perivascular spaces White matter signal changes Parenchymal volume loss Ventriculomegaly Dysostosis multiplex affecting the spine (spinal canal stenosis, endplate irregularities, platyspondyly, bullet-shaped vertebrae/anterior beaking, and dehydrated disks)
Zellweger	Peroxisomal disorder	White matter	Abnormal myelination Polymicrogyria Periventricular germinolytic cysts May have associated liver and kidney abnormalities

CSF, Cerebrospinal fluid; *MRS*, magnetic resonance spectroscopy; *NAA*, N-acetylaspartate.

ATYPICAL TERATOID RHABDOID TUMOR

ATRTs are highly malignant tumors that tend to occur in young children, most commonly before the age of 3 years. Posterior fossa location is more common than supratentorial, pineal, or spinal. On imaging, ATRT is characterized by a hypercellular heterogeneous tumor demonstrating diffusion restriction (Fig. 8-101A and B). Intratumoral hemorrhage is also common. It may be difficult to differentiate ATRT from a medulloblastoma. ATRT should be considered in the differential diagnosis of medulloblastoma in patients below the age of 3 years.

BRAINSTEM GLIOMA

Brainstem gliomas are part of a group of astrocytomas involving the midline structures known as diffuse midline gliomas. They occur most often in the pons (diffuse intrinsic pontine glioma—DIPG). Unlike other posterior fossa masses, the lesions tend to present with cranial nerve abnormalities, pyramidal tract signs, or cerebellar dysfunction rather than with signs of hydrocephalus. The lesions usually cause circumferential enlargement of the brainstem. The lesions often surround the basilar artery when centered in the pons (Fig. 8-102A and B). Less commonly, the lesions can grow in an exophytic fashion. On MRI, the lesions tend to demonstrate a homogeneous high signal on T2-weighted images. Before treatment, enhancement is rare (see Fig. 8-102B). Exophytic lesions more commonly enhance. Approximately 10% of lesions have a cystic component. If displaced, the fourth ventricle is pushed posteriorly (see Fig. 8-102A). In the vast majority of these tumors, complete surgical resection is not possible. Radiation therapy remains the primary mode of therapy, although different types of chemotherapy agents and vaccines are currently being used in research trials.

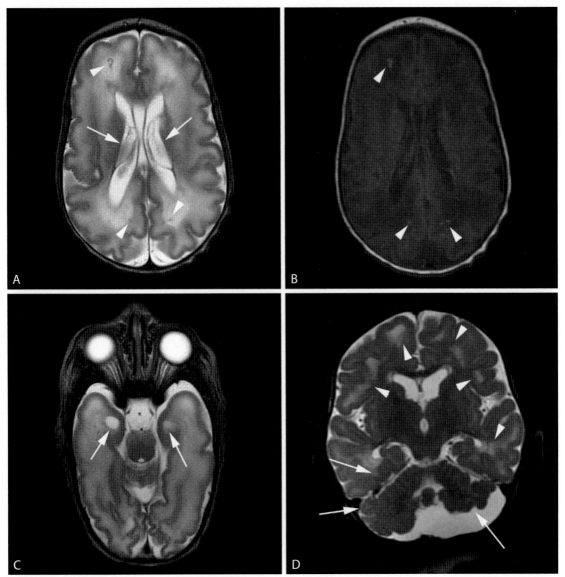

■ **FIGURE 8-91** **Sequelae of cytomegalovirus infection. A,** Axial T2-weighted sequence shows bilateral subependymal cysts (*arrows*) and few white matter calcifications (*arrowheads*). **B,** Axial T1-weighted sequence again shows scattered white matter calcifications (*arrowheads*). **C,** Lower image shows increased subcortical T2 signal within the bilateral temporal lobes with cystic changes (*arrows*). This finding is highly suggestive of CMV when congenital infection is suspected. **D,** Coronal T2-weighted sequence of a different patient shows patchy white matter signal abnormalities (*arrowheads*) and polymicrogyria (*arrows*).

EPENDYMOMA

Ependymomas are relatively slow-growing tumors that arise from the ciliated ependymal cells that line the ventricles. Two thirds occur in the fourth ventricle. When they occur in the fourth ventricle, ependymomas arise from and have a broad connection with the floor of the fourth ventricle, opposite from the more common roof involvement seen in medulloblastoma. Therefore, the border between the lesion and floor of the fourth ventricle is often poorly defined (Fig. 8-103A and B). The lesions may fill and grow out of the fourth ventricle via the foramina into the cisterna magna and spinal canal ("soft" or "plastic" tumor) (Fig. 8-104A and B). The lesions appear very heterogeneous and enhance heterogeneously on CT and MRI. Ependymomas have well-defined, lobulated margins. Calcifications are seen on CT in 50% −70% of cases (Fig. 8-103A).

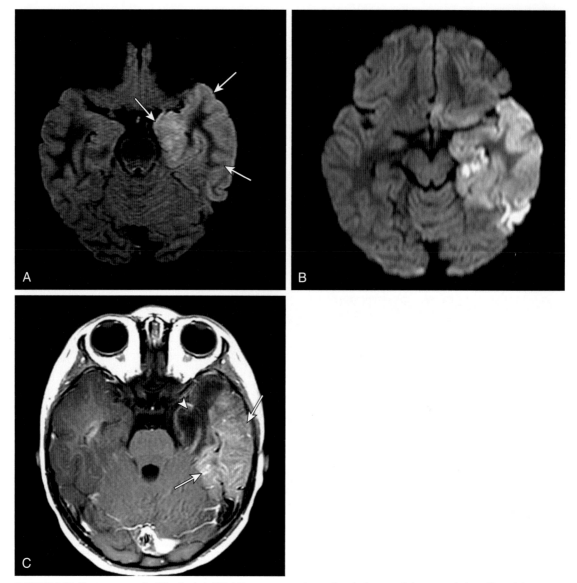

■ **FIGURE 8-92** **Herpes encephalitis.** **A,** Axial FLAIR sequence shows focal abnormal, increased signal involving most of the left temporal lobe (*arrows*). **B,** Restricted diffusion was noted on DWI sequence. **C,** Axial postcontrast T1-weighted sequence from a follow-up MRI demonstrates focal area of encephalomalacia (*arrowhead*) and abnormal peripheral enhancement of the reminder of the left temporal lobe (*arrows*), sequelae of prior infarct, and ischemia from herpes encephalitis.

Supratentorial Tumors

In children, supratentorial tumors are much less common than those of the posterior fossa. Most cerebral tumors affecting children are glial in origin (astrocytoma, oligodendroglioma, glioblastoma). Astrocytomas are the most common, varying from low to high grade and from well circumscribed to infiltrative. Imaging appearance does not always correlate with histologic grade. Low-grade, peripherally located tumors that involve the cerebral cortex and may act as an epileptogenic focus include ganglioglioma (Fig. 8-105A and B), Dysembryoplastic Neuro-epithelial Tumor (Fig. 8-106A and B), pleomorphic xanthoastrocytoma, angiocentric glioma, and less commonly oligodendroglioma. Desmoplastic infantile ganglioglioma (DIG) are large, solid-cystic tumors usually in children less than 1 year of age (Fig. 8-107A and B). Less common supratentorial tumors include embryonal tumors and ependymoma. Approximately half of the supratentorial ependymomas are extraventricular.

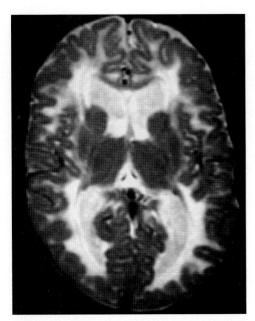

■ FIGURE 8-93 **Subacute sclerosing panencephalitis.** Axial T2-weighted MR image shows abnormal increased signal throughout periventricular white matter. There is associated volume loss and dilatation of the lateral ventricles.

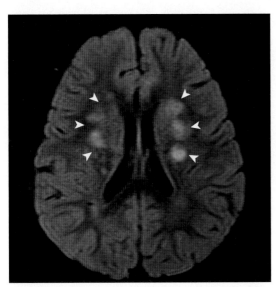

■ FIGURE 8-94 **Acute disseminated encephalomyelitis (ADEM) in a young child presenting with focal neurological symptoms and recent respiratory illness.** Axial FLAIR MR image shows multiple foci of abnormal, increased signal in the bilateral deep cerebral white matter (*arrowheads*). Other demyelinating diseases, such as multiple sclerosis, can have similar findings, and differentiation may be impossible based solely on imaging. Demographics, clinical history, and course of disease are usually necessary to reach a final diagnosis.

Intraventricular Tumors

Choroid plexus tumors are the most common intraventricular tumors in pediatrics and occur most commonly in the lateral ventricles. They are benign and slow growing in most cases (choroid plexus papilloma). However, there are malignant choroid plexus tumors (choroid plexus carcinoma) that often have similar imaging appearance to its benign counterpart but may demonstrate infiltration of the surrounding parenchyma or metastatic disease. These lesions are markedly vascular and demonstrate marked enhancement at imaging (Fig. 8-108). As previously mentioned, SEGAs are slow-growing tumors arising near the foramen of Monro in patients with TS and can cause hydrocephalus (Fig. 8-75). Intraventricular meningiomas are rare in pediatrics; however, they may mimic choroid plexus papilloma. Approximately half of the supratentorial ependymomas are located within the ventricles. Central neurocytomas and subependymomas are uncommon in children.

Sellar and Suprasellar Tumors

Although there is a long list of sellar and suprasellar tumors, the most common types in children include optic and hypothalamic astrocytoma, craniopharyngioma, and germ cell tumors.

OPTIC AND HYPOTHALAMIC ASTROCYTOMA

Optic and hypothalamic astrocytoma is one of the most common suprasellar tumors in childhood. They are typically low-grade pilocytic tumors, with pilomyxoid variant being less common. It can involve any or all portions of the visual pathway and hypothalamus. There is an increased incidence of optic pathway tumors in patients with NF-1 (Fig. 8-109). Optic nerve involvement is demonstrated as bulbous enlargement of the optic nerves with increased enhancement on MRI (see Fig. 8-69A−C). It is often difficult to differentiate optic gliomas of the chiasm from hypothalamic gliomas on MRI. Tumors arising in either location commonly extend into the other location. Both optic nerve and hypothalamic astrocytomas tend to be hyperintense on T2-weighted images and demonstrate heterogeneous enhancement of solid portions, sometimes difficult to differentiate from craniopharyngioma.

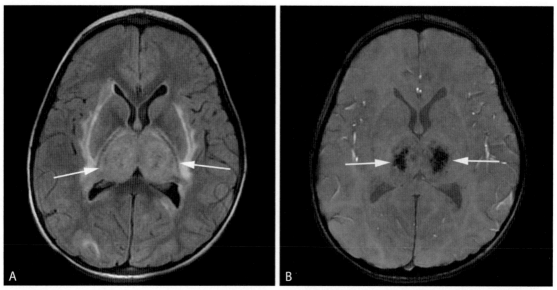

■ **FIGURE 8-95 Acute necrotizing encephalopathy. A,** Axial FLAIR sequence shows marked enlargement and signal abnormality within the bilateral thalami. Note also abnormal signal within the bilateral PLIC and extreme capsule. **B,** Gradient echo sequence shows associated bilateral thalamic hemorrhages (*arrows*).

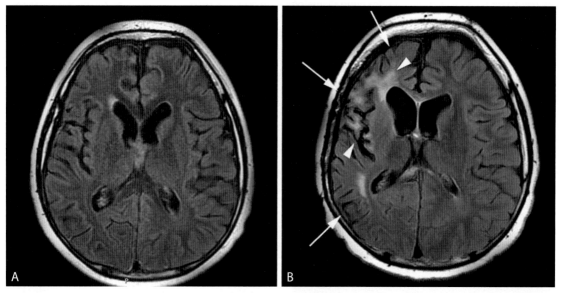

■ **FIGURE 8-96 Rasmussen encephalitis. A,** Axial FLAIR sequence shows mild diffuse volume loss without focal signal changes in a patient with refractory seizures. **B,** Follow-up imaging 1 year later shows marked progressive focal right anterior hemisphere volume loss (*arrows*) with abnormal underlying white matter signal (*arrowheads*).

GERM CELL TUMORS

Germ cell tumors of the CNS most commonly occur in the region of the pineal gland and/or suprasellar region (Fig. 8-110). Rarely they can be seen within the basal ganglia when metastatic. The most common histologic type is germinoma. Nongerminomatous types include teratoma, embryonal carcinoma, yolk sac tumor, and

TABLE 8-7	Posterior Fossa Tumors
Tumor	**Imaging Characteristics**
Cerebellar astrocytoma	Cystic and/or solid Most common presentation: cystic with mural nodule Mostly within cerebellar hemisphere, off-midline Well defined Fourth ventricle displaced, with well-defined interface No calcification or hemorrhage No diffusion restriction
Medulloblastoma	Mostly arises from fourth ventricle; poorly defined fourth ventricular roof interface Mostly a solid midline mass, but it can present off-midline Increase attenuation on CT Restricted diffusion on DWI sequences CSF metastasis may be present Elevated Tau at 3.3 ppm on spectroscopy
ATRT	Heterogeneous mostly solid mass Increase attenuation on CT Restricted diffusion on DWI sequences CSF metastasis may be present Younger age of presentation compared to medulloblastoma, mostly before 3 years of age
Brainstem glioma	Circumferential enlargement or exophytic mass of brainstem (most commonly pons), engulfing basilar artery Mostly nonenhancing Fourth ventricle pushed posteriorly Hydrocephalus uncommon
Ependymoma	Arises mostly from floor of fourth ventricle; poorly defined interface Mostly heterogeneous (hemorrhage, necrosis) midline mass "Plastic" tumor, tendency to extend through foramens magnum, Luschka, and Magendie Calcifications in 50%–70%

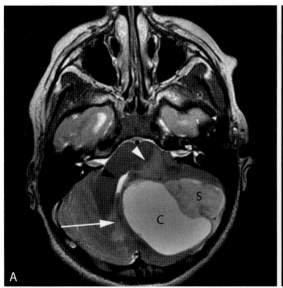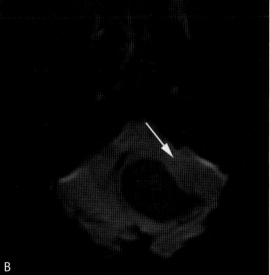

■ FIGURE 8-97 **Cerebellar pilocytic astrocytoma. A,** Axial T2-weighted sequence shows a large left-sided posterior fossa mass (*arrow*) with a cystic component (*c*) and a solid peripheral nodule (*s*). Note surrounding edema (*white arrowhead*) and laterally displaced fourth ventricle (*black arrowhead*) w. **B,** DWI sequence shows no diffusion restriction within the solid component of the mass (*arrow*).

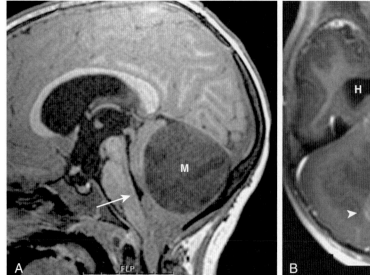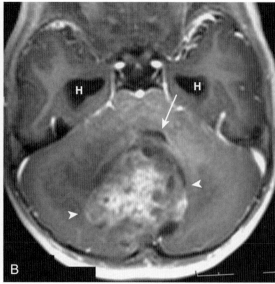

■ **FIGURE 8-98 Predominantly solid cerebellar pilocytic astrocytoma. A,** Sagittal T1-weighted MRI shows large, heterogeneous, relatively low-signal mass (*M*) seen within the cerebellar vermis. Note anterior displacement of fourth ventricle (*arrow*). The third ventricle is dilatated secondary to obstructive hydrocephalus. **B,** Axial postcontrast T1-weighted MRI shows heterogeneous enhancement of mass (*arrowheads*) and anterior displacement of fourth ventricle (*arrow*). Note the dilatated temporal horns of lateral ventricles (*H*), consistent with secondary obstructive hydrocephalus.

choriocarcinoma. Teratomas may demonstrate fatty tissue or calcifications. Germinomas are seen on MRI as an enhancing mass that may demonstrate diffusion restriction and CSF seeding. Sellar and suprasellar germinomas may present initially with an absent posterior pituitary T1 bright spot with or without thickening of pituitary stalk. Clinical symptoms may predate any findings on imaging. A synchronous enhancing mass in the pineal and suprasellar regions is highly suggestive of a germ cell tumor. Diabetes insipidus is a common clinical presentation in this scenario, and differential diagnoses including Langerhans cell histiocytosis (LCH) (Fig. 8-111). Other rare lesions presenting with homogeneous thickening or enhancing mass at the pituitary stalk include lymphocytic hypophysitis, lymphoma or leukemia, neurosarcoidosis, and pituicytoma.

CRANIOPHARYNGIOMA

Craniopharyngiomas arise from the persistence and proliferation of squamous epithelial cells within the tract of an embryologic structure, the craniopharyngeal duct. They account for 7% of all intracranial tumors in children. They are benign and slow-growing lesions. Typically, they are intrasellar and suprasellar in location. Rarely they can be infrasella/pharyngeal in location.

Calcifications are present in up to 80% of pediatric cases. Typically, CT shows a large, partially calcified suprasellar mass with both cystic and solid enhancing portions. On MRI, the cystic components tend to be high signal on all sequences because they contain proteinaceous and cholesterol-laden fluid (Fig. 8-112A–C). The signal characteristics of the solid portions are variable on MRI. If small and mostly intrasellar, it may be difficult to differentiate from a benign Rathke's cleft cyst. CT may be used to look for calcifications, not seen in Rathke's cleft cyst.

HYPOTHALAMIC HAMARTOMA

Hypothalamic hamartomas are actually considered a congenital gray matter heterotopia in the region of the tuber cinereum and mammillary bodies. It is described in this section because it presents as a suprasellar mass that should be differentiated from other neoplastic processes. This lesion may be sessile or pedunculated and presents clinically with seizures or precocious puberty. Gelastic seizures are classically associated with this lesion; however, this is not necessary the most common presentation. On imaging, this lesion is mostly isointense to gray matter and does not enhance (Fig. 8-113). If enhancement is seen, consider other pathologies such as a glioma.

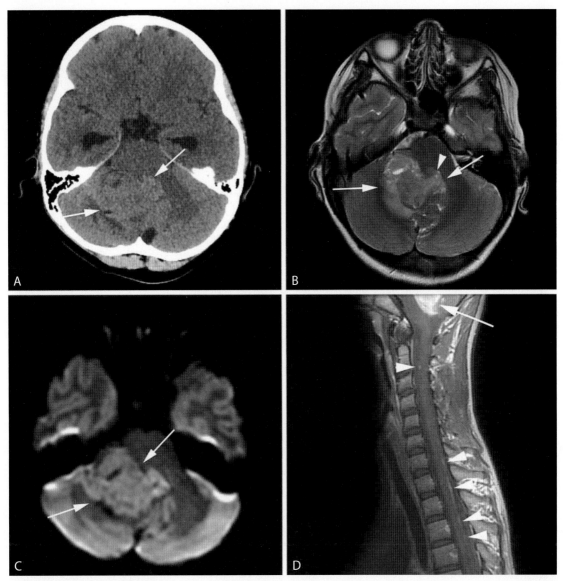

■ **FIGURE 8-99** **Medulloblastoma. A,** Noncontrasted axial CT shows a mostly solid mass within the posterior fossa (*arrows*). Note the increased attenuation suggestive of a high cellularity tumor. **B,** Axial T2-weighted MRI again demonstrates the large mass (*arrows*) which is located within rather than displacing the fourth ventricle (*arrowhead*). **C,** DWI sequence shows tumor diffusion restriction, suggesting a high cellularity/high-grade tumor (*arrows*). **D,** T1 postcontrast sagittal image of the cervical spine shows multiple linear and nodular foci of leptomeningeal enhancement compatible with drop metastasis (*arrowheads*). Partially imaged is the enhancing posterior fossa mass (*arrow*).

PINEAL TUMORS

The majority of pineal region neoplasms arise from germ cells (60%) or from pineal parenchyma (15%). Rarely ATRT, astrocytoma, ependymoma, and trilateral retinoblastoma may occur at this region. Pineal tumors arising from the pineal parenchyma range from benign pineocytomas to highly malignant pineoblastomas (Fig. 8-114A–C). Clinical presentation is most often related to mass effect and hydrocephalus with symptoms of headache, nausea, vomiting, or Parinaud syndrome. Pineal germ cell tumors are

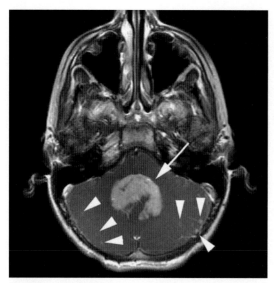

■ **FIGURE 8-100 Metastatic medulloblastoma.** Axial T1 postcontrast sequence of a patient with a medulloblastoma (*arrow*) showing multiple additional foci of leptomeningeal enhancement (*arrowheads*) compatible with leptomeningeal metastasis.

classified as germinomas or nongerminomatous. Symptoms may include precocious puberty. Germinomas and pineoblastomas are highly cellular tumors and often have similar imaging findings: isointense to hypointense T2 signal compared with gray matter, diffusion restriction on DWI, and CSF spread.

MISCELLANEOUS

Newly described "diffuse leptomeningeal glioneuronal tumor" does not conform to an anatomical location and therefore is described here separately. This tumor tends to involve the leptomeningeal surface of the brain and spine without intraparenchymal lesions. On imaging, it is characterized by leptomeningeal enhancement and innumerable cystic leptomeningeal lesions (Fig. 8-115A–D).

■ TRAUMA

Children with minor head trauma usually require no imaging. The evaluation of significant pediatric head trauma is usually performed by CT. New fast MRI sequences have been recently adopted for trauma evaluation in some organizations. Skull radiographs offer little useful information. The presence of a skull fracture does not necessarily indicate intracranial injury, and the absence of a skull fracture certainly does not exclude it. Finally, the presence or absence of a skull fracture usually does not affect the management of a child with head trauma.

Most of the CT findings in intracranial trauma, including subdural hematoma, epidural hematoma, subarachnoid hemorrhage, and parenchymal contusion, are similar in appearance in adults and children and are not discussed here.

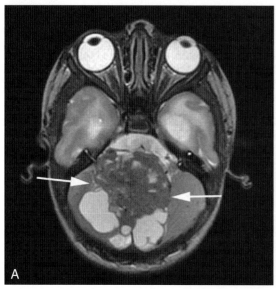
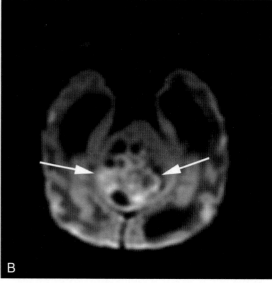

■ **FIGURE 8-101 Atypical teratoid rhabdoid tumor (ATRT) in a 2 month-old patient. A,** Axial T2-weighted sequence shows a large heterogeneous posterior fossa mass (*arrows*). **B,** DWI sequence shows diffusion restriction (*arrows*) compatible with a high-grade tumor. Imaging findings are indistinguishable from a medulloblastoma. The early age of presentation is highly suggestive of an ATRT.

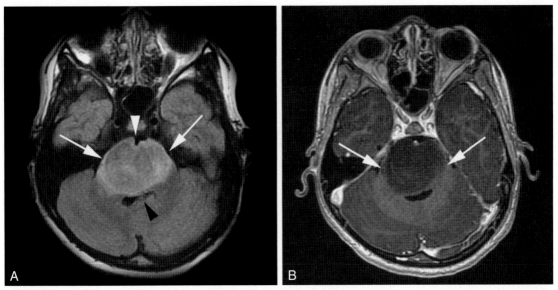

■ FIGURE 8-102 **Brainstem glioma. A,** Axial FLAIR sequence shows a large mass occupying and expanding the pons (*arrows*). Note the lesion engulfing the basilar artery (*white arrowhead*). Note compression of fourth ventricle (*black arrowhead*). **B,** Axial postcontrast T1-weighted MR image shows no enhancement (*arrows*).

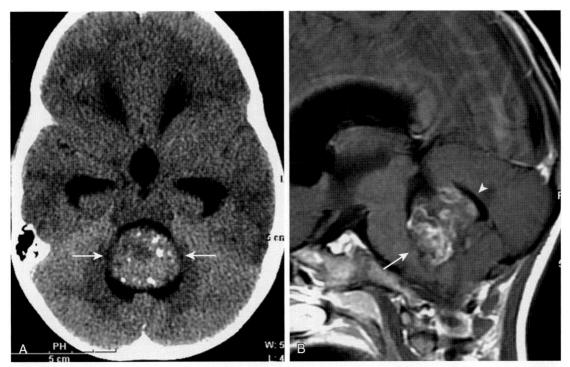

■ FIGURE 8-103 **Ependymoma in a 2-year-old child with headaches. A,** Axial, noncontrast CT shows heterogeneous but well-defined mass (*arrows*) with calcifications filling the fourth ventricle. **B,** Sagittal contrast-enhanced T1-weighted MR image shows mass with heterogeneous enhancement. The border between the brainstem and mass (*arrow*) is poorly defined, whereas the outline of the roof of the fourth ventricle (*arrowhead*) is well defined.

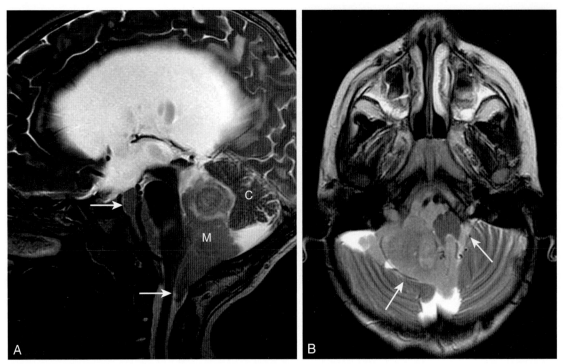

■ FIGURE 8-104 **Ependymoma. A,** Sagittal T2-weighted sequence shows a large midline posterior fossa mass (*M*) occupying the inferior fourth ventricle and displacing the cerebellum posteriorly (*C*). Note the tumor "plasticity" characterized by inferior extension through the foramen magnum and anterior extension via foramen of Luschka (*arrows*). **B,** Axial T2-weighted sequence of the same patient demonstrating the bilateral tumor extension thought the foramen of Luschka (*arrows*), right greater than left.

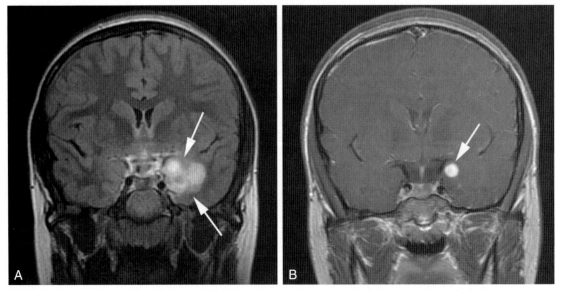

■ FIGURE 8-105 **Ganglioglioma. A,** Coronal FLAIR sequence shows a peripherally located cortically based hyperintense mass within the left mesial temporal lobe (*arrows*). **B,** T1 postcontrast shows nodular enhancement (*arrow*).

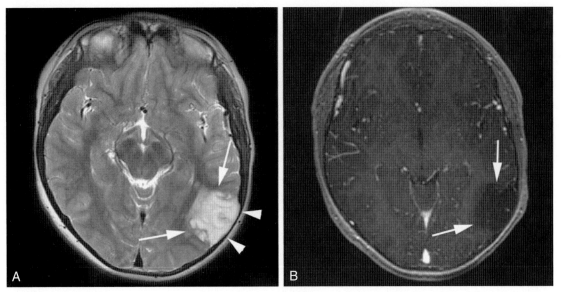

■ **FIGURE 8-106 Dysembryoplastic Neuroepithelial Tumor (DNET). A,** Axial T2-weighted sequence shows a cortically based mass (*arrows*) within the left temporoparietal region, demonstrating increased T2 signal. Note the "bubbly" appearance of the lesion and associated skull bony remodeling (*arrowheads*). **B,** T1 postcontrast shows no enhancement within the mass (*arrows*).

Abuse

For the most part, the imaging appearance of intracranial trauma that occurs secondary to abusive head injury (child abuse) is similar to that seen with accidental trauma. Therefore, imaging findings should be interpreted in the context of the clinical history. Intracranial injury is the number one cause of death in abused children. Types of injury that should increase the degree of suspicion for abuse include multiple/complex fractures and fractures crossing sutures, inter-hemispheric subdural hematoma (caused by shaking) (Fig. 8-116), and the combination of traumatic subdural or subarachnoid hematoma with anoxic–ischemic injury (Fig. 8-117A and B). Bridging veins thrombosis along the para-sagittal vertex is a frequent finding in child abuse, although nonspecific. When a bridging vein is thrombosed and there is a small collection of subarachnoid blood adjacent to it, this is known as the "tadpole sign" or "lollipop sign" (Fig. 8-118). Subdural hemorrhages of varying ages, as shown on CT or MRI, are also highly suggestive of abuse (Fig. 8-119A–C). Spine imaging have become an important part of the evaluation of child abuse. MRI is the imaging modality of choice demonstrating mostly ligamentous injury (more commonly at the craniocervical junction due to whiplash injury while shaking) and

subdural blood (Fig. 8-120), which can extend inferiorly from intracranial compartment. Other findings include spinal fractures, epidural hematomas (reflecting focal injury), and spinal cord/ nerve injury.

■ HYDROCEPHALUS AND VENTRICULAR SHUNTS

Hydrocephalus is a problem commonly encountered in pediatric neuroimaging. It may be secondary to overproduction (choroid plexus papilloma or choroid villous hyperplasia), disturbances of CSF flow or absorption (tumors or cysts, infection, hemorrhage, or genetic causes), or the result of loss of ventricular wall compliance. A common cause of prenatally diagnosed hydrocephalus is aqueduct stenosis, which can be acquired or developmental (Fig. 8-121A–C). Patients with hydrocephalus are often treated by the placement of ventricular shunts. The most commonly used shunt is the ventriculoperitoneal (VPS), in which the proximal portion of the shunt is positioned in one of the lateral ventricles, and the distal end is positioned in the peritoneal cavity. When a patient with a VPS presents with headaches, vomiting, or lethargy, increased intracranial pressure resulting from VPS malfunction should be investigated.

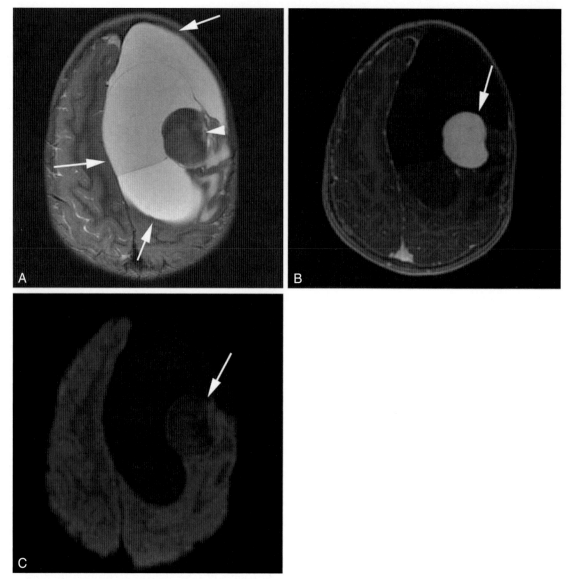

■ FIGURE 8-107 **Desmoplastic infantile ganglioglioma (DIG). A,** Axial T2-weighted sequence shows a large cystic mass (*arrows*) with a hypointense solid component (*arrowhead*) near the meningeal surface. **B,** T1 postcontrast shows avid enhancement within the solid component (*arrow*). **C,** DWI sequence shows no diffusion restriction in this low-grade tumor (*arrow*).

Imaging includes radiographs of the shunt from cranium to abdomen (shunt series) to ensure that there is no evidence of shunt disconnection or kinking. The most common site for shunt dislocation is at the connection between the shunt tubing and shunt reservoir (Fig. 8-122), which usually overlies the cranium. The shunt may still function if there is chronic disconnection lined by fibrin sheath. Therefore, clinical correlation and evaluation of ventricular size is important to determine shunt malfunction. Familiarity with the various types of commercially available shunts is important because some types have radiolucent portions that could be mistaken for areas of disconnection.

Fast MRI utilizing single shot fast spin echo sequences is the exam of choice in the evaluation of shunt malfunction, looking for interval changes in ventricular size (Fig. 8-123A and B). Low-dose head CT may be an alternative if MRI is

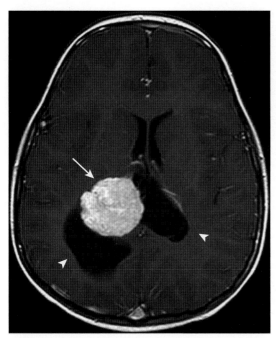

■ FIGURE 8-108 **Choroid plexus papilloma.** Axial post-contrast T1-weighted image shows homogeneously enhancing mass (*arrow*) within the posterior horn of the right lateral ventricle. There is associated enlargement of the bilateral posterior lateral ventricles (*arrowheads*).

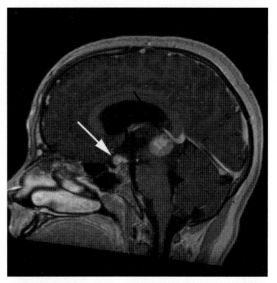

■ FIGURE 8-110 **Germ cell tumor.** Sagittal T1postcontrast sequence shows synchronous enhancing masses within the suprasellar region (*white arrow*) and pineal region (*black arrow*).

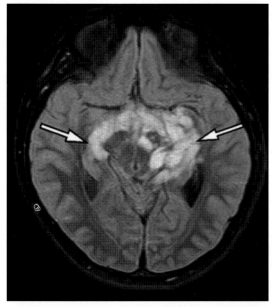

■ FIGURE 8-109 **Optic pathway glioma.** Axial FLAIR sequence shows a large mass involving the optic chiasm and optic radiations (*arrows*) in a patient with NF-1.

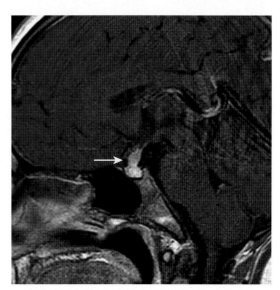

■ FIGURE 8-111 **Langerhans cell histiocytosis.** Sagittal postcontrast T1-weighted sequence shows an enlarged pituitary stalk (*arrow*). This patient was confirmed to have LCH. Aside from classic skull lesions and pituitary stalk abnormalities, intracranial findings of LCH also include choroid plexus masses and cerebellar white matter demyelination (not shown).

contraindicated or not available. Symptoms are most often related to insufficient shunting with interval increase in ventricular size but can occasionally be secondary to overshunting, which produces slit-like ventricles. An abdominal pseudocyst

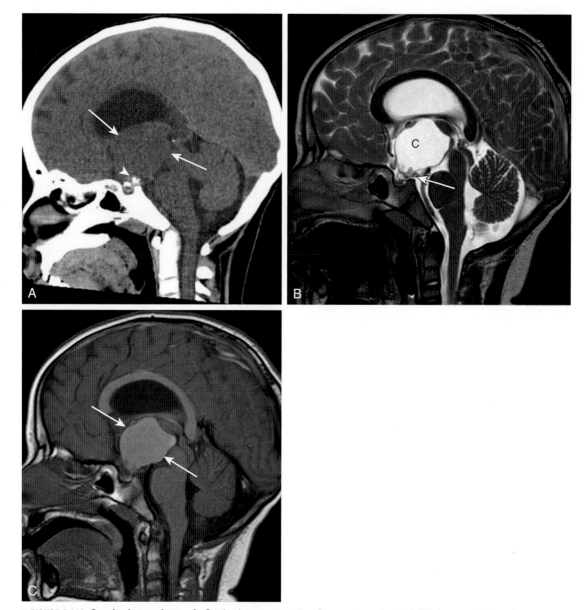

■ **FIGURE 8-112 Craniopharyngioma. A,** Sagittal reconstruction from noncontrasted CT demonstrates a large supra-sellar mass extending into the superior aspect of the sella. The mass is composed of a large cyst with proteinaceous components (*arrows*) and a smaller solid component inferiorly with internal calcifications (*arrowhead*). **B,** Sagittal T2-weighted sequence MR image again shows the large cystic component (*C*) and smaller solid component (*arrow*). **C,** Note the increased signal on noncontrasted T1-weighted sequence due to proteinaceous contents (*arrows*).

surrounding and obstructing the intraabdominal tip of the VPS is also a possibility. This may be suspected when interval radiographs demonstrate a static position of the distal shunt tubing. Further investigation for VPS pseudocysts is usually performed using ultrasound.

■ CRANIOSYNOSTOSIS

Craniosynostosis is the premature closure of the skull sutures. It can occur as an idiopathic, primary condition, or it can be secondary to a number of genetic disorders. The sagittal suture

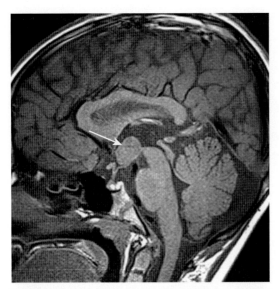

■ FIGURE 8-113 **Hypothalamic hamartoma.** Sagittal noncontrast T1-weighted sequence shows a midline hypothalamic mass (*arrow*) centered at the expected location of the tuber cinereum and mammillary bodies. The mass is isointense to the brain parenchyma and did not enhance after contrast administration (postcontrast not shown).

is most common suture involved in isolated primary synostosis. Because the skull stops growing in the direction of the closed suture and continues to grow in the directions of the open sutures, craniosynostosis of a particular suture leads to a predictable abnormal head shape on physical exam and on imaging. With sagittal suture synostosis, the head becomes long and narrow (dolichocephaly or scaphocephaly) (Fig. 8-124A and B). With bilateral coronal or lambdoid suture synostosis, the head becomes short from anterior to posterior and is wide from left to right (brachycephaly). The orbits in coronal synostosis assume an oval, oblique lateral margin that is referred to as a harlequin eye appearance (Fig. 8-125). With metopic suture craniosynostosis, the forehead assumes a pointed or triangular appearance (trigonocephaly; Fig. 8-126A and B), and the eyes are usually hypoteloric. The metopic suture can be fused normally as early as 6 months of age. Plagiocephaly refers to an asymmetric skull shape that can be seen with unilateral coronal and unilateral lambdoid suture synostosis (Fig. 8-127A) or, more commonly, the result of positional molding with no synostosis (Fig. 8-127B). Positional

molding occurs due to preferential sleep positions in young infants. Synostosis of all of the sutures results in cloverleaf skull (kleeblattschädel). There is severe deformity of the skull, with bulging in the squamosal areas and in the bregma. It is associated with thanatophoric dysplasia.

When multiple sutures are fused, a genetic cause is suspected. Genetic causes of craniosynostosis are largely due to mutations affecting the fibroblast growth factor receptor (FGFR) and include the following syndromes: Apert (Fig. 8-128A and B), Crouzon (see Fig. 8-130), Pfeiffer, Muenke, Beare—Stevenson, and Jackson—Weiss syndromes as well as Thanatophoric dysplasia. FGFR mutations also cause abnormal gyration of the temporal lobes. Syndromic craniosynostosis may present also with narrowing of the skull base/foramen magnum, hydrocephalus, and venous hypertension.

The screening examination for craniosynostosis may be done by radiography, although low-dose CT with three-dimensional surface-rendered reconstruction of the skull is the preferred method of evaluation. In addition to the characteristic skull shapes, imaging may demonstrate complete or partial closure of the suture, bony ridging, and perisutural sclerosis.

■ LACUNAR SKULL

Lacunar skull, or lückenschädel, is a defect in the mesenchymal formation of the skull that is associated with myelomeningocele. The radiographic findings include multiple oval lucencies that occur secondary to the thinning of the inner table of the skull (Fig. 8-129) and are more prominent in the occipital and parietal regions. It is present in patients with myelomeningocele under 3 months of age. The imaging findings typically resolve by 6 months of age. Lacunar skull should not be confused with the skull changes related to increased intracranial pressure (Fig. 8-130A—D). With increased intracranial pressure, there is marked accentuation of the normal convolutional markings. The appearance has been likened to hammer-beaten silver. Personally, the authors think that they appear rather similar, with lacunar skull appearing more severe. Other radiographic findings of increased intracranial pressure include sutural diastasis, sellar enlargement, and demineralization.

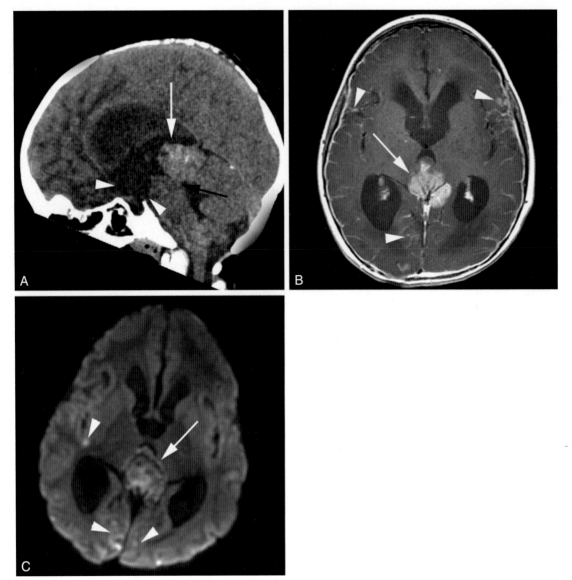

■ **FIGURE 8-114 Pineoblastoma. A,** Sagittal view of a noncontrast head CT shows a large hyperdense mass within the pineal region (*withe arrow*). The mass is causing marked narrowing of the cerebral aqueduct (*black arrow*). Note findings of obstructed ventriculomegaly characterized by dilatation of the inferior third ventricular recesses (*arrowheads*). **B,** Postcontrast sequence of the same patient shows the mass (*arrow*) and diffuse leptomeningeal metastasis with few leptomeningeal nodules marked by *arrowheads*. **C,** DWI sequence shows diffusion restriction within the mass (*arrow*) and leptomeningeal metastasis (*arrowheads*) compatible with a high-grade tumor.

■ CONGENITAL EAR MALFORMATIONS

External Auditory Canal Atresia

External auditory canal atresia (aural atresia) is characterized by partial or complete atresia of the external auditory canal associated with different degrees of microtia. The atresia can be osseous or membranous depending on the presence or absence of a bony plate at the expected level of the external auditory canal. Associated abnormalities may include variable hypoplasia of the middle ear cavity, ossicular dysplasia, ossicular fusion to the atretic plate, and anterior anomalous course of the facial nerve. It can be isolated or syndromic.

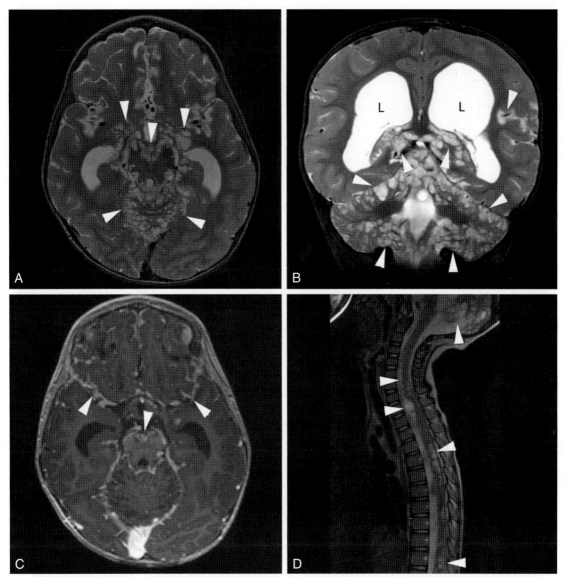

■ FIGURE 8-115 **Diffuse leptomeningeal glioneuronal tumor (DLGNT). A,** Axial T2-weighted sequence shows innumerous cystic lesions along the leptomeningeal surface of the brain, a few of them marked here by *arrowheads*. **B,** Coronal T2-weighted sequence again showing the multiple leptomeningeal lesions (*arrowheads*) and enlarged lateral ventricles (*L*). **C,** Postcontrast sequence shows diffuse leptomeningeal enhancement (*arrowheads*). **D,** Note similar lesions extending along the spinal leptomeningeal surfaces, few lesions marked by *arrowheads*.

Inner Ear Anomalies

The severity of inner ear abnormalities depends on the gestational age in which the insult happened. The spectrum of inner ear malformations includes cochlear aplasia, common cavity deformity, incomplete partitioned type I, incomplete partitioning type II, and incomplete

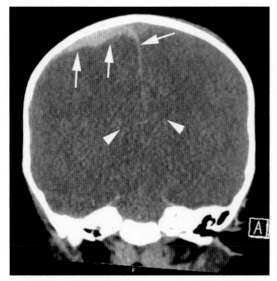

■ FIGURE 8-116 **Child abuse.** Coronal noncontrasted CT image shows increased attenuation along the falx and right convexity (*arrows*), compatible with subdural blood. This is nonspecific, but subdural hemorrhage is frequently seen in child abuse. Note also the small size of the lateral ventricles (*arrowheads*) due to cerebral edema.

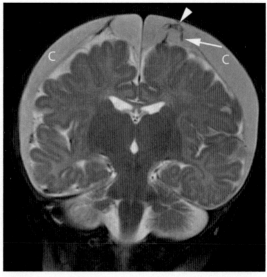

■ FIGURE 8-118 **Child abuse.** Coronal T2-weighted sequence shows bilateral subdural collections (*c*) and thrombosis of bridging veins, one (*arrow*) of which has adjacent focal hemorrhage (*arrowhead*). This appearance has been described as "tadpole" sign.

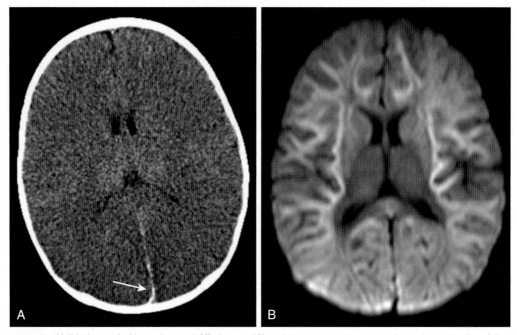

■ FIGURE 8-117 **Child abuse. A,** Nonenhanced CT shows diffuse low attenuation throughout the majority of the brain parenchyma with loss of gray–white matter differentiation. Findings are consistent with edema and infarction, related to asphyxia. There is also high attenuation along the right aspect of the posterior falx (*arrow*), consistent with subdural hemorrhage. **B,** Diffusion MR image shows diffuse parenchymal diffusion restriction.

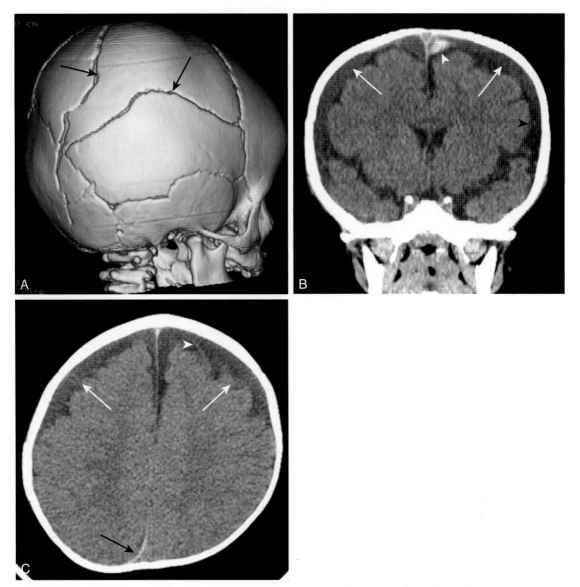

■ FIGURE 8-119 **Child abuse, subdural hematomas of varying ages. A,** Volume-rendered, three-dimensional reformat from noncontrasted CT shows a complex parietal skull fracture (*arrows*). **B,** Coronal reformat demonstrates bilateral subacute subdural hemorrhage along the convexities (*arrows*). There is also a more acute hemorrhage along the left parasagittal subdural space (*white arrowhead*). Note the medially displaced cortical vein (*black arrowhead*), a finding that may help in the detection of a low attenuation or chronic subdural collection. **C,** Axial CT image of the same patient again shows bilateral subacute subdural hemorrhages (*white arrows*), as well as a small amount of acute blood along the posterior falx (*black arrow*). Note a bridging vein traversing the subdural collection on the right frontal region (*arrowhead*). Bridging veins drain into the superior sagittal sinus and transverse the subdural space; therefore, they can be seen within a subdural collection, usually along the superior and anterior midline regions. This should not be confused with the smaller and more numerous cortical vessels present in the subarachnoid spaces that do not transverse the subdural space and are usually displaced medially by a subdural collection (see **B**).

partitioning type III. Cochlear aplasia is characterized by complete absence of cochlear structures with different degrees of dysplasia of the vestibule and semicircular canals. Differential diagnosis of cochlear aplasia includes labyrinthitis ossificans, a complication of meningitis leading to progressive ossification of the labyrinthine structures (Fig. 8-131). Common cavity

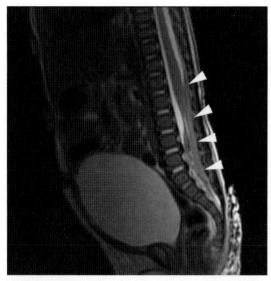

■ FIGURE 8-120 **Child abuse.** Sagittal T2-weighted sequence of the spine of an infant with intracranial findings of child abuse showing blood (*arrowheads*) along the posterior lumbar subdural space.

deformity demonstrates lack of separation between the cochlea and the vestibule. Incomplete partitioning type I is characterized by a cystic featureless cochlear (Fig. 8-132). Incomplete partitioning type II (formerly known as Mondini deformity) is often associated with an enlarged vestibular aqueduct. It is the most common cause of sensorineural hearing loss (SNHL) in the pediatric population. On imaging, there is incomplete cochlear partitioning with an absent interscalar septum and spiral lamina leading to a bulbous coalescent middle and apical turns (Fig. 8-133A and B). This malformation can be associated with Pendred syndrome. Incomplete partitioning type III is a rare genetic inner ear malformation also known as X-linked deafness. On imaging, there is absence of the modiolus with a present interscalar septa and a dilated distal internal auditory canal (IAC) (Fig. 8-134).

Cochlear Nerve Aplasia/Hypoplasia

Cochlear nerve aplasia or hypoplasia is an important cause of congenital profound SNHL. On CT, there is small size of the IAC and small or absent cochlear aperture (Fig. 8-135A). On MRI, there is absent or hypoplastic size of the cochlear nerve, best seen on oblique sagittal steady-state free precession sequences (axial view of the IAC) (Fig. 8-135B and C).

■ ORBITAL AND FACIAL DEVELOPMENTAL ANOMALIES

The most common orbital and facial developmental anomalies and their imaging findings are listed on Table 8-8. Representative images are shown in (Figs. 8-136—8-143).

■ HEAD AND NECK INFLAMMATORY AND INFECTIOUS PROCESSES

Orbital Cellulitis

Orbital cellulitis is the most common abnormality of the pediatric orbit. It is most commonly due to a bacterial infection that arises from extension of sinus disease. Orbital cellulitis is categorized anatomically as being preseptal or postseptal on the basis of the relationship between the inflamed tissue and the orbital septum. Preseptal tissue is limited to the eyelid. When inflammation extends posterior to the septum, it is considered to be postseptal and typically involves the extraconal tissues, sometimes with the formation of a subperiosteal abscess (Fig. 8-144A and B). Almost all cases of postseptal cellulitis are associated with ethmoid sinus disease (see Fig. 8-144) and may present clinically with ophthalmoplegia and visual loss. The presence of a drainable abscess is suggested on CT when rim enhancement is present surrounding an area of fluid attenuation with or without gas. Drainable abscesses are typically treated surgically. Cellulitis without abscess is treated with antibiotics alone. Less frequent complications of postseptal cellulitis include thrombosis of the ophthalmic vein and cavernous sinus (Fig. 8-145A and B). When sinus disease involves the frontal sinus, complications may include frontal bone osteomyelitis with frontal soft tissue abscess formation ("Pott puffy tumor"; Fig. 8-146A and B) and intracranial empyema.

Acute Otomastoiditis

Acute otomastoiditis is a complication of otitis media. Clinical presentation may include fever, otalgia, otorrhea, mastoid tenderness, and auricular proptosis. Imaging findings include middle ear and mastoid opacification with associated edema of the superficial retroauricular soft tissues (Fig. 8-147A and B). Complications include retroauricular subperiosteal abscess,

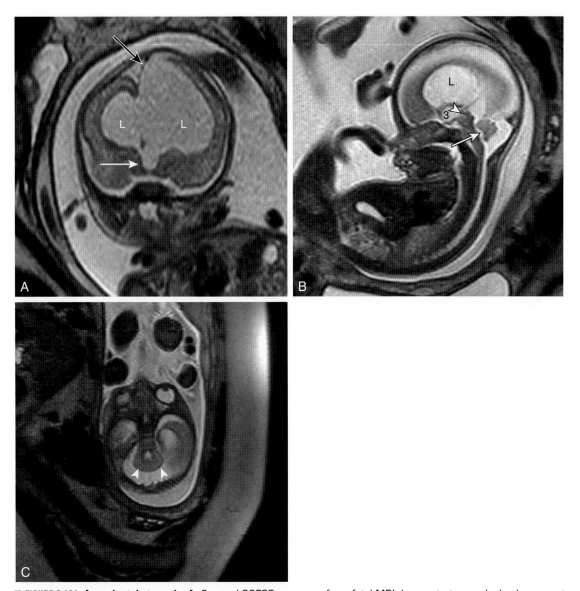

■ **FIGURE 8-121** **Aqueductal stenosis. A,** Coronal SSFSE sequence from fetal MRI demonstrates marked enlargement of the lateral (*L*) and third (*white arrow*) ventricles. Note also the focal absence of left high parasagittal cerebral parenchyma covering the enlarged lateral ventricle (*black arrow*). This is compatible with a ventricular diverticulum often seen in cases of marked prenatal hydrocephalus, most commonly due to aqueductal stenosis. **B,** Sagittal view of a different fetus shows also an enlarged lateral (*L*) and third (*3*) ventricles with normal size of the fourth ventricle (*arrow*). Note also the "funnel" shape of the aqueduct (*arrowhead*) due to inferior aqueductal obstruction or stenosis. **C,** Axial image from same fetal MRI as shown in **B** also shows posterior fossa findings of rhombencephalosynapsis (RES). Note the small transverse cerebellar diameter, absence of cerebellar vermis, and cerebellar hemisphere fusion (*arrowheads*). Although the etiology of aqueductal stenosis is multifactorial and may be secondary to infection and/or hemorrhage, careful evaluation of other fetal anatomical structures, especially the posterior fossa, is important to exclude associated malformations and genetic syndromes. RES is not uncommonly associated with aqueduct stenosis. Cobblestone malformations and X-linked hydrocephalus (in a male fetus) are also potential associated abnormalities.

erosion of mastoid septations (coalescent otomastoiditis) or bony walls, intracranial empyema or abscess, and dural sinus thrombosis (see Fig. 8-147A and B). Isolated opacification of middle ear and mastoid air cells without soft tissue edema or other complications is a common finding in pediatrics and should not be interpreted as acute otomastoiditis. More aggressive

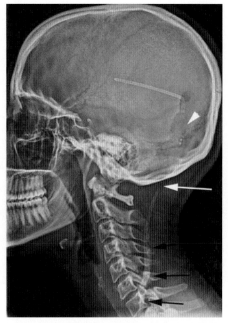

FIGURE 8-122 Ventriculoperitoneal shunt disconnection. A, Lateral view of skull from shunt series shows normal radiolucent shunt reservoir (*arrowhead*) and a focal area of shunt disconnection (*white arrow*) just below the reservoir. Note also fibrin sheet surrounding the shunt tubing within the proximal neck (*black arrows*).

pathologies presenting with soft tissue attenuation and mastoid bony erosions include disorders such as LCH (Fig. 8-148A and B), rhabdomyosarcoma, and cholesteatoma and are part of the differential diagnosis of acute coalescent otomastoiditis.

Suppurative Adenitis

Acute suppurative adenitis in the cervical region is a complication of upper respiratory tract bacterial infection, resulting in lymph node enlargement and suppurative changes that can evolve to abscess formation (Fig. 8-149). Abscess as a result of suppurative adenitis occurs commonly in the lateral retropharyngeal spaces (see Chapter 2). Ultrasound is often the initial imaging study to determine whether a drainable fluid collection is present in superficial neck lymphadenopathy. CT can also be used and is the imaging test of choice for suspected retropharyngeal adenitis or abscess. Acute bacterial suppurative adenitis demonstrates marked associated inflammatory changes of the surrounding soft tissues. This is an important differentiating characteristic from mycobacterial infections, especially atypical mycobacteria. Atypical mycobacteria infection also demonstrates central lymph node necrosis; however, it tends to have

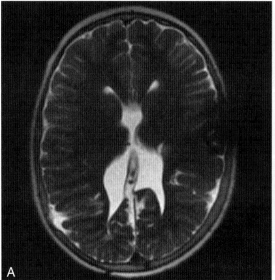

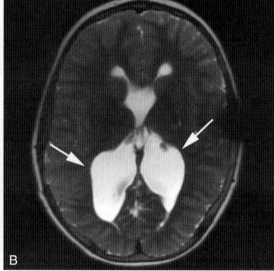

FIGURE 8-123 Ventriculoperitoneal shunt malfunction. A, Axial T2 Single Shot Fast Spin Echo sequence shows the baseline size of the lateral ventricles in a patient with ventriculoperitoneal shunt in place. **B,** Follow-up exam shows interval increase in size of lateral ventricles (*arrows*) in a symptomatic patient, consistent with shunt malfunction.

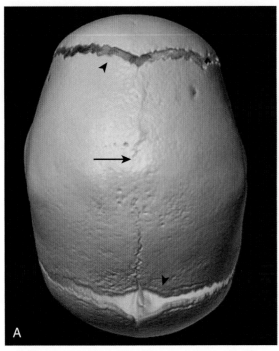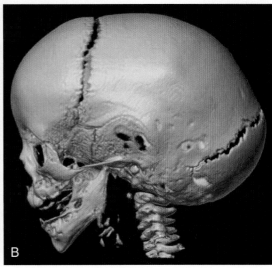

■ FIGURE 8-124 **Sagittal suture synostosis. A,** Volume-rendered, three-dimensional CT image of the skull shows early fusion of sagittal suture (*arrow*), as well as diastatic coronal and lambdoid sutures (*arrowheads*). **B,** Note the increased anteroposterior dimension of the skull (scaphocephaly or dolichocephaly).

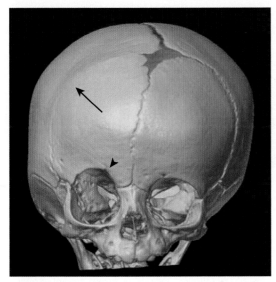

■ FIGURE 8-125 **Unilateral coronal synostosis.** Volume-rendered, three-dimensional CT image shows early fusion of the right coronal suture (*arrow*). Note also "harlequin eye" (*arrowhead*).

minimal associated inflammatory changes. When present, the inflammation tends to involve mostly the superficial soft tissues and has a typical skin discoloration (Fig. 8-150A and B).

■ RETINOBLASTOMA

Retinoblastoma is a malignant tumor that arises in the retina and may invade the optic nerve. It typically presents in children younger than 5 years of age. It is bilateral in as many as 25% of cases and can also rarely involve the pineal region (trilateral retinoblastoma) and suprasellar region (quadrilateral retinoblastoma). In bilateral cases, there is often a genetic predisposition. Patients with retinoblastoma are also predisposed to secondary osteosarcoma after radiation therapy. On CT, retinoblastoma typically appears as a calcified, intraocular mass (Fig. 8-151A–C). MRI demonstrates a heterogeneous intraocular mass of variable enhancement.

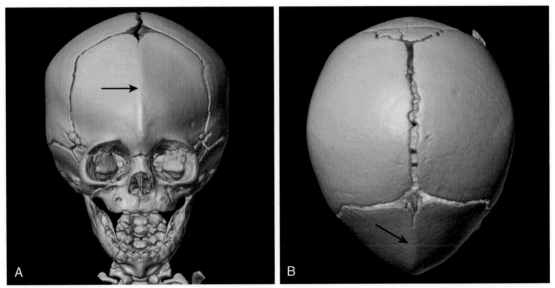

■ FIGURE 8-126 **Metopic synostosis. A,** Volume-rendered, three-dimensional CT shows fusion of the metopic suture with associated bony ridging (*arrow*). **B,** Superior view again shows fusion of the metopic suture (*arrow*), as well as triangular shape of the forehead (trigonocephaly).

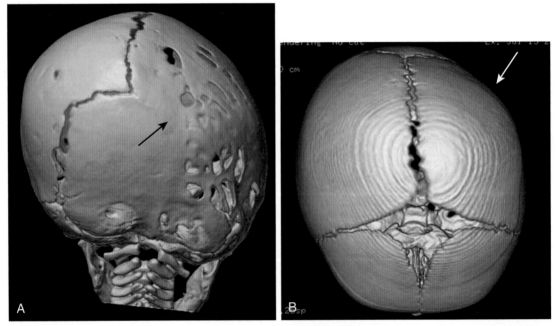

■ FIGURE 8-127 **Plagiocephaly. A,** Volume-rendered, three-dimensional CT image shows unilateral lambdoid suture synostosis (*arrow*) causing asymmetric posterior skull flattening of the involved side. **B,** Different patient showing positional plagiocephaly seen as an asymmetric flattening of the left occipital region (*arrow*) with no craniosynostosis (note patent skull sutures).

There are a variety of other causes of intra-orbital masses, the most common of which are listed in Table 8-9. The differential diagnosis can be limited on the basis of the location of the mass: globe, intraconal, or extraconal. Aggressive lesions involving the orbital rim include metastatic neuroblastoma (Fig. 8-152A and B), rhabdomyosarcoma, and LCH.

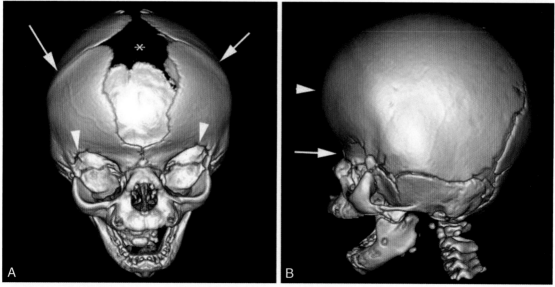

■ FIGURE 8-128 **Syndromic craniosynostosis, Apert syndrome. A,** Volume-rendered, three-dimensional CT shows fusion of the bilateral coronal sutures (*arrows*) in this patient with Apert syndrome (FGFR 2 gene mutation). Note also bilateral "harlequin eyes" (*arrowheads*). **B,** Lateral view of volume-rendered three-dimensional reconstruction shows deep nasal bridge (*arrow*) and an elongated forehead with frontal bossing (*arrowhead*). This patient had also syndactyl (not shown), another characteristic of Apert syndrome.

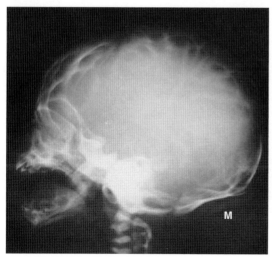

■ FIGURE 8-129 **Lacunar skull in an infant with ence-phalocele.** Radiograph shows multiple oval lucencies. The encephalocele can be seen as a subtle posterior soft tissue mass (*M*).

■ NECK MASSES

There are a large number of causes of pediatric neck masses (Table 8-10). The most common cause is suppurative lymphadenitis (see Fig. 8-149).

Of pediatric malignancies, 5% occur in the head and neck. Most malignant lesions present as painless masses. The head and neck area is one of the most common sites, along with the genito-urinary tract, for rhabdomyosarcoma to occur. Rhabdomyosarcoma typically presents in the preschool age child. In older children, lymphoma is most common, presenting with malignant lymphadenopathy.

A number of congenital lesions can present with palpable neck masses, including branchial cleft cyst (Figs. 8-153 and 8-154), thyroglossal duct cyst (Fig. 8-155A and B), lingual thyroid (Fig. 8-156), laryngocele, thymic cyst, lymphatic malformation, and dermoid or epidermoid. Branchial cleft cysts can persist from any of the developmental branchial arches, but those arising from the second branchial cleft are the most common. Typically, second branchial cleft cysts occur near the angle of the mandible—posterolateral to the submandibular gland, lateral to the carotid space, and anterior or anteromedial to the sternocleidomastoid muscle (see Fig. 8-153).

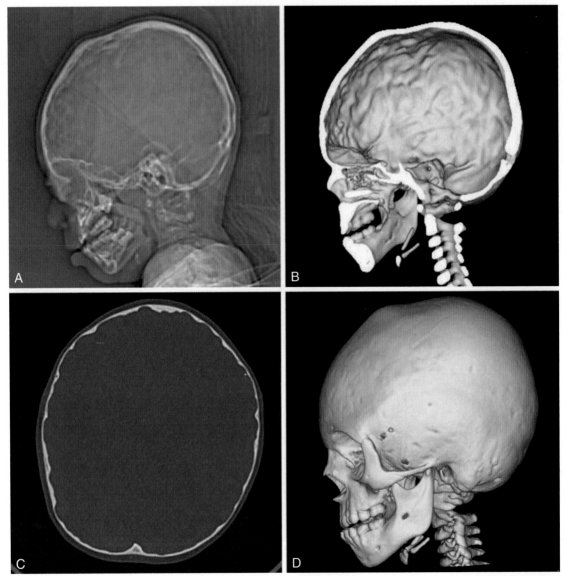

■ **FIGURE 8-130 Skull changes in increased intracranial pressure. A–C,** Head CT shows accentuation of convolutional markings on scout view (**A**), volume-rendered three-dimensional reconstruction (**B**) and axial bone windows (**C**). **D,** Volume-rendered three-dimensional reconstruction also shows complete fusion of all cranial suture in this patient with Crouzon syndrome.

■ CONGENITAL VERTEBRAL ANOMALIES

A number of fairly common anomalies of the vertebral bodies occur as the result of abnormal development. There may be lack of fusion of the two cartilaginous centers of the vertebral bodies that results in a cleft in the sagittal plane. This is referred to as a butterfly vertebra. When one of the lateral cartilaginous centers fails to form, a hemivertebra results. It may be associated with scoliosis, rib anomalies, and other vertebral anomalies. Anterior and posterior hemivertebrae are also possible. If there is failure of separation of two or more adjacent vertebral bodies, a fusion

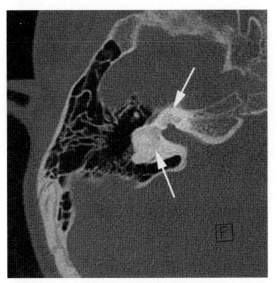

■ FIGURE 8-131 **Labyrinthitis ossificans.** Axial CT of the right temporal bone shows complete ossification of the right cochlea, vestibule, and semicircular canals (*arrows*) in a patient with prior history of meningitis.

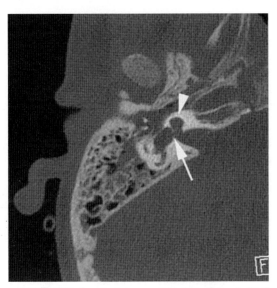

■ FIGURE 8-132 **Incomplete partitioning type I (IP-I).** Axial CT of the right temporal bone shows a cystic featureless cochlea (*arrowhead*). There is partial membranous partition between the cochlea and dysplastic vestibule with only a small communication (*arrow*), helping differentiate from a common cavity. Note also near complete opacification of the mastoid air cells and middle ear cavity.

anomaly with block vertebra is formed. The fusion of multiple cervical vertebral bodies can be seen in Klippel–Feil syndrome. A number of other associated anomalies may be seen in Klippel–Feil syndrome: a low posterior hairline, a short webbed neck, genitourinary anomalies, and congenital heart disease. A Sprengel deformity (high-riding scapula) in association with a bridging omovertebral bone is present in 25% of patients with Klippel–Feil syndrome.

■ SPINAL DYSRAPHISM

Spinal dysraphism is a group of disorders of the spine in which the posterior bony and neuronal tissues fail to fuse, due to abnormal neurulation (Table 8-11). The abnormalities are categorized as open (neural tissue exposed through bone and skin defect) or closed (abnormality covered by skin).

The most common types of the open dysraphism are myelomeningoceles and myeloschisis. Myelomeningoceles contain the meninges, neuroplacode, and nerve roots protruding through the skin defect (see Fig. 8-37B). Myeloschisis is a flat defect with neuroplacode and meninges contained within the dysraphic spinal canal. Although the lesions are most common in the lower lumbar spine, they can occur at any level. Encephaloceles occur through defects in the cranium. As previously discussed, essentially all patients with myelomeningoceles have associated Chiari II malformations, and the vast majority have hydrocephalus. Hydromyelia is also often present. On radiography, the posterior elements of the spine are absent, and there is widening of the spinal canal and interpedicular distances (Fig. 8-157). Typically, multiple contiguous vertebral levels are involved. MRI is often used to look for delayed complications after primary surgical repair, such as syrinx, dermoid, or postoperative tethering.

With closed dysraphisms, children may be asymptomatic or may present with subcutaneous masses or dermal tracts, bladder dysfunction, lower extremity neurologic abnormalities, or orthopedic deformities of the feet or legs.

Lipomyelomeningocele is a closed dysraphic defect characterized by a lipomatous mass and

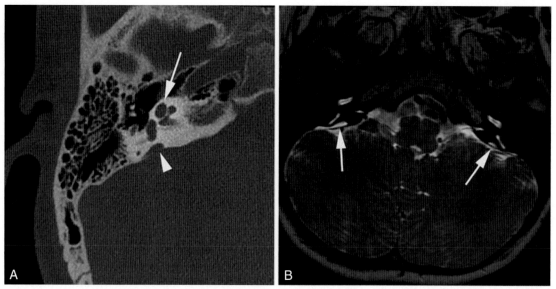

■ **FIGURE 8-133 Incomplete partitioning type II (IP-II) with enlarged vestibular aqueduct. A,** Axial CT of the right temporal bone shows lack of separation between the middle and apical turns of the cochlear (*arrow*) with a deficient modiolus compatible with (IP-II). There is also enlargement of the vestibular aqueduct (*arrowhead*). **B,** Axial T2 steady-state free precession sequence of the temporal bones shows dilated bilateral endolymphatic sac/duct (*arrows*), the MRI finding of an enlarged vestibular aqueduct seen on CT.

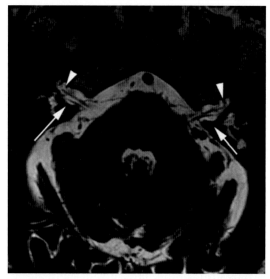

■ FIGURE 8-134 **Incomplete partitioning type III.** Axial T2 steady-state free precession sequence of the internal auditory canals/temporal bones shows dilated bilateral internal auditory canals (*arrows*) and cochlear aperture with absent modiolus (*arrowheads*).

neural elements extending from the low-lying cord through a defect in the bone and contiguous with the subcutaneous fat (Fig. 8-158). A palpable mass may be present, but the overlying skin is intact. Other less common closed defects include lipomyelocele, myelocystocele, and meningocele. A dermal sinus is an epithelium-lined tract that extends from the skin to the deep spinal soft tissues. If a true open tract is present, immediate surgical attention is necessary, given the risk of meningitis. The tract may connect to the spinal canal and be associated with a dermoid, epidermoid, or lipoma (Fig. 8-159A and B) or no associate mass. When findings of occult dysraphism are found on ultrasound or are highly suspected clinically, definitive evaluation is performed using MRI.

In infants who demonstrate a high skin dimple, patch of hair, or other findings suspicious for an occult dysraphism, the initial screening examination is often ultrasound. In a normal infant, the conus medullaris is located superior to or at the level of L2–L3 (Fig. 8-160). The cord and nerve

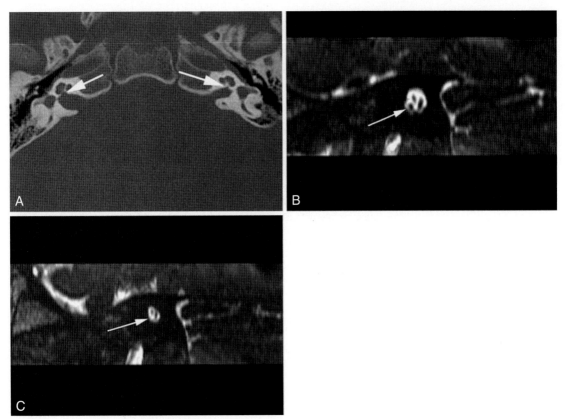

■ FIGURE 8-135 **Cochlear nerve hypoplasia/aplasia. A,** Axial CT of the temporal bones shows a left atretic cochlear aperture in comparison with the normal right side (*arrows*). **B,** Sagittal oblique view of the same patient MRI showing an axial cut of the right internal auditory canal. See normal right-sided cochlear nerve within the anteroinferior IAC (*arrow*). **C,** Left side showed absent cochlear nerve (*arrow*).

✳ TABLE 8-8 Orbital and Facial Developmental Anomalies

Developmental Anomaly	Causes and Imaging Characteristics
Coloboma	Congenital ocular defect characterized by a focal ocular globe outpunching through a chorioretinal gap Part of many genetic syndromes CHARGE, Aicardi, Treacher–Collins, trisomies, and others
Persistent hyperplastic primary vitreous	Lack of regression of embryonic hyaloid artery On imaging, there is a linear soft tissue connecting the posterior lens with the optic disk The lens is triangular in shape The globe is small in size May have vitreous or subretinal hemorrhage May be isolated or syndromic Differential diagnosis includes retinopathy of prematurity, Coats disease, retinal detachment, and retinoblastoma
Morning glory disk anomaly	Optic disk malformation resembling a morning glory flower on fundoscopic exam. On imaging, there is a funnel-shaped outpouching of the optic disk with elevation of the adjacent retina, abnormal soft tissue, and enhancement within the distal optic nerve May be associated with stenoocclusive vasculopathy (moyamoya like), cephaloceles, and PHACES syndrome

Continued

✳ **TABLE 8-8**	
Developmental Anomaly	**Causes and Imaging Characteristics**
Nasofrontal dermoid/glioma	Congenital defect in nasofrontal neural tube closure with persistent embryonic connection between the dorsal nose and the foramen cecum, with or without sequestered tissue Spectrum of imaging findings includes nasal dermal sinus tract, nasal and/or intracranial dermoid or glioma, and nasofrontal encephalocele. The intracranial component when present is located at the level of the foramen cecum. A bifid crista galli can sometimes be associated
Nasolacrimal mucocele	Congenital nasolacrimal duct mucocele is due to lack of distal duct canalization On imaging, there is a tubular cystic structure extending from the orbital medial canthus into the inferior nasal meatus
Choanal atresia	Congenital choanal obstruction Presents clinically with neonatal respiratory distress if bilateral or failure to pass NG tube On imaging, there is narrowing of the choana (unilateral or bilateral) with either osseous or membranous atresia. Accumulated secretions within the posterior nasal cavity are a common finding May be associated with CHARGE syndrome
Pyriform aperture stenosis	Congenital narrowing of the nasal apertures presenting with neonatal respiratory distress May have associated single central maxillary incisor May be associated with holoprosencephaly
Cleft lip and palate	Abnormal facial development with lack of fusion of the medial frontonasal process with the maxillary process of the first pharyngeal arch during fetal life May be unilateral or bilateral May involve the lip and primary palate (midline palate in front of the foramen incisor), extend into the secondary palate (complete cleft lip and palate), or be isolated to the secondary palate Mostly isolated but it may be associated with genetic syndromes

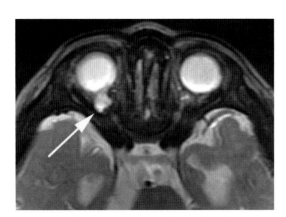

■ **FIGURE 8-136 Coloboma.** Axial T2-weighted sequence of the orbits shows posterior right ocular globe outpouching compatible with a coloboma (*arrow*). This can be seen as an isolated finding or genetic in nature. This patient also had absent corpus callosum and extensive malformation of cortical development (not shown here—see Fig. 8-45C) compatible with Aicardi syndrome.

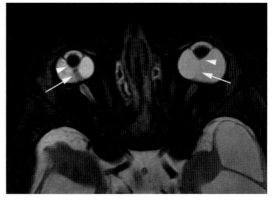

■ **FIGURE 8-137 Persistent hyperplastic primary vitreous.** Axial T2-weighted sequence of the orbits shows dysmorphic small ocular globes with bilateral linear retrolental soft tissue extending from the lens to the optic disk (*arrows*) compatible with the hyaloid remnant of Cloquet canal. Note also the triangular shape of the lens (*arrowheads*).

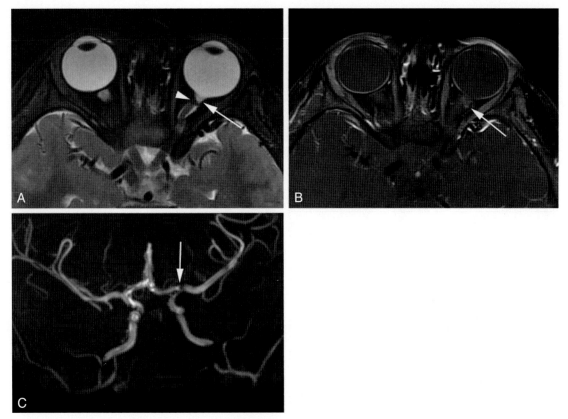

■ **FIGURE 8-138 Morning glory disk anomaly/syndrome. A,** Axial T2-weighted sequence of the orbits shows funnel-shaped excavation of the left optic disk (*arrow*) with associated abnormal tissue within the distal intraorbital distal optic nerve (*arrowhead*). **B,** Postcontrast image shows abnormal enhancement within the distal optic nerve (*arrow*). **C,** MR angiogram shows focal arterial narrowing of the left carotid terminus compatible with associated steno-occlusive vasculopathy (*arrow*).

roots are seen to be freely moving during real-time ultrasound evaluation. With tethered cord, the tip of the spinal cord is low lying, below the level of L2–L3 (see Fig. 8-159), and nerve roots do not float freely in the CSF space and are often posteriorly positioned.

Tethered cord may occur as a primary problem or may be associated with a tethering lesion, such as a terminal lipoma (see Fig. 8-159) or multiple other dysraphic defects. With a tethered cord, the filum terminale may be abnormally thick (>1–2 mm) and demonstrate fibrofatty infiltration.

Caudal regression syndrome is a complex spinal dysraphism that results from abnormal formation of the caudal mesoderm. The most severe form of caudal regression syndrome results in sirenomelia with fusion of lower extremities. Potential etiologies include toxic, ischemic, infectious, or genetic causes. There is a high association with maternal diabetes, VACTERL, and OEIS (omphalocele, exstrophy of the cloaca, imperforate anus, and spinal defect) complex. There is lack of formation of the distal spinal cord and vertebrae. Associated abnormalities of the anal opening, genitalia, bladder, and kidneys are common. Findings on imaging include a blunted high conus medullaris, usually above L1, and sacral hypogenesis (Fig. 8-161).

■ SPINAL TRAUMA

Injury to the spine is much less common in infants and young children than it is in adults. Most injuries that occur in older children and

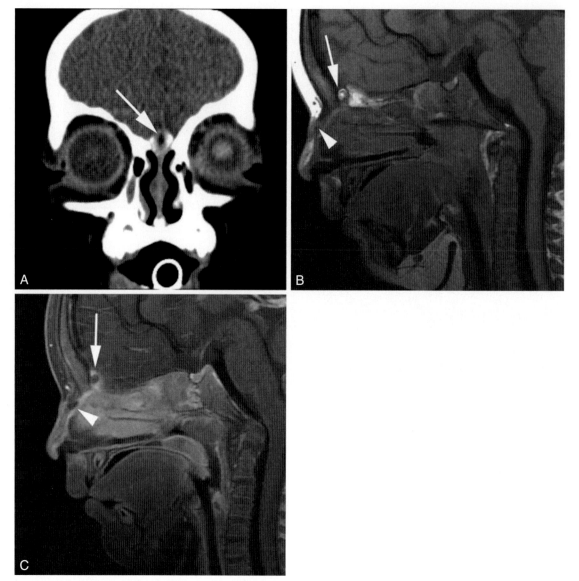

■ FIGURE 8-139 **Nasofrontal dermoid. A,** Coronal CT shows a bifid crista galli with an associated fatty lesion (*arrow*). **B,** Sagittal T1-weighted sequence of the same patient shows a small oval-shaped dermoid cyst along the dorsal soft tissues of the nose (*arrowhead*) and an intracranial fatty lesion (*arrow*), also compatible with a dermoid. **C,** Post-contrast sagittal MRI shows enhancement surrounding the nasal (*arrowhead*) and intracranial (*arrow*) dermoid lesions. No obvious patent sinus tract connecting these two lesions although fibrous tract is difficult to exclude.

teenagers have the same appearances and locations as those seen in adults and are not discussed here. In infants and young children, the majority of cervical spine injuries involve the superior cervical spine, as opposed to the lower cervical spine injuries seen in adults. This is thought to be related to the relatively large head size of young

children and the immaturity of the spinal column. As with all cervical spine trauma, one must be diligent concerning the technical factors and the interpretation of radiographs.

Fractures of the upper cervical spine in infants and young children often involve the atlas and axis. With flexion injuries, there can be a fracture

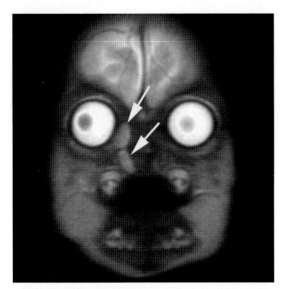

■ FIGURE 8-140 **Nasolacrimal mucocele**. Coronal T2-weighted sequence shows fluid enlargement of the right nasolacrimal duct extending from the orbital medial canthus into inferior nasal meatus (*arrows*).

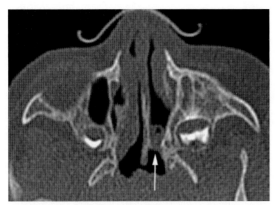

■ FIGURE 8-141 **Choanal atresia**. Axial CT shows narrowing of the left choana with associated membranous atresia (*arrow*) and retained secretions along the posterior nasal cavity.

through the base of the dens (at the synchondrosis between the dens and body of C2) (Fig. 8-162A and B). With this injury, there is typically anterior displacement of C1 in association with soft tissue swelling. Extension injuries in this region may result in fractures of the posterior arch of C1, the dens, or a "hangman fracture" (a fracture through the posterior arch of C2) (Fig. 8-163). Atlantooccipital dislocations can also occur (Fig. 8-164A and B). Atlantooccipital dislocation is a severe injury that may result in death. On radiographs, the distance between the occiput and C1 is increased, and there is marked soft tissue swelling. Atlantoaxial instability can also occur and is discussed subsequently.

Lap belt injuries occur in children who are restrained by lap belts but not by shoulder belts. Anterior compression fractures of the lumbar vertebral bodies may occur in association with disruption of the posterior processes (Chance fractures; Fig. 8-165A and B). These fractures are not commonly associated with neurologic injury but are frequently associated with intra-abdominal injuries, particularly of the bowel.

■ NORMAL VARIANTS AND CONGENITAL ANOMALIES OF THE CERVICAL SPINE

There are a number of normal variants of the cervical spine that should not be misinterpreted as traumatic injury. One of the more common normal variants that may lead to confusion is cervical pseudosubluxation. In normal children, there may be a slightly anterior position of C2 in relation to C3 (Fig. 8-166). However, in contrast to ligamentous injury, with pseudosubluxation, the posterior cervical line (a line drawn along the

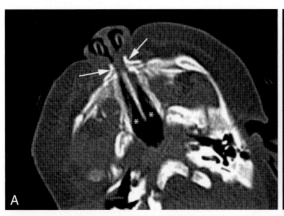
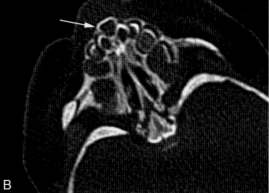

■ FIGURE 8-142 **Pyriform aperture stenosis**. **A,** Axial CT shows narrowing of the nasal aperture (*arrows*) with lack of air column. Please note patent choana bilaterally (***). **B,** Lower imaging plane shows a single central maxillary incisor (*arrow*).

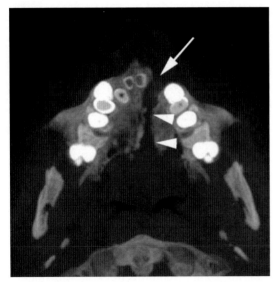

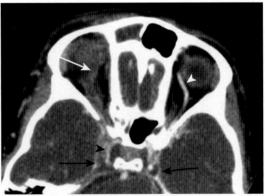

■ FIGURE 8-145 **Ophthalmic vein and cavernous sinus thrombosis.** Axial contrast-enhanced CT in a patient with postseptal orbital cellulitis shows an enlarged and nonenhancing right superior ophthalmic vein compatible with thrombosis (*white arrow*). Note normal enhancement of the contralateral vein (*white arrowhead*). There is also lack of normal enhancement within the bilateral cavernous sinus (*black arrows*) due to thrombosis. Note also the small size of the cavernous portion of the right internal carotid artery due to spasm (*black arrowhead*).

anterior aspect of the posterior processes) remains straight. Pseudosubluxation may also be seen at the C3 to C4 level.

There are a number of age-related variations in C1 and C2. The ossification centers that make up the atlas fuse posteriorly by 1 year of age and laterally by 3 years of age. Before fusion, a lucent synchondrosis is seen radiographically. In addition, there may be a congenital defect in of the posterior portion of C1 that should not be

confused with a fracture (Fig. 8-167). C2 also has multiple ossification centers. These nonossified synchondroses should not be mistaken for fractures. The synchondrosis between the dens and body of C2 typically fuses between 3 and 6 years of age. Before fusion, the lucent synchondrosis is seen through the base of the dens. The ossiculum terminale (tip of the dens) fuses to the body of the dens by 12 years of age. The dens may also be normally tilted slightly posteriorly in young children.

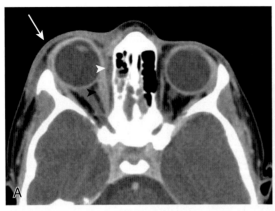
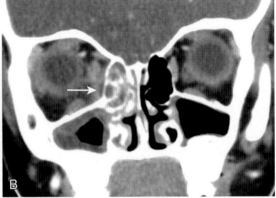

■ FIGURE 8-144 **Preseptal and postseptal cellulitis. A,** Axial, contrast-enhanced CT of the orbits shows asymmetric thickening of the right preseptal soft tissues (*arrow*). There is also involvement of the medial extraconal postseptal soft tissues (*white arrowhead*). The medial rectus muscle is enlarged (*black arrowhead*) due to reactive myositis. Note partial ethmoid sinus opacification. **B,** Coronal contrast-enhanced CT of a different patient also showing right medial postseptal cellulitis with a small subperiosteal collection representing an early abscess (*arrow*). Note again ethmoid sinusitis as the cause of orbital cellulitis.

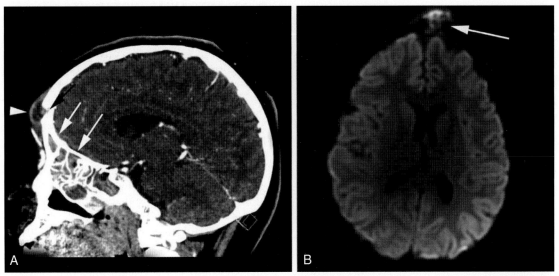

■ FIGURE 8-146 **Pott's puffy tumor. A,** Sagittal CT of the head shows complete opacification of the paranasal sinuses (*white arrows*). An abscess is seen along the frontal soft tissues (*arrowhead*) as complication of sinus disease known as "Pott's Puffy Tumor." Note also involvement of the underlying frontal bone compatible with osteomyelitis (*black arrow*). **B,** Axial DWI sequence shows diffusion restriction within the frontal abscess (*arrow*).

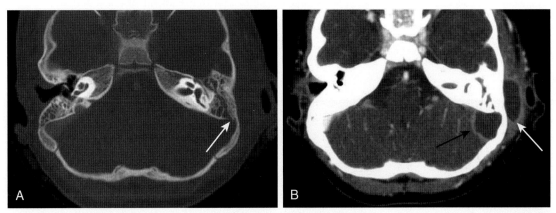

■ FIGURE 8-147 **Otomastoiditis. A,** Axial CT image in bone window shows complete fluid opacification of the left mastoid air cells and middle ear cavity. There is a focal area of bony disruption along the posterior mastoid wall (*arrow*). **B,** Soft tissue window demonstrates large retroauricular (*white arrow*) and intracranial (*black arrow*) ring-enhancing fluid collections compatible with abscesses.

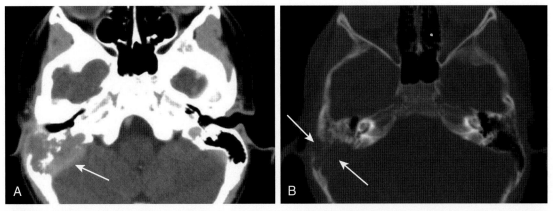

■ FIGURE 8-148 **Langerhans cell histiocytosis. A,** Axial contrast-enhanced CT of the temporal bones demonstrates an enhancing soft tissue lesion involving the right mastoid (*arrow*). **B,** Bone window shows marked bony destruction (*arrows*), not typical for otomastoiditis. Biopsy of the lesion confirmed LCH.

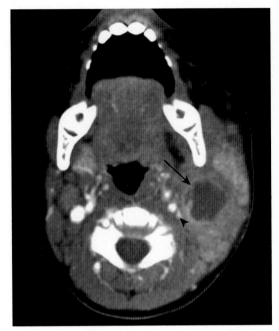

■ FIGURE 8-149 **Suppurative adenitis.** Left neck ring-enhancing fluid collection, lateral to the carotid space, with surrounding inflammatory changes, compatible with suppurative adenitis and abscess formation (*arrow*). Note compression of left internal jugular vein (*arrowhead*) due to mass effect from abscess.

■ ATLANTOAXIAL INSTABILITY

The atlantoaxial joint, or the articulation between the C1 and C2 vertebral bodies, is a unique joint that allows for lateral rotation of the cervical spine. The joint is stabilized by a number of ligaments. The transverse ligament is responsible for stabilizing the relationship between the dens of C2 and anterior arch of C1. In children, the space between the dens and anterior arch of C1 should not exceed 5 mm. Atlantoaxial subluxation leads to an abnormal increase in this distance (Fig. 8-168) and decrease in the diameter of the spinal canal with potential cord compression (see Fig. 8-168). Causes of atlantoaxial instability include trauma, inflammation (juvenile idiopathic arthritis, retropharyngeal abscess), and congenital predisposition (Down syndrome, hypoplasia of the dens, os odontoideum [Fig. 8-169], absence of the anterior arch of C1). Patients with Down syndrome are typically screened for atlantoaxial instability with flexion and extension radiographs before participation in physical activities.

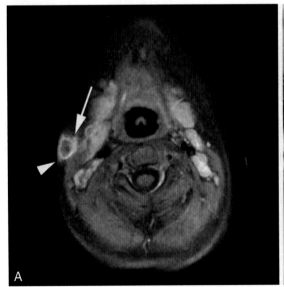
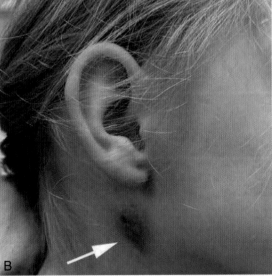

■ FIGURE 8-150 **Atypical mycobacteria infection. A,** Axial T1 postcontrast shows a ring-enhancing lesion compatible with a necrotic lymph node adjacent to the skin surface (*arrow*). There are only minimum inflammatory changes, helping differentiate from acute bacterial suppurative adenitis. **B,** Patient's image shows typical skin discoloration (*arrow*).

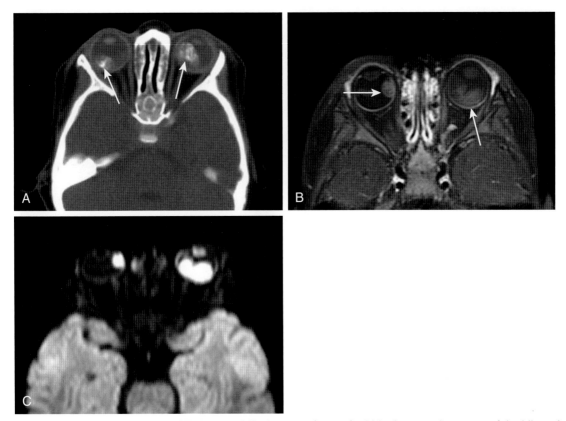

■ **FIGURE 8-151** **Retinoblastoma. A,** CT shows calcified masses (*arrows*) within the posterior aspect of the bilateral globes. **B,** Axial contrast-enhanced T1-weighted sequence of a different patient shows bilateral enhancing intraocular masses (*arrows*). **C,** Same patient as **B**; DWI sequence demonstrates diffusion restriction seen in highly cellular tumors.

TABLE 8-9 Common Causes of Pediatric Orbital Masses (Extraocular)
• Dermoid
• Orbital cellulitis or abscess
• Orbital pseudotumor
• Infantile hemangioma
• Lymphatic or venous malformation
• Optic nerve glioma
• Rhabdomyosarcoma
• Lymphoma or leukemia
• Retinoblastoma
• Langerhans cell histiocytosis
• Metastatic neuroblastoma
• Hematoma

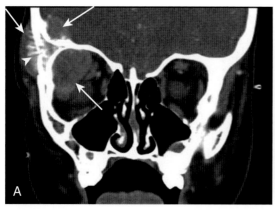 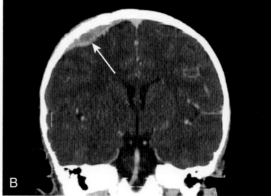

■ FIGURE 8-152 **Metastatic neuroblastoma. A,** Contrast-enhanced CT of the orbits in coronal plane demonstrates a large soft tissue mass (*arrows*) at the right superolateral orbital wall with associated "hair-on-end" periosteal reaction of involved bone (*arrowhead*), characteristic of metastatic neuroblastoma. **B,** Contrast-enhanced CT of the head in coronal view of a different patient shows an enhancing subdural mass (*arrow*).

✳ **TABLE 8-10** Common Causes of Pediatric Neck Masses	
Congenital	Thyroglossal duct cyst
	Branchial cleft cyst
	Lingual thyroid
	Dermoid or epidermoid
Inflammatory	Lymphadenitis
	Abscess
	Inflamed salivary gland
	Ranula
Neoplastic	Rhabdomyosarcoma
	Lymphoma
	Metastatic disease
Vascular	Venous malformation
	Lymphatic malformation
	Infantile hemangioma

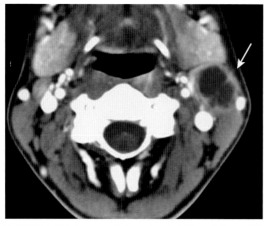

■ FIGURE 8-153 **A second branchial cleft cyst in an 18-year-old girl with a tender mass.** CT shows a low attenuation cystic lesion (*arrow*) just inferior to the left angle of the mandible. The lesion has an enhancing rim.

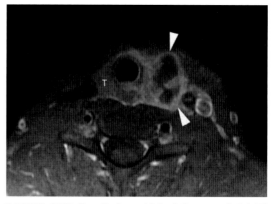

■ FIGURE 8-154 **Fourth branchial cleft cyst.** Axial T1 postcontrast sequence of the neck shows a heterogeneous ring-enhancing fluid collection involving the left lobe of the thyroid gland (*arrowheads*). Findings compatible with an infected fourth branchial cleft cyst. Note normal right lobe of the thyroid gland (*T*).

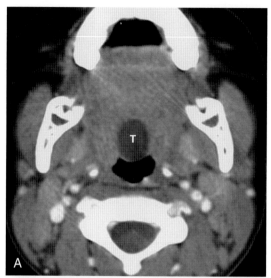

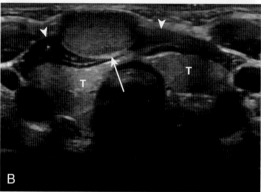

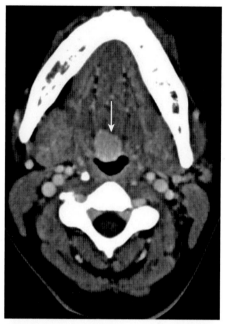

■ FIGURE 8-156 **Lingual thyroid.** Contrast-enhanced CT of the neck shows a hyperdense mass at the base of the tongue (*arrow*), compatible with a lingual thyroid. High attenuation is not related to enhancement; it is secondary to thyroid tissue iodine content.

■ FIGURE 8-155 **Thyroglossal duct cyst. A,** Contrast-enhanced CT shows well-defined, nonenhancing mass (*T*) in the midline, just inferior to the base of the tongue. **B,** Ultrasound of the neck in a different patient shows an oval-shaped lesion (*arrow*) embedded in the strap muscles (*arrowheads*), as demonstrated by presence of a "claw sign." The lesion is just to the right of midline and causing mild mass effect upon the right lobe of the thyroid gland (*T*). Note homogeneous internal echos compatible with proteinaceous contents (pseudosolid lesion), as well as enhanced through-transmission.

■ SPONDYLOLYSIS AND SPONDYLOLISTHESIS

The most common abnormality identified on radiography in children who present with lower back pain is spondylolysis. Spondylolysis refers to a defect in the pars interarticularis of the posterior vertebral arch. It usually occurs bilaterally and at a single level. The overwhelming majority of cases (93%) occur at the L5 level, the second most common location is L4. It is a common lesion, affecting approximately 7.1% of adolescents. Symptoms usually present in late

✳ TABLE 8-11 Common Types of Spinal Dysraphism	
Open spinal dysraphism	Myelomeningocele
	Myeloschisis
Closed spinal dysraphism with a subcutaneous mass	Lipomyelomeningocele
	Lipomyelocele
	Myelocystocele
	Meningocele
Closed spinal dysraphism without a subcutaneous mass	Caudal regression syndrome
	Split notochord syndrome (dorsal enteric fistula and neurenteric cyst)
	Split cord malformation (diastematomyelia)
	Segmental spinal dysgenesis
	Dermal sinus tract
	Tethered cord syndrome
	Intraspinal lipoma

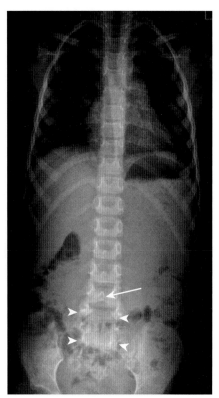

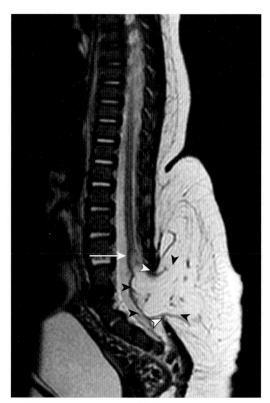

■ FIGURE 8-157 **Dysraphic changes within the lumbosacral spine.** Radiograph shows absence of the posterior elements and widening of the interpeduncular distance (*arrowheads*). The posterior elements superior to the level of the dysraphism appear normal (*arrow*).

■ FIGURE 8-158 **Lipomyelomeningocele.** Sagittal T2-weighted sequence of the lumbar spine shows a low-lying conus medullaris (*white arrow*). The neuroplacode terminates into a fatty mass (*black arrowheads*) that extends through a lumbosacral dysraphic defect (*white arrowheads*) and is in continuity with the subcutaneous fat tissues.

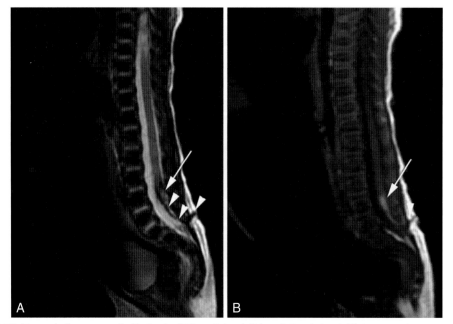

■ FIGURE 8-159 **Dermal sinus tract. A–B,** Sagittal T2-weighted (**A**) and T-weighted (**B**) images showing a tract connecting the skin with the thecal sac compatible with a dermal sinus tract (*arrowheads*). Note also low-lying spinal cord terminating in a terminal lipoma (*arrow*).

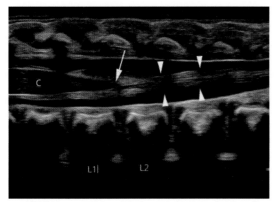

■ FIGURE 8-160 Normal infant spinal ultrasound. Midline sagittal image shows tip of conus medullaris (*arrow*) to be located at the level of *L1–L2*, which is normal position. The cord (*C*) is shown as a hypoechoic structure, and nerve roots (*arrowheads*) are more echogenic. Note that the cord and nerve roots lay anteriorly, with gravity. On real-time ultrasound in a normal patient, the cord and nerve roots float freely in the CSF and show motion.

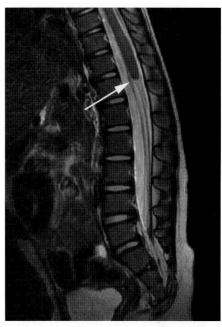

■ FIGURE 8-161 Caudal regression syndrome. Sagittal T2-weighted sequence of the lumbar spine shows a truncated conus medullaris (*arrow*). Note also hypoplastic sacrum.

childhood, although many of these children are asymptomatic. There is debate concerning whether the cause is traumatic, congenital, or some combination of the two.

Spondylolisthesis refers to anterior displacement of the more superior vertebral body as related to the inferior vertebral body (Fig. 8-170). Spondylolisthesis is graded from one through five on the basis of increments of one quarter of the vertebral body. Grade 1 refers

to anterior displacement of up to one quarter of the superior vertebral body beyond the anterior border of the inferior vertebral body. In grade 2, the displacement is up to one half; in grade 4, it is the entire vertebral body. Grade 5 is complete anterior displacement and inferior migration

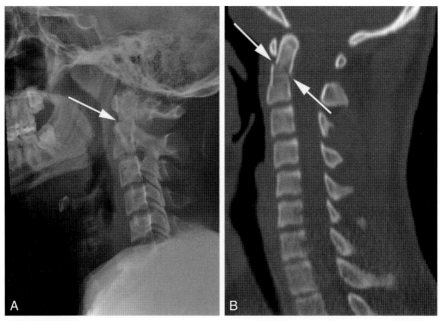

■ FIGURE 8-162 Fracture through base of dens. Lateral radiograph (**A**) and sagittal reconstructed CT (**B**) of the cervical spine shows a fracture line (*arrows*) through base of dens.

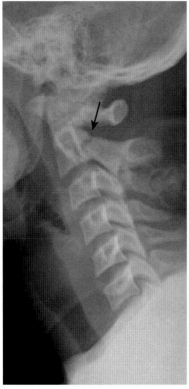

■ FIGURE 8-163 **Hangman fracture.** Radiograph shows linear fracture (*arrow*) through the posterior elements of C2.

such that the superior vertebral body is anterior to the inferior vertebral body.

On lateral radiographs, spondylolysis appears as a lucent defect through the region of the pars interarticularis, with or without associated anterior slippage (spondylolisthesis). Oblique views demonstrate the lucency through the pars. The pars defect has been likened to a lucent broken neck of what appears to look like a Scottish terrier on the oblique views. Personally, the authors find the defect easier to see on the straight lateral films. In cases in which confirmation is necessary, CT or MRI can be used.

Spinal Tumors

Spinal tumors are extremely rare in the pediatric population. Similarly to adults, they can be classified based on location as follows: intradural intramedullary, intradural extramedullary, and extradural extramedullary. The most common intradural intramedullary tumor in pediatric is a low-grade astrocytoma. On imaging, astrocytomas show as an expansile intramedullary mass with T2 hyperintense signal and mild-to-moderate enhancement (Fig. 8-171A and B). The tumor may have cystic areas. The second and third most common intramedullary tumors are ependymomas and gangliogliomas. Ependymomas are more commonly hypervascular/

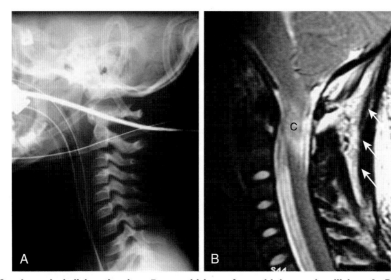

■ FIGURE 8-164 **Craniocervical dislocation in a 5-year-old boy after a high-speed collision. A,** Radiograph shows increased distance between the skull base and C1 vertebral body. **B,** Sagittal T2-weighted MR image shows high signal within the cord (*C*), representing a cord contusion. There is high-signal edema within the posterior soft tissues (*arrows*) secondary to ligamentous injury.

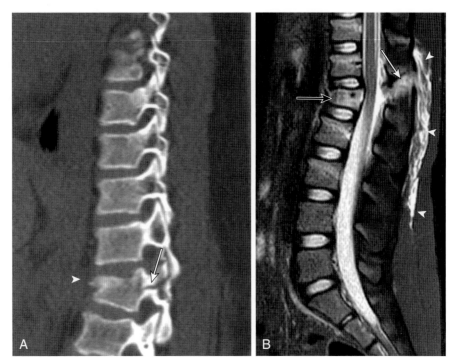

■ FIGURE 8-165 **Chance fracture. A,** Radiograph shows fracture (*arrow*) through posterior elements of the spine and compression fracture of the vertebral body (*arrowhead*). **B,** STIR MR sequence again shows the fracture through the posterior elements (*white arrow*) and vertebral body compression fracture (*black arrow*). Note also subcutaneous edema (*arrowheads*).

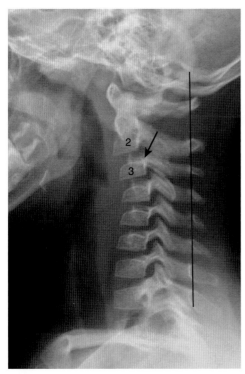

■ FIGURE 8-166 **Pseudosubluxation of C2 onto C3.** Radiograph shows that the posterior aspect of C2 vertebral body is slightly more anteriorly positioned than is that of C3 (*arrow*). However, the posterior cervical line shows that the posterior elements of C2 are not more anterior than the posterior elements of C3, consistent with pseudosubluxation rather than true injury.

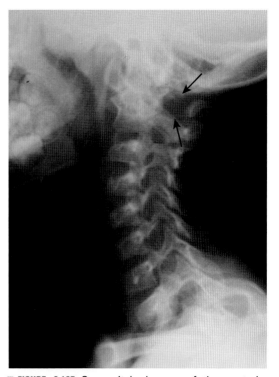

■ FIGURE 8-167 Congenital absence of the posterior portion of C1 is shown in the lucent area (*arrows*) on radiography.

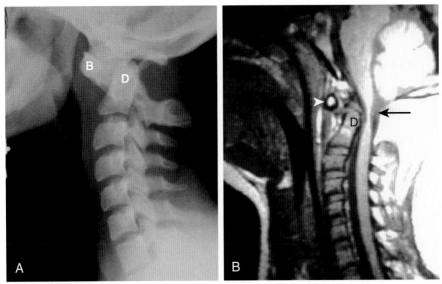

■ **FIGURE 8-168 Atlantoaxial instability in a 20-year-old patient with down syndrome. A,** Radiograph shows increased distance between the anterior arch of C1 (*B*) and the dens of C2 (*D*). **B,** Sagittal T1-weighted MR image again shows increased distance between the anterior arch of C1 (*arrowhead*) and the dens of C2 (*D*). There is also narrowing of the spinal canal and severe spinal cord compression (*arrow*).

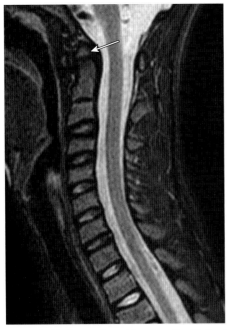

■ **FIGURE 8-169 Os odontoideum.** Sagittal STIR sequence shows an ossicle at the tip of the odontoid process of C2 (*arrow*), which is separated from the remaining of the odontoid process. This is compatible with an orthotopic os odontoideum. There is no associated edema or ligamentous injury to suggest an acute fracture.

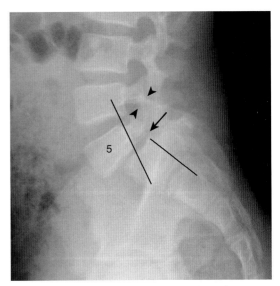

■ **FIGURE 8-170 L5-S1 spondylolysis with grade 2 spondylolisthesis.** Lateral radiograph shows anterior displacement of L5 vertebral body in relationship to the S1 vertebral segment. Lines are drawn parallel to the posterior aspect of L5 and S1, demonstrating the anterior displacement of L5. The normal, intact pars is seen at L4 (*arrowheads*) and resembles a "dog collar on a Scotty dog." There is lucency through the pars (*arrow*) at the L5 level, consistent with the spondylolysis.

hemorrhagic and frequently central in location. Less common intradural intramedullary spinal tumors include ATRT, diffuse midline glioma, and oligodendroglioma. Intradural extramedullary

lesions include myxopapillary ependymoma (Fig. 8-172 A and B), leptomeningeal metastasis (see Fig. 8-99D), nerve sheet tumors (neurofibromas or schwannomas), meningioma, lipoma, dermoid/

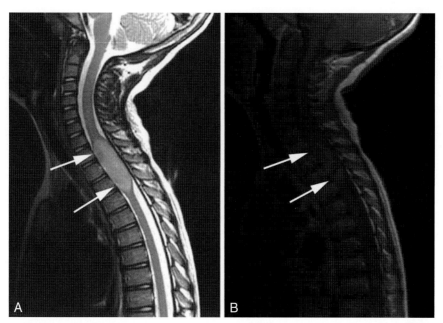

■ **FIGURE 8-171 Spinal astrocytoma. A,** Sagittal T2-weighted sequence shows a homogenous expansile T2 hyperintense intradural intramedullary cervicothoracic spinal mass (*arrows*). **B,** Postcontrast T1-weighted sequence shows mild diffuse enhancement within the mass (*arrows*).

epidermoid, and arachnoid cyst. Myxopapillary ependymoma is a subtype of ependymoma characteristically arising from conus medullary or filum terminale (Fig. 8-172A and B). Extradural extramedullary lesions include bony lesions and intraspinal extension of paraspinal tumors such

as neuroblastoma and sarcomas (most commonly rhabdomyosarcoma and extraosseous Ewing sarcoma). Spinal bone lesions include osteoid osteoma (Fig. 8-173), osteoblastoma (osteoid osteoma larger than 2 cm), aneurysm bone cyst, osteochondroma, rarely giant cell tumor, and

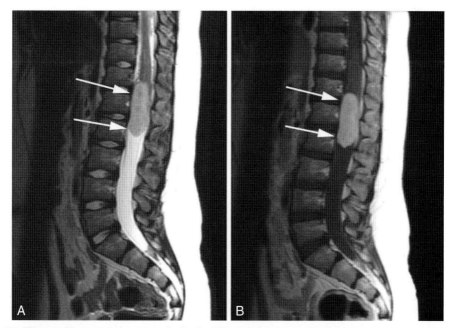

■ **FIGURE 8-172 Mixopapillary ependymoma. A,** Sagittal T2-weighted sequence shows a homogenous expansile T2 hyperintense mass at the level of the conus medullaris (*arrows*). **B,** Postcontrast T1-weighted sequence shows marked diffuse enhancement within the mass (*arrows*). Differential diagnosis includes other avidly enhancing intradural extramedullary lesions such as nerve sheet tumors and meningioma.

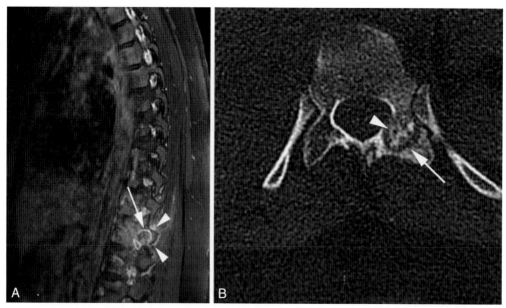

■ **FIGURE 8-173 Osteoid osteoma. A,** Sagittal T1-weighted postcontrast sequence shows enhancement surrounding a rounded T1 hypointense lesion (*arrow*) within thoracic vertebrae posterior elements. Note also enhancement of the paravertebral soft tissues (*arrowheads*). **B,** Axial CT imaging shows a lucent nidus (*arrow*) within the left vertebral pedicle with internal sclerotic changes (*arrowhead*).

the very aggressive malignant chordoma. Other pathologies involving the vertebrae include metastasis or lymphoma and leukemia—either as focal or diffuse bone marrow infiltration.

SUGGESTED READING

Barkovich A, Raybaud C: *Pediatric neuroimaging*, Sixth Edition, Philadelphia, PA, 2019, Wolters Kluwer.

Brandao LA, Mukherji SK: MR spectroscopy of the brain, *Neuroimaging Clin N Am.* 23(3):359−562, August 2013.

Cruz LCH, Mukherji SK: Clinical applications of diffusion imaging of the brain, *Neuroimaging Clin N Am* 21(1):1−196, February 2011.

Pillai JJ, Mukherji SK: Clinical applications of functional MRI, *Neuroimaging Clin N Am* 24(4):557−728, November 2014.

Lowe LH, Balley Z: State-of-the-art cranial sonography: part 1, modern techniques and imaging interpretation, *Am J Roentgenol* 196(5):1028−1033, May 2011.

Lowe LH, Balley Z: State-of-the-art cranial sonography: part 2, pitfalls and variants, *Am J Roentgenol* 196(5):1034−1039, May 2011.

Dinan D, Daneman A, Guimaraes CV, et al.: Easily overlooked sonographic findings in the evaluation of neonatal encephalopathy: lessons learned from magnetic resonance imaging, *Semin Ultrasound CT MR* 35(6):627−651, December 2014.

Kline-Fath B, Bulas D, Lee W: *Fundamental and advanced fetal imaging—ultrasound and MRI*, Philadelphia, PA, 2020, Wolters Kluwers.

Welker K, Patton A: Assessment of normal myelination with magnetic resonance imaging, *Semin Neurol* 32:15−28, 2012.

Severino A, Geraldo AF, Utz N, et al.: Definitions and classification of malformations of cortical development: practical guidelines, *Brain* 174:1−21, 2020. awaa.

Shekdar KV, Bilaniuk LT: Imaging of pediatric hearing loss, *Neuroimaging Clin N Am* 29:103−115, 2019.

Note: Page numbers followed by *f* indicate figures and *t* indicate tables.